Diagnostic Devices with Microfluidics

Devices, Circuits, and Systems

Series Editor

Krzysztof Iniewski
Emerging Technologies CMOS Inc.
Vancouver, British Columbia, Canada

PUBLISHED TITLES:

PUBLISHED TITLES:

PUBLISHED TITLES:

Optical, Acoustic, Magnetic, and Mechanical Sensor Technologies
Krzysztof Iniewski

Optical Fiber Sensors: Advanced Techniques and Applications
Ginu Rajan

Optical Imaging Devices: New Technologies and Applications
Ajit Khosla and Dongsoo Kim

Organic Solar Cells: Materials, Devices, Interfaces, and Modeling
Qiquan Qiao

Physical Design for 3D Integrated Circuits
Aida Todri-Sanial and Chuan Seng Tan

Power Management Integrated Circuits and Technologies
Mona M. Hella and Patrick Mercier

Radiation Detectors for Medical Imaging
Jan S. Iwanczyk

Radiation Effects in Semiconductors
Krzysztof Iniewski

Reconfigurable Logic: Architecture, Tools, and Applications
Pierre-Emmanuel Gaillardon

Semiconductor Devices in Harsh Conditions
Kirsten Weide-Zaage and Malgorzata Chrzanowska-Jeske

Semiconductor Radiation Detection Systems
Krzysztof Iniewski

Semiconductors: Integrated Circuit Design for Manufacturability
Artur Balasinski

Smart Grids: Clouds, Communications, Open Source, and Automation
David Bakken

Smart Sensors for Industrial Applications
Krzysztof Iniewski

Soft Errors: From Particles to Circuits
Jean-Luc Autran and Daniela Munteanu

Solid-State Radiation Detectors: Technology and Applications
Salah Awadalla

Structural Health Monitoring of Composite Structures Using Fiber Optic Methods
Ginu Rajan and Gangadhara Prusty

Technologies for Smart Sensors and Sensor Fusion
Kevin Yallup and Krzysztof Iniewski

Diagnostic Devices with Microfluidics

Edited by
Francesco Piraino • **Šeila Selimović**

Managing Editor
Krzysztof Iniewski

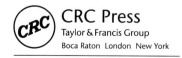

CRC Press
Taylor & Francis Group
Boca Raton London New York

CRC Press is an imprint of the
Taylor & Francis Group, an **informa** business

CRC Press
Taylor & Francis Group
6000 Broken Sound Parkway NW, Suite 300
Boca Raton, FL 33487-2742

© 2017 by Taylor & Francis Group, LLC,
CRC Press is an imprint of Taylor & Francis Group, an Informa business

No claim to original U.S. Government works

Printed on acid-free paper

International Standard Book Number-13: 978-1-4987-7293-8 (Hardback)

Contents

Section I Microfluidic Devices for Diagnostics

Section II Applications in Disease Detection

Section III   Practical Aspects of Developing a Commercial Diagnostic Device

Preface

This book provides insight into the latest developments in point-of-care (POC) and laboratory diagnostic devices that are based on microfluidic principles. Microfluidic techniques and devices have had a steadily growing influence on research in life sciences and bioengineering, leading to their adoption in modern diagnostic solutions. The goal of this book is to highlight this growing field and present a selection of important topics, making it an excellent introductory reading for graduate students in bioengineering and related disciplines. The book is also suitable for advanced researchers, as a review of the latest published studies.

The three sections of the book are devoted to the devices for diagnostics, applications for specific diseases, and practical aspects of developing a diagnostic device.

Chapter 1 provides the description of a handheld microfluidic device for POC in vitro diagnostics. In Chapter 2, recent developments in wearable microfluidic sensors are highlighted, with a special focus on microfluidic devices for monitoring physical and physiological activity and noninvasive collection and analysis of biological fluids, such as breath condensates, sweat, saliva, and tears. The chapter discusses paper-based microfluidics, which is an emerging and rapidly developing technology. It harnesses the material merits of paper as well as the basic concepts of microfluidics. This synergistic combination not only leverages analytical functions and transforms them into a POC technique, but also renders the configuration of the assay as simple as possible. It is advantageous to address technical bottlenecks in current diagnostic assays and to develop novel POC tests. Consequently, paper-based microfluidics is capable of enhancing the delivery of healthcare interventions to patients, especially in resource-limited settings, showing potential to revolutionize first-line clinical practice. Chapter 3 provides a background of paper-based microfluidics, reviews the recent advances in fabrication techniques, and emphasizes its critical applications in a few specific clinical scenarios, including immunoassay, blood typing, and sickle disease detection. Chapter 4 describes a method for fabricating paper analytical devices (PADs) containing wax-ink valves to control the timing of reagent delivery in multistep assays. Wax-ink valves are printed onto membranes in defined patterns and can be actuated by applying localized heat to the valves to allow fluid to flow. Here, the authors describe how to use these valves to enhance the lateral flow immunoassay detection signal water test kit to detect microbiological contamination. Chapter 5 briefly describes some of the established methods of mycotoxin analysis and highlights the limitations of these methods. The need to develop rapid, portable analytical platforms is emphasized. These platforms must be able to compete with the gold standard techniques in areas such as sensitivity and specificity so that analysis can be moved from the laboratory to "on-site" monitoring. Current research on microfluidics-based devices is examined and examples of devices utilizing microfluidic platforms to offer potential solutions for rapid analysis are described throughout the chapter. Chapter 6 describes a device and its technology underpinnings that are capable of revolutionizing clinical breath diagnostics based on a combination of its small size, low power requirements, ease of use, and applicability to a broad range of clinically relevant biomarker signatures. This technology, based upon the principle of ion mobility spectrometry, generates signature spectral patterns as distinctive as mass spectrometry (MS) but with far greater simplicity and adaptability. The differential mobility spectrometer (DMS) is a portable, handheld device that generates multidimensional biological spectra from volatile compounds found in exhaled breath. Current prototype models of the DMS fit in the palm of the hand, are highly durable, operate at atmospheric pressure, and can be operated with standard batteries.

Due to numerous advantages, there is great potential for microfluidic technology to be applied in the development of disposable, inexpensive, portable, and easy-to-use devices for the detection of infectious diseases in resource-limited settings. Chapter 7 reviews the application of microfluidic device and chips for detecting infectious diseases. While no microfluidic diagnostic platform has been rolled out for TB in endemic countries, significant strides have been made in the development and implementation of molecular diagnostics, which now set the scene for POC microfluidic platforms. Chapter 8 details these molecular diagnostic platforms and follows this with a discussion on the state of the art for TB microfluidic diagnostics that are in development. It also outlines the challenges in scaling up of these interventions and integrating them into healthcare systems.

Chapter 9 highlights considerations for designing a diagnostic device for use on individual patients or populations by assessing and incorporating the answers to two fundamental questions—who is asking for the test and how do test results guide a treatment decision. The methodology described is a best practice for assessing and ensuring that user needs are central to the design, development, and evaluation of a new diagnostic tool. The assessment starts with a clear intended-use statement that is centered on an actionable decision and justifies the time and cost to obtain a diagnosis. This definition is used to frame use-cases and user scenarios that identify users and describe how the test will be implemented, as well as the criteria for generating an actionable test result. All three of these assessments are then used to create a list of product attributes that are required to meet the needs of an end user.

Finally, ensuring that a POC test is designed so that the user can correctly operate and interpret results is paramount to obtaining a correct diagnosis. Designing with end user needs in mind allows researchers to mitigate potential errors and device failures early in the development process. Yet, too often, a lack of knowledge in how to meaningfully engage device users during the research and design process is a roadblock to progress in early diagnostic development. This is especially true in designing for global health settings where resources to access end users may be limited. Chapter 10 outlines techniques to incorporate the needs of users into device development using a framework of human-centered design (HCD). HCD provides a set of methods to engage with users even before a verified diagnostic device has been created to develop tests that have improved clinical diagnoses, regulatory approval, and commercialization outcomes. Two case studies focused on incorporating HCD into early-stage diagnostic test development provide specific examples of methods in use. Finally, common misconceptions about when and how HCD can be used in diagnostic development are addressed.

We sincerely hope that this book will be a source of inspiration for new applications and stimulate further development of microsystems technologies.

Francesco Piraino
Lausanne, Switzerland

Šeila Selimović
Washington, DC

MATLAB® and Simulink® are registered trademarks of The MathWorks, Inc. For product information, please contact:

The MathWorks, Inc.
3 Apple Hill Drive
Natick, MA, 01760-2098 USA
Tel: 508-647-7000
Fax: 508-647-7001
E-mail: info@mathworks.com
Web: www.mathworks.com

Series Editor

Krzysztof (Kris) Iniewski is managing R&D at Redlen Technologies Inc., a start-up company in Vancouver, Columbia, Canada. Redlen's revolutionary production process for advanced semiconductor materials enables a new generation of more accurate, all-digital, radiation-based imaging solutions. Kris is also a founder of Emerging Technologies CMOS Inc. (www.etcmos.com), an organization of high-tech events covering communications, microsystems, optoelectronics, and sensors. In his career, Dr. Iniewski held numerous faculty and management positions at the University of Toronto, University of Alberta, SFU, and PMC-Sierra Inc. He has published over 100 research papers in international journals and conferences. He holds 18 international patents granted in the USA, Canada, France, Germany, and Japan. He is a frequent invited speaker and has consulted for multiple organizations internationally. He has written and edited several books for CRC Press, Cambridge University Press, IEEE Press, Wiley, McGraw-Hill, Artech House, and Springer. His personal goal is to contribute to healthy living and sustainability through innovative engineering solutions. In his leisurely time, Kris can be found hiking, sailing, skiing, or biking in beautiful British Columbia. He can be reached at kris.iniewski@gmail.com.

Editors

Francesco Piraino is currently a research scientist at the Swiss Federal Institute of Technology in Lausanne (Switzerland). He uses microscale technologies to develop next-generation microfluidic diagnostics platforms. Following his graduate studies in Biomedical Engineering at Politecnico di Milano (Italy) and at Harvard-MIT Division of Health Science & Technology (USA), he joined the Broad Institute of MIT and Harvard (USA) to develop devices for single-cell genomics. Dr. Piraino is a trained bioengineer who has also attended programs at the Universitat de Barcelona (Spain), the City College of the City University of New York (USA), and the Massachusetts Institute of Technology (USA). His work aims to solve problems at the intersection of biomedical engineering and medicine. His research interests include in vitro diagnostics, tissue engineering, and biomaterials.

Šeila Selimović is director of the NIBIB programs in tissue chips/tissue preservation technologies and biosensors. Her other scientific interests include lab-on-a-chip platforms, paper microfluidics, and point-of-care diagnostics. In 2015, she was selected as one of the "50 Leaders of Tomorrow" from among hundreds of young biotech leaders in the Mid-Atlantic region. Prior to her current position, she was chosen by the American Association for the Advancement of Science to serve as a Science and Technology Policy Fellow at the U.S. Department of State, where she covered science diplomacy issues related to energy security, climate, and innovation. Previously, she was a postdoctoral research fellow at Harvard Medical School and Brigham and Women's Hospital in Boston, Massachusetts. Dr. Selimović's research has focused on the development of microfluidic platforms for applications in biophysics and biological engineering, and her research interests include the physics of microscale flows, protein crystallization, colloidal suspensions, and rheology and microrheology. Dr. Selimović earned her PhD and MSc in physics from Brandeis University, with National Science Foundation support, and her BA in physics and German from Wellesley College. She is a member of Sigma Xi.

Contributors

Jeffrey T. Borenstein
Biomedical Engineering Centre
    Draper
Cambridge, Massachusetts

Richard S. Conroy
Office of Strategic Coordination
Division of Program Coordination,
    Planning, and Strategic Initiatives
Office of the NIH Director
National Institutes of Health
Bethesda, Maryland

Mohamed Shehata Draz
Department of Medicine
Harvard Medical School
Brigham and Women's Hospital
Cambridge, Massachusetts

Bhavna G. Gordhan
DST/NRF Centre of Excellence for
    Biomedical TB Research
School of Pathology
Faculty of Health Sciences
University of the Witwatersrand
    and the National Health
    Laboratory Service
Johannesburg, South Africa

Elizabeth Johansen
Diagnostics For All
Salem, Massachusetts

and

Spark Health Design
Hanover, Massachusetts

Bavesh D. Kana
DST/NRF Centre of Excellence for
    Biomedical TB Research
School of Pathology
Faculty of Health Sciences
University of the Witwatersrand
    and the National Health
    Laboratory Service
Johannesburg, South Africa

and

Centre for the AIDS Programme of
    Research
Durban, South Africa

Gregor S. Kijanka
Biomedical Diagnostics Institute
Dublin City University
Dublin, Ireland

Sophia Koo
Division of Infectious Diseases
Department of Medicine
Brigham and Women's Hospital
Boston, Massachusetts

Ashok A. Kumar
Jana Care
Boston, Massachusetts

and

Department of Chemistry and
    Chemical Biology
Harvard University
Cambridge, Massachusetts

Baichen Li
Department of Biomedical
    Engineering
School of Engineering and Applied
    Sciences
The George Washington University
Washington, DC

Zhenyu Li
Department of Biomedical
    Engineering
School of Engineering and Applied
    Sciences
The George Washington University
Washington, DC

Mark David Lim
Diagnostics, Global Health
    Bill and Melinda Gates Foundation
Seattle, Washington

Jacqueline C. Linnes
Weldon School of Biomedical
    Engineering
Purdue University
West Lafayette, Indiana

Jonathan H. Loftus
School of Biotechnology
Dublin City University
Dublin, Ireland

Kenneth Markoski
Mechanical Engineering Draper
Cambridge, Massachusetts

Xuan Mu
Division of Engineering in Medicine
Brigham and Women's Hospital
Harvard Medical School
Cambridge, Massachusetts

Erkinjon G. Nazarov
BioMEMS Centre Draper
Tampa, Florida

Richard O'Kennedy
School of Biotechnology and
    Biomedical Diagnostics Institute
Dublin City University
Dublin, Ireland

Vinay M. Pai
National Institute of Biomedical
    Imaging and Bioengineering
National Institutes of Health
Bethesda, Maryland

Hardik Jeetendra Pandya
Department of Medicine
Harvard Medical School
Brigham and Women's Hospital
Cambridge, Massachusetts

Elizabeth Phillips
Weldon School of Biomedical
    Engineering
Purdue University
West Lafayette, Indiana

Timothy Postlethwaite
Biomedical Solutions Program
    Office Draper
Tampa, FL

Mary M. Rodgers
National Institute of Biomedical
    Imaging and Bioengineering
National Institutes of Health
Bethesda, Maryland

Hadi Shafiee
Department of Medicine
Harvard Medical School
Brigham and Women's Hospital
Cambridge, Massachusetts

Majid Ebrahimi Warkiani
School of Mechanical and
    Manufacturing Engineering
University of New South Wales
and
Garvan Institute for Biomedical
    Research
Sydney, New South Wales, Australia
and
School of Medical Sciences
Edith Cowan University
Perth, Western Australia, Australia

Yu Shrike Zhang
Division of Engineering in Medicine
Brigham and Women's Hospital
Harvard Medical School
Cambridge, Massachusetts

Section I

Microfluidic Devices for Diagnostics

1

Handheld Microfluidics for Point-of-Care In Vitro Diagnostics*

Baichen Li and Zhenyu Li

CONTENTS

1.1 Introduction

In vitro diagnostics (IVD) influences 70% of all healthcare decisions according to a study (Lewin Group 2005). However, such a universally demanded service is still largely centralized partly due to the fact that current IVD technologies are still too complicated, expensive, bulky, and slow for point-of-care (POC) settings such as emergency rooms, physicians' offices, patients' homes, and ultimately on (or in) human bodies. One important goal of

---

* Part of this chapter was published in *Lab on a Chip* as a peer-reviewed article (Li et al. 2014).

lab-on-a-chip research is to miniaturize conventional medical diagnostic instruments, including IVD systems (Manz et al. 1992, Whitesides 2006). One common feature of traditional IVD instruments is that they all require complex manipulations of liquid samples such as blood, urine, saliva, and liquid reagents, and so on. Therefore, it is essential for POC IVD systems to have built-in liquid-handling capabilities comparable to robotic pipetting and centrifugation used in conventional clinical labs in order to achieve truly automated sample-to-answer operations. In the past three decades, there have been extensive efforts on miniaturizing liquid-handling components on chip, such as MEMS valves and pumps (Kwang and Chong 2006, Laser and Santiago 2004), elastomeric on-chip valves and pumps (Unger et al. 2000), and droplet manipulation systems (Pollack et al. 2000). However, due to various material, fabrication, integration, and reliability challenges, few handheld (not to mention fully on-chip) self-contained microfluidic systems capable of sophisticated liquid handling exist in the market today except for capillary-driven microfluidics such as lateral flow tests (Wong and Tse 2009). Most lab-on-a-chip systems still rely on bulky off-chip components such as compressed pressure sources, syringe pumps, and electronics to achieve their liquid manipulation functions, which severely limits the applicability of such systems for POC diagnostics, environmental monitoring, and bioterrorism detection. Recently, a handheld instrument was developed that can actuate on-chip elastomeric microvalves using solenoid-containing actuation units (Addae-Mensah et al. 2010). Another promising technique is digital microfluidics, in which droplets are manipulated by electrowetting (Pollack et al. 2000); however, to our knowledge a handheld digital microfluidic system has not been demonstrated. Braille display devices have also been used to build portable microfluidic systems (Gu et al. 2004). In this chapter, we present a smartphone-controlled handheld microfluidic liquid-handling system recently developed by us. It combines elastomeric on-chip microfluidic valves, a handheld pneumatic system, and a smartphone-based control and data processing system. The handheld pneumatic system provides onboard multiple pressure generation, stabilization, and control by using a miniature pump, pressure-storage reservoirs, and small solenoid valves. This system is applicable to both single-layer, pressure-driven microfluidics and multilayer, elastomeric microfluidics (Grover et al. 2003, Hansson et al. 1994, Hosokawa, Maeda 2000, Hansen et al. 2004, Thorsen et al. 2002 and Unger et al. 2000), although the main focus is on the latter. Elastomeric microfluidics refers to microfluidic systems with on-chip valves based on the mechanical deformations of elastomeric membranes or structures, such as multilayer PDMS microfluidics (Hosokawa and Maeda 2000, Unger et al. 2000), glass/PDMS/glass devices (Grover et al. 2003), and other hybrid devices (Hansson et al. 1994).

In a typical elastomeric microfluidic system, often two different pressure sources are needed: one for actuating on-chip valves, which typically require a relatively high pressure level (5–10 psi, depending on the membrane property and valve geometry); and the other for driving reagents into micro-fluidic channels (for typical microfluidic channel dimensions, e.g., 10 μm high, 100 μm wide, 1–5 psi is sufficient for many applications). Traditionally, this is achieved by using two pressure regulators connected to a compressed gas (often nitrogen or air) tank (Unger et al. 2000). However, the sizes and nature of these components make them unsuitable for building a handheld system. Although it is possible to use two separate diaphragm pumps to build such a system, the significant fluctuations of the output pressure of a diaphragm pump limit its applications.

To address these challenges, we have recently developed a handheld microfluidic liquid-handling system controlled by a smartphone (Figure 1.1), which can provide two different stable pressure sources and an array of eight pneumatic control lines for operating elastomeric microfluidic chips (Li et al. 2014). One pressure source (P1) is set to above 10 psi (maximum 20 psi) to operate on-chip elastomeric valves, while the other (P2) can be set to any value between 0 psi and P1 to drive liquid flow, with a precision of ±0.05 psi. Eight independent pneumatic control lines are available to handle eight dif-ferent liquid reagents. The size of the resulting system is 6 × 10.5 × 16.5 cm, and the total weight is 829 g (including battery). The system can operate con-tinuously for 8.7 h while running a sandwich immunoassay liquid-handling protocol when powered by a 12.8 V, 1500 mAh lithium battery. This technol-ogy can serve as a general-purpose, handheld small-volume liquid-handling

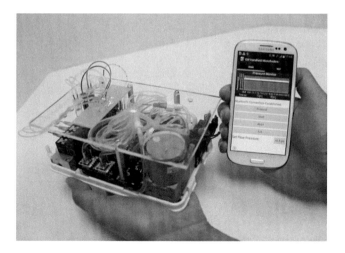

FIGURE 1.1
Picture of the smartphone-controlled handheld microfluidic liquid-handling system. The foot-print of the instrument is 6 × 10.5 × 16.5 cm. Powered by a 12.8 V 1500 mAh lithium battery, the instrument consumes 2.2 W on average for a typical sandwich immunoassay and lasts for 8.7 h. A multilayer PDMS device with on-chip elastomeric valves is on top of the handheld instrument.

platform for many biochemical and cell-based assays such as immunoassay, fluorescence in situ hybridization (FISH), polymerase chain reaction (PCR), flow cytometry, DNA/RNA/protein microarrays, and sequencing. The integration of this system with biosensors may help realize the long-sought dream of handheld multianalyte in vitro diagnostic (IVD) systems, that is, something that can be called a medical tricorder (Qualcomm Tricorder XPRIZE 2014).

1.2 Design of the Handheld Microfluidic System

The overall handheld microfluidic system consists of three subsystems: (1) a pneumatic pressure generation, stabilization, and control subsystem (*pneumatic* subsystem); (2) an electronic printed circuit board (PCB) with two microcontrollers, a Bluetooth wireless communication module, pressure sensors, and power component drivers (*electronic* subsystem); and (3) an elastomeric microfluidic chip (*microfluidic* chip). The system can be controlled by a Bluetooth-enabled Android smartphone (e.g., Galaxy SIII). Each subsystem will be described in more detail in the following sections.

1.2.1 *Pneumatic* Subsystem

The *pneumatic* subsystem is designed to generate two compressed air pressure sources at different levels (P1: >10 psi; P2: 0 to P1) for operating elastomeric microfluidic chips (or cartridges). Two pressure reservoirs, labeled as Reservoir 1 and Reservoir 2 (Figure 1.2), are used to store compressed air. A miniature DC diaphragm pump is used to pump air into Reservoir 1 to generate the primary pressure source for actuating on-chip elastomeric valves (Grover et al. 2003, Hansson et al. 1994, Hosokawa and Maeda 2000, Unger et al. 2000). A secondary pressure source, stored in Reservoir 2, is derived from Reservoir 1 and stabilized by a feedback control system with a precision of ±0.05 psi for driving liquid reagents through microfluidic channels. The system can be easily extended to have multiple secondary pressure sources of different pressures if needed.

Each pressure reservoir is made of four segments of 1/8″ ID Tygon tubing connected with a four-way barbed cross-connector, leaving four open ports. Each open port of a reservoir is connected to a functional part of the pneumatic subsystem (such as a pump, a solenoid valve, or a pressure sensor, as shown in Figure 1.2 and described in more detail in the following) via a barbed connector. The volume of each reservoir is determined by the total length of tubing used. In this work, the volumes of Reservoirs 1 and 2 are 6.2 and 16.2 mL, respectively.

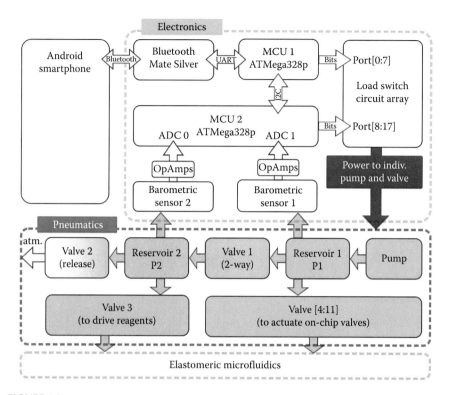

FIGURE 1.2
Block diagram of the handheld microfluidic system. The whole system consists of an Android smartphone, an *electronic* subsystem with microcontrollers and a Bluetooth module, a *pneumatic* subsystem capable of generating two different pressure outputs, and elastomeric *microfluidic* chips. Valve 1 is a two-way normally closed solenoid valve and valves 2–11 are three-way solenoid valves. (Adapted from Li, B.C. et al., *Lab Chip*, 14(20), 4085, August 2014. With permission.)

The four open ports of Reservoir 1 are connected to the following components, respectively:

1. A miniature DC diaphragm pump (Parker, H004C-11), used to generate the primary pressure source for the system. A check valve in-between is used to prevent air leakage when the pump is off.

2. Barometric sensor 1, to monitor the pressure level in Reservoir 1.

3. The normally open (N.O.) port of a solenoid valve manifold with eight channels (Pneumadyne, MSV10-8); each common port of this manifold is connected to an on-chip elastomeric valve.

4. The common port of a solenoid valve (valve 1, Pneumadyne, S10MM-30-12-3) with base (Pneumadyne, MSV10-1), to generate the secondary pressure source (P2, between 0 and P1, typically 0–5 psi). A plastic needle valve restrictor (Poweraire, F-2822-41-B85-K) is placed before the common port of valve 1 to limit the airflow into Reservoir 2.

The four open ports of Reservoir 2 are connected to the components, as follows, respectively:

1. The normally closed (N.C.) port of valve 1, described earlier. Once the pressure in Reservoir 2 drops to below the lower bound of the target pressure range, valve 1 will be opened to increase the Reservoir 2 pressure gradually. Another plastic needle valve restrictor (Poweraire, F-2822-41-B85-K) is used to fine-tune the flow rate of air to reduce excessive pressure overshoot in Reservoir 2. The N.O. port of valve 1 is completely sealed with PDMS to mimic a two-way N.C. valve.

2. The N.C. port of a solenoid valve (valve 2), to release pressure in Reservoir 2. The common port of valve 2 is sealed with PDMS, resulting in a small internal air volume (~250 μL). By toggling the state of valve 2, its internal volume is connected to either Reservoir 2 or atmosphere. When Reservoir 2 is connected to valve 2's internal volume, the pressure in Reservoir 2 drops by a small amount due to volume expansion. Immediately following this, the pressure in valve 2's internal volume is released by connecting it to atmosphere. By choosing the appropriate Reservoir 2 volume, we can control the pressure release precisely to achieve the desired pressure resolution. Design details can be found in Li et al. (2014 ESI).

3. Barometric sensor 2, to monitor the pressure level in Reservoir 2.

4. The N.C. port of a solenoid valve (valve 3), to drive reagents into a microfluidic chip. The common port of valve 3 is divided into multiple lines, each connected to a reagent container (a modified microcentrifuge tube). Once it is actuated, the pressure stored in Reservoir 2 is applied to every reagent container in the system.

1.2.2 Pressure Stabilization in Reservoirs 1 and 2

The pressure levels in the two reservoirs of the *pneumatic* subsystem are automatically adjusted by a feedback control algorithm programmed in the second microcontroller, with the barometric sensor as the feedback sensor, and the diaphragm pump and solenoid valves (valves 1 and 2) for pressure control. A user only needs to set the upper and lower bounds of both pressure levels through the smartphone interface.

Reservoir 1, which contains higher pressure (>10 psi) to actuate on-chip valves and serves as the pressure source for Reservoir 2, is directly pressurized by the diaphragm pump. If the pressure level drops to below the chosen lower bound detected by barometric sensor 1, the pump starts to run until the pressure is restored to the target upper bound.

The pressure in Reservoir 2 is used to drive liquid reagents through microfluidic channels, and the required pressure level is relatively low (normally below 5 psi for typical microfluidic channel dimensions of 10–100 μm). However, it is desirable to be able to precisely change the Reservoir 2 pressure in seconds. In order to obtain a stable Reservoir 2 pressure, instead of directly using the diaphragm pump as the pressure source, we used Reservoir 1 as a buffered pressure supply, connected to Reservoir 2 via a two-way N.C. solenoid valve (valve 1). As already described, another three-way solenoid valve (valve 2) is used to precisely release pressure in a stepwise fashion. If a pressure below the set lower bound is sensed, valve 1 will be opened. Conversely, if the pressure exceeds the higher bound, valve 2 starts to operate to decrease the pressure in Reservoir 2.

1.2.3 Microcontroller-Based *Electronic* Subsystem

We used two ATMega328p 8-bit microcontrollers in the electronics design. The first microcontroller is responsible for four tasks: (1) receive commands from a smartphone via Bluetooth 2.1 (Bluetooth Mate Silver, Sparkfun, WRL-12576), (2) pass commands to the second microcontroller, (3) request real-time barometric sensor data from the second microcontroller and send it to the smartphone at a frequency of 50 Hz, and (4) control the status of 6 load switch circuits for pump and solenoid valve operation. The second microcontroller also has four functions: (1) control the status of the other 12 load switch circuits (making the system capable of operating 18 electromechanical components [valves or pumps]), (2) monitor the barometric sensor data with the built-in 10-bit ADCs, (3) automatically adjust pressure levels in the two pressure reservoirs, and (4) send barometric sensor data to the first microcontroller on request. Communication between these two microcontrollers is realized with the Wire Library provided by Arduino, which enables bidirectional communication via only two wires using the I2C protocol.

Two barometric sensors (Measurement Specialties, 1240-015D-3L) are used to acquire real-time pressure data in the pneumatic subsystem. Electrical sensor output data are amplified by two instrumentation amplifiers (Texas Instruments, INA114). We also used two general-purpose rail-to-rail operation amplifiers (Texas Instruments, OPA2171) to shift the signal level to between 0 and 5 V before connecting to the 10-bit ADCs of the second microcontroller. Each barometric sensor is calibrated with a commercial-grade sanitary pressure gauge (Ashcroft, 1035). The calibration curve is saved in the microcontroller's flash memory. Detailed calibration procedure and results can be found in Li et al. (2014).

Our PCB circuit is powered by a 12.8 V LiFePO4 battery pack with a capacity of 1500 mAh. This battery is directly used as the power supply to an array of 18 load switch circuits to power solenoid valves and the diaphragm pump. Each output of the load switch circuit is wired to a screw terminal block (Sparkfun, PRT-08084), into which the power wires of the valves and pump are mounted. The battery is also regulated by a 5 V regulator to power the PCB (microcontrollers, Bluetooth module, barometric sensors, and OpAmps).

1.2.4 Android Application

An Android (version 4.2) app with a graphical user interface (GUI) was written to allow user control of the system, and the display and analysis of collected data. We designed a straightforward application protocol (details can be found in Li et al. (2014 ESI), and implemented it in, both, the smartphone app and the ATMega328 microcontrollers. This application protocol has three basic functions: (1) set the status of each solenoid valve, (2) set the target pressure range of each reservoir, and (3) request barometric sensor readings from the microcontroller. The protocol of the bead-based fluorescence immunoassay is programmed in this Android application, using these three fundamental functions, to achieve liquid manipulation and monitor the pressure levels of the reservoirs.

1.2.5 Microfluidic Device Design and Fabrication, Reagent Containers, and Interfaces

We fabricated a PDMS elastomeric microfluidic chip using conventional multilayer soft lithography (Unger et al. 2000) for microbead-based sandwich florescence immunoassays. The on-chip valves were operated in a push-down configuration (flow layer on the bottom). Briefly, we first fabricated the master molds using standard UV photolithography with AZ50XT positive photoresist. The control layer was made by pouring a PDMS mixture (RTV615 A:B at a 5:1 ratio) onto the mold and baking it for 1 h at 65°C. For the flow layer, a PDMS mixture at a 20:1 ratio was spin coated onto the flow layer mold at 3000 rpm for 1 min and baked at 65°C for 30 min. After curing of these two layers, we peeled off the control layer from the mold, aligned and placed it on top of the flow layer, followed by a 2 h bake. Then the device was peeled off the flow layer mold and bonded to a glass slide by air plasma treatment. The design of the microfluidic device is given in the section 1.3.2.

The reagent containers were modified 1.5 mL disposable microcentrifuge tubes (Ted Pella MC-6600, polypropylene). The lid of every tube was punched by a 21 gauge needle to form two holes. Two 21 gauge needles of different lengths were inserted into the holes. The longer needle was immersed in the liquid reagent, while the shorter one was above the liquid surface for pressurization. By storing the reagents in the tubes, and applying air pressure through the shorter needle, the reagents were pushed out from the longer needle. Interfaces between the pneumatic subsystem, the reagent containers, and the microfluidic devices were made of Tygon tubings and 21 gauge needles. Details can be found in Li et al. (2014 ESI).

1.2.6 Simulated Bead-Based Fluorescence Immunoassay Liquid Handling

As a demonstration, we used the system to perform all the liquid-handling steps of a microbead-based sandwich fluorescence immunoassay (FIA) (Wild 2005). We used three colored food dyes to simulate the reagents used

TABLE 1.1

Simulated Immunoassay Liquid-Handling Protocol

1. Fill the device with blocking buffer (green, 5 s).
2. Incubate (5 min).
3. Load washing buffer (clear, 5 min).
4. Load beads (red, 10 s).
5. Load washing buffer (clear, 5 min).
6. Load sample (red, 5 s) and incubate (1 min). Repeat step 6 ten times.
7. Load washing buffer (clear, 5 min).
8. Load detection antibody (green, 5 s) and incubate (1 min). Repeat step 8 ten times.
9. Load washing buffer (clear, 5 min).
10. Ready for detection.

in this immunoassay. The detailed 10-step FIA protocol (liquid-handling sequences) is shown in Table 1.1. Briefly, the microfluidic channels are first blocked by a blocking buffer to reduce nonspecific binding. Then, capture antibody-coated polystyrene microbeads are loaded and immobilized by the microfluidic hydrodynamic traps (Tan and Takeuchi 2007, Xu et al. 2013a,b). Microbeads of different sizes can be immobilized at different locations for multiplexed detections. Then after a washing step, sample solution is loaded into the reaction chamber and allowed to incubate. During the incubation, the liquid flow is controlled to move back and forth to facilitate mixing and target binding. The sample loading and incubation step is repeated 10 times. After another washing step, fluorescently labeled detection antibodies will be loaded and allowed for incubation. Finally, excess detection antibodies and other reagents will be washed away, and the microbeads are then ready for fluorescence readout.

1.3 System Performance

1.3.1 Pneumatic Subsystem

We first characterized the pneumatic performance of the system, including achievable pressure range, pressure stability, response time, and leakage rate. Reservoir 1 was tested under no loading conditions, with a target pressure range of 13–14 psi. The maximum achievable pressure was ~20 psi, limited by the diaphragm pump. Starting from 0 psi, it took about 0.3 s to rise to 14 psi (Figure 1.3a). The pressure dropped by about 1 psi every minute, and the pump automatically started to restore the pressure in Reservoir 1. This level of pressure leakage, although preventable by better sealing, does not affect the actuation of on-chip valves, nor the pressure level in Reservoir 2 due to the feedback pressure stabilization mechanism described earlier.

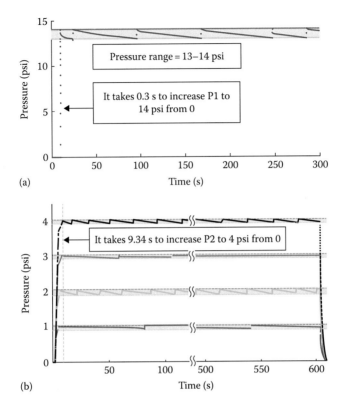

(a)

(b)

FIGURE 1.3
Pneumatic subsystem performance. (a) Performance test of pressure source 1: P1. The target pressure range of P1 was set to 13–14 psi. The plot shows the reading from barometric sensor 1 over 300 s. (b) Performance test of pressure source 2: P2. P2 was tested under four different target pressure levels: 1, 2, 3, and 4 psi (four colored curves), with a tolerance of ±0.05 psi. Meanwhile, one on-chip valve was opened to allow a reagent (colored food dye) to be driven into the microfluidic chip. Every test lasted for 10 min. The target pressure was set to 0 psi at the end of each test. (Adapted from Li, B.C. et al., *Lab Chip*, 14(20), 4085, August 2014. With permission.)

Reservoir 2 was tested and characterized with a simple one-channel pressure-driven microfluidic chip as the load. Colored food dye was pushed into the microfluidic channel (500 × 20 μm, W × H) continuously. We tested four integer pressure levels below 4 psi (1, 2, 3, 4 psi), with a tolerance of ±0.05 psi. The measured results are shown in Figure 1.3b. It took about 10 s for the pressure in Reservoir 2 to rise to 4 psi, which is much longer compared with that of Reservoir 1. This is because we used two needle valve restrictors to limit the flow rate between Reservoir 1 and Reservoir 2 to improve stability. During the 10 min test, the pressure was completely controlled in the target pressure ranges. At the end of the tests, we set the target pressure to 0 psi to examine the performance of pressure release. The results were comparable to theoretical calculations from ideal gas law.

During the tests, we found that the volume of a reservoir, especially Reservoir 2, had a significant influence on the performance. Whenever the system opens a valve, the effective volume of a reservoir will increase, which leads to a pressure drop inside the reservoir. When reagents are driven into a microfluidic device, the effective volume of Reservoir 2 is also increased (Figure 1.3b). Increasing the volume of a reservoir will make it less sensitive to volume changes. However, this will increase the size of the system, which is undesirable for a handheld system. Moreover, increasing the volume of Reservoir 2 makes it respond slower when changing the target pressure settings. We found the parameters listed earlier gave sufficient performance for our immunoassay applications, but there is still room for improvements by optimizing the airflow rate and volumes of reservoirs.

Improving the sealing of the pneumatic system will also improve the overall performance of the system, in terms of pressure and power. In this work, no special effort was made to ensure that the system was completely airtight, as the pressure performance was sufficient for our applications. However, it is desirable and feasible to improve the sealing in the future with better pneumatic connections and components, so that the system can be more stable and consume less power.

Next, we tested the operation of on-chip valves under a bright field optical microscope. We validated that the on-chip valves could be fully closed without leakage by driving colored food dye into the flow layer at P2 = 2 psi, and toggling the state of the controlling solenoid valve multiple times. The on-chip valve was completely closed when P1 was set to 13–14 psi. We also tested other PDMS devices with different valve geometries and configurations (both push-up and push-down), and found that it is possible to operate properly designed push-up valves with even lower actuation pressure down to 5 psi, as already reported (Studer et al. 2004).

1.3.2 Microbead-Based HIV p24 Immunoassay

A real HIV p24 antigen detection immunoassay was performed to demonstrate the system liquid-handling performance;15 μm carboxylated polystyrene beads were used as the solid phase, and immobilized at predefined locations by the microfluidic hydrodynamic traps. Monoclonal anti-p24 antibodies (Abcam) were covalently attached to the beads by standard EDC (Carbodiimide) coupling chemistry (Bangs PolyLink Protein Coupling Kit). FITC labeled polycolonal anti-p24 were used as the detection antibodies. HIV-1 p24 antigen standard (ZeptoMetrix) with known concentrations serially diluted in 1X PBS Tween-20 buffer were used as the samples. Blocking buffers (Superblock, Pierce) and washing buffers (PBS + 0.1% Tween-20, Pierce) were filtered using 0.2 μm filters to remove any debris that might clog the microfluidic device. The liquid-handling protocol was the same as the simulated protocol given in Table 1.1. The fluorescence readout was performed on an Olympus IX71 fluorescence microscope at 20× magnification

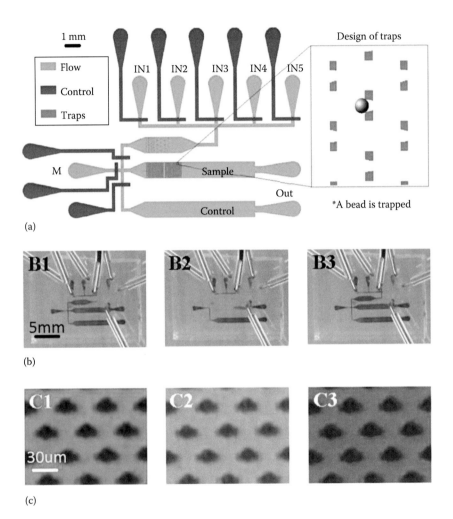

FIGURE 1.4

Two-layer PDMS elastomeric *microfluidic* chip for bead-based immunoassays and demonstration of immunoassay liquid handling. (a) Design layout of the microfluidic chip for bead-based immunoassays. Inset: Magnified view of the hydrodynamic trap arrays with one trapped microbead. (b1–b3) Washing and incubating the immobilized microbeads with different reagents. Two colored dyes and water were used to simulate different reagents in an immunoassay. (c1–c3) Optical micrographs of an array of microbeads in the traps. Microbeads of 15 μm diameter are loaded before the experiment. Optical micrographs showing the trapped microbeads being washed (or incubated) with different colored liquids. Two videos showing the operations of the system and the microfluidic traps are available in Li et al. (2014). (Adapted from Li, B.C. et al., *Lab Chip*, 14(20), 4085, August 2014. With permission.)

equipped with an FITC filter set and an Andor iXon+ EMCCD with an electron multiplication gain of 300 and 10 s integration time. The fluorescence readout can be miniaturized into a handheld system by using low-noise photodiodes, or avalanche photodiodes (APDs) or miniature photomultiplier tubes (PMTs).

The design layout of the PDMS microfluidic device is shown in Figure 1.4a. The device has five inlet ports, two reaction chambers (sample and control), and one outlet port. Each inlet port is supplied with one of the following reagents: blocking buffer (e.g., PBS + 0.1% Tween-20 + 0.5% BSA), washing buffer (e.g., PBS + 0.1% Tween-20), capture antibody-coated polystyrene microbeads, sample, and fluorescently labeled detection antibodies. Inside the reaction chambers, arrays of hydrodynamic traps with openings of different sizes are used to immobilize individual capture antibody-coated microbeads at predefined locations (Wild 2005, Xu et al. 2013b). Sequential traps of different sizes (larger sizes upstream) can be used to trap different-sized microbeads for multiplexed detection. In addition, such bead trapping based assays are naturally reconfigurable by changing the capture-molecule coated bead species without modifying the microfluidic chips. Once the microbeads are immobilized, subsequent mixing, washing, and incubation steps can be easily performed on them under well-controlled flow conditions. During the incubation steps, the liquid flow can be controlled to move back and forth by pressurizing port M (Figure 1.4a) and the output port alternatively to facilitate mixing and target binding. For every test, all reagents except for the sample solution are loaded into both reaction chambers, following the sequence of a typical sandwich florescence immunoassay protocol. Sample solution will be loaded only into the sample chamber, leaving the other chamber as a control. All waste is discharged from the outlet port, and collected by a disposable microcentrifuge tube. We designed a 10-step simulated fluorescence immunoassay protocol (Table 1.1), which took about 50 min to complete. This protocol was programmed in the Android application, and could be easily modified by the user. Two different colored food dyes and water were used to simulate various reagents. Screenshots of various liquids flowing inside the microfluidic device are shown in Figure 1.4b. A video showing the system operating in real time is available in Li et al. (2014).

After the on-chip liquid handling, the real HIV p24 immunoassay was read out on an Olympus IX 71 microscope. The lower limit of detection (LoD) was about 2 pg/mL (background + 3std of the noise floor), comparable to commercially available HIV1 p24 ELISA tests (e.g., ZeptoMetrix RETRO-TEK HIV-1 p24 Antigen ELISA 2.0). The system dynamic range was tested from 2 to 130 pg/mL.

1.3.3 Power Consumption

Power consumption is a critical performance metric of a handheld system. We used a digital multimeter (Keithley, Model 2000) to record the voltage

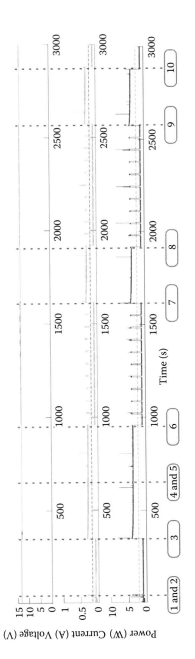

FIGURE 1.5

Power consumption for running the simulated immunoassay protocol (Table 1.1). A digital multimeter (DMM) was connected to the system to measure the voltage (V) and current (I) of the battery at a frequency of 10 Hz. Power consumption was then calculated as P = VI. The immunoassay protocol took about 50 min to complete. Horizontal dashed lines (black) indicate the average values of the measured parameters. Vertical dashed lines (marked with numbers in a box) indicate the starting points of the various immunoassay steps. (Adapted from Li, B.C. et al., *Lab Chip*, 14(20), 4085, August 2014. With permission.)

and current changes at a sampling rate of 10 Hz while running the simulated immunoassay protocol. Power consumption was obtained by multiplying the voltage with the current (Figure 1.5). The average power consumption during the simulated immunoassay was 2.2 W. As the capacity of the battery used was 19.2 Wh, the system could last for 8.7 h on one full charge.

The average power consumption of 2.2 W can be further reduced by 0.65 W by replacing the normally closed (N.C.) solenoid valve (valve 3) at the output of Reservoir 2 with a normally open (N.O.) one. Additionally, if we replace the solenoid valves with latching solenoid valves or use a "Spike and Hold" circuit (Lee Company, 2006), the power consumption can be further reduced to less than 1 W. We also found that when our system was idle (no solenoid valves are operating), it still consumed 0.98 W of power, which can be reduced by redesigning the circuit with low-power microcontrollers (TI MSP430) and electronic components (e.g., TI CC2540 or CC2640 Bluetooth low-energy SoC). The system operation time can also be extended by using a higher capacity battery. For example, four 2600 mAh cell phone Li batteries (3.7 V) can theoretically power the device for 25 h on a full charge, thus permitting full-day operation.

The current system measures 6 × 10.5 × 16.5 cm (H × W × L), and the total weight is 829 g (including the battery). By improving the design and choosing more compact components such as integrating miniature solenoid valves (LHL series valves, The Lee Company) on a PCB and using surface mounted (SMD) microcontrollers (TI MSP430) and smaller PCBs, we believe it is feasible to reduce the weight to below 1 pound (454 g), and reduce the size by a half in the future. With better designed microfluidic devices, we can also decrease the pressure required for actuating on-chip valves, and consequently, further reduce the power consumption, size, and weight of the whole system.

1.4 Summary

In this chapter, we have described a smartphone-operated, fully automated handheld microfluidic liquid-handling system for POC IVDs. In addition to traditional multilayer PDMS microfluidics, this system is also applicable to other types of elastomeric microfluidics such as devices similar to GE's Biacore™ SPR chips (Hansson et al. 1994), glass/PDMS/glass devices (Grover et al. 2003), and other hybrid devices (Webster 1987). We believe this general-purpose, handheld liquid-handling system is an enabling technology that can find broad applications in point-of-care medical diagnostics, environmental testing, food safety inspection, biohazard detection, and fundamental biological research. Several practical challenges such as handling of complex biological samples like whole blood, chip-to-world interface, low-cost manufacture, onboard reagent storage, and disposable cartridges remain to be demonstrated. If successfully addressed, the integration of this technology with readout biosensors may help enable the realization of handheld IVD systems with performance comparable to those of clinical lab instruments.

Acknowledgments

This work was partially supported by the National Institute of Biomedical Imaging and Bioengineering (NIBIB) of the National Institutes of Health (NIH) under award number U01EB021986, and by the National Science Foundation under Grant No. 0963717.

References

Addae-Mensah K.A., Cheung Y.K., Fekete V., Rendely M., and Sia S.K., *Lab on a Chip*, 2010, 10, 1618–1622.

Grover W.H., Skelley A.M., Liu C.N., Lagally E.T., and Mathies R.A., *Sensors and Actuators B: Chemical*, 2003, 89(3), 315–323.

Gu W., Zhu X., Futai N., Cho B.S., and Takayama S., *Proceedings of the National Academy of Sciences of the United States of America*, 2004, 101(45), 15861–15866.

Hansen C.L., Sommer M.O., and Quake S.R., *Proceedings of the National Academy of Sciences of the United States of America*, 2004, 101(40), 14431.

Hansson T. et al., US Patent 5,593,130, 1994.

Hosokawa K. and Maeda R., *Journal of Micromechanics and Microengineering*, 2000, 10, 415.

Kwang W.H. and Chong H.A., *Journal of Micromechanics and Microengineering*, 2006, 16, R13.

Laser D.J. and Santiago J.G., *Journal of Micromechanics and Microengineering*, 2004, 14, R35–R64.

Lee Company, *Electro-Fluidic Systems Handbook*, 2006, Release7.1, Westbrook, CT.

Lewin Group, *The Value of Diagnostics*, 2005, Falls Church, VA.

Li B.C., Li L., Guan A., Dong Q., Ruan K.C., Hu R.G., and Li Z.Y., A smartphone controlled handheld microfluidic liquid handling system, *Lab on a Chip*, August 2014, 14(20), 4085–4092.

Manz A., Harrison D.J., Verpoorte E.M., Fettinger J.C., Paulus A., Lüdi H., and Widmer H.M., *Journal of Chromatography*, 1992, 593, 253–258.

Pollack M.G., Fair R.B., and Shenderov A.D., *Applied Physics Letters*, 2000, 77(11), 1725–1726.

Qualcomm Tricorder XPRIZE, http://tricorder.xprize.org/ (accessed August 2016), 2014.

Studer V., Hang G., Pandolfi A., Ortiz M., Anderson W.F., and Quake S.R.J., *Applied Physics*, 2004, 95(1), 393–398.

Tan H. and Takeuchi S., *Proceedings of the National Academy of Sciences of the United States of America*, 2007, 104, 1146–1151.

Thorsen T., Maerkl S.J., and Quake S.R., *Science*, 2002, 298, 580–584.

Unger M.A., Chou H.P., Thorsen T., Scherer A., and Quake S.R., *Science*, 2000, 288, 113–116.

Webster M.E., US Patent, 4,858,883, 1987.

Whitesides G.W., *Nature*, 2006, 442, 368–373. Arpe, H.J. 2007. *Industrielle Organische Chemie*. Weinheim, Germany: Wiley VCH.

Wild D. ed., *The Immunoassay Handbook*, 3rd edn., Elsevier, 2005.

Wong R. and Tse H. ed., *Lateral Flow Immunoassay*, Humana Press, 2009.

Xu X.X., Li Z.Y., Kotagiri N., Sarder P., Achilefu S., and Nehorai A., *Proceedings of SPIE*, 2013a, 8615, 86151E.

Xu X.X., Sarder P., Li Z.Y., and Nehorai A., *Biomicrofluidics*, 2013b, 7, 014112.

2

Body-Worn Microfluidic Sensors

Mary M. Rodgers, Vinay M. Pai, and Richard S. Conroy

CONTENTS

2.1 Introduction

Body-worn microfluidic sensors have the potential to impact global health for many reasons. The rising cost of monitoring, management, and treatment of chronic diseases and conditions with current approaches, coupled with the aging of the global population, has precipitated a critical need for better healthcare management. Increasingly discussed, precision medicine is an approach that customizes healthcare for an individual and is greatly assisted by tailored monitoring and tracking of an individual's physiological and molecular biomarkers. Strategies for diagnosing conditions at an early stage will potentially lead to better outcomes and prognostic power that can lead to possible avoidance of disease with effective interventions.

Body-worn sensors that provide unobtrusive, regular measurement of specific physiological parameters and biomarkers from bodily fluids noninvasively and comfortably for extended periods of time are important for realizing affordable precision healthcare. In this chapter, we will highlight recent developments in wearable microfluidic sensors with a focus on microfluidic devices for two purposes: (1) monitoring physical and physiological activity and (2) for the noninvasive collection and analysis of biological fluids such as breath condensates, sweat, saliva, and tears. This chapter is not a comprehensive review of the field, but a preview of the potential role wearable microfluidic systems may play in precision medicine.

2.2 Methods and Technologies for Collecting, Sensing, and Detection

Noninvasive, body-worn microfluidic devices that are unobtrusive can provide repetitive measurements and are user-friendly, have the potential to significantly improve our understanding of the different time courses of chronic diseases, causes of idiopathic diseases, or improve selection of treatment choices. Additionally, they can potentially help in early diagnosis of biomedical or behavioral health issues. Microfluidic devices offer two configurations that can be used for sensing biomarkers related to human health. In a sealed system, where there is no path from fluid in the sensor to the human wearing the device, the fluid can be used for sensing physical activity such as movement or physiological measures such as pulse rate. The second configuration is as an open system, in which the microfluidic channels are configured to sample exogenous biofluids secreted by the body. An additional design consideration for the devices that are used to study biofluids is whether to include detection and readout as part of an integrated package, or whether to just sample and store specimens. Both of these general configurations provide their own opportunities and challenges for monitoring health and will be discussed in more detail later in this chapter.

The inclusion of detection and readout is advantageous for providing rapid analysis; however, it comes with high manufacturing and power requirements. There is a wide diversity of methods for detecting biomarkers of interest that can be integrated into a microfluidic system, including biochemical, electrochemical, electroluminescence or chemiluminescence, fluorescence, spectroscopy, and colorimetry that can measure different properties such as intensity, rate of change, changes in spectra or voltage, or presence of specific molecules, for example from enzymatic action on a substrate. With the recognition that it is often desirable to measure multiple biomarkers, there is increasing interest in developing multiplex assays using regionally labeled surfaces, nanoparticles, or synthetic biological systems. Despite the advantages of integrating sensors, there are practical limitations to maintaining reliably, sensitivity, and specificity for a significant length of time in daily life. The following two sections provide more detailed description of recent advances in the design of closed and open systems, highlighting recent advances for making them wearable.

2.2.1 Closed System Designs

Microfluidic interfacial capacitive sensing (MICS) has been utilized in a variety of sensors for detection of force and pressure. There are a number of advantages of MICS over conventional sensors, including ultrahigh pressure sensitivity, ultraprecise mechanical resolution, optical transparency, excellent mechanical flexibility, outstanding adaptability and compatibility, fast response time (>1 kHz), ultrathin microstructure (<200 microns), massive scalability, and manufacturability (Nie et al. 2014). A device developed by Nie et al. (2014) provides three-dimensional (3D) contact force measurement utilizing MICS principles. Consisting of common and differential microfluidic sensing elements and topologically microtextured surfaces, the microfluidic sensing device measures both normal mechanical loads and forces tangential to the surface upon contact. In response to normal or shear loads, the membrane surface deforms the underlying sensing elements either uniformly or differentially. The corresponding variation in interfacial capacitance can be detected from each sensing unit, from which the direction and magnitude of the original load can be determined. Benefiting from the highly sensitive and adaptive MICS principle, the microfluidic sensor is capable of detecting normal forces with a device sensitivity of 29.8 nF N^{-1} in a 7 mm × 7 mm × 0.52 mm package, which is at least a thousand times higher than its solid-state counterparts. In addition, the microfluidic sensing elements enable facilitated relaxation response/time in the millisecond range (up to 12 ms). This 3D microfluidic sensor has been configured into a fingertip-mounted setting for continuous tracing of the fingertip movement and contact force measurement.

A wearable artificial skin was developed by Chossat et al. (2015) to detect hand motion (Figure 2.1). The skin has an array of embedded soft train sensors for detecting various hand gestures by measuring joint motions of the five fingers. The skin is composed of an elastomer material with embedded microchannels filled with two different liquid conductors, an ionic liquid and a liquid metal. The ionic liquid microchannels detect the mechanical strain changes of the sensing material, and the liquid metal microchannels are used as flexible and stretchable electrical wires connecting the sensors to an external control circuit. Flexible conductive threads provide an electrical interface that prevents the two liquid conductors from mixing.

Body-worn microfluidic sensors have also been developed to monitor hemodynamic pressure. Digiglio et al. (2014) combined microfluidics and electronics to produce a miniature, flexible, transparent, highly sensitive, and wearable pressure sensor with microfluidic elements (Figure 2.2). The microflotronic sensor is comprised of an array of sensors positioned over the target artery to provide noninvasive and continuous blood pressure measurement. The ultraflexible and thin plastic construct of the microflotronic sensor (of 270 microns in height) can be worn comfortably for extended

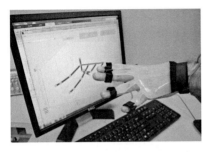
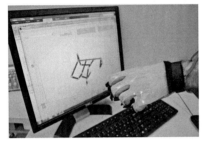
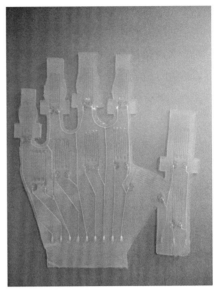

FIGURE 2.1

Shown is a soft and compliant microfluidic skin used to capture hand motion. The artificial skin is filled with microfluidic channels embedded with two different conductive liquids: one is a room temperature ionic liquid (RTIL) and the other a low-temperature melting alloy (eGaIn). The use of multiple liquids effectively decouples the sensing from the signal routing function as each liquid's impedance is several orders different from the other. As the skin moves, the channels' cross-sectional areas change, thus changing each channel's impedance. The two different liquids are connected through sewn-in conductive thread. (Photo courtesy of Jean-Baptiste Chossat.)

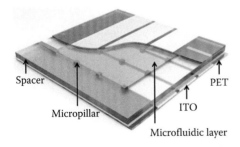
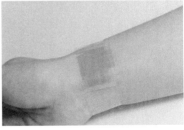

FIGURE 2.2

Construction of the microfluidic pressure sensor element is shown along with a demonstration of the sensing array placement over the radial artery. Tonometry can be performed by applying minimal pressure over the artery using the microflotronic device. (Photo courtesy of Ruya Li.)

periods of time. This microflotronic sensor has been utilized to perform arterial tonometry using noninvasive real-time monitoring of arterial blood pressure waveforms.

2.2.2 Open System Designs for Biofluid Analysis

The ideal, wearable microfluidic device for bodily fluids can be envisaged as a smart, noninvasive, flexible device that can work with unprocessed samples, can multiplex the analysis of several biomarkers quickly and measure over a large dynamic range, can self-calibrate and fault-check, minimizes crosstalk or false positives, and can communicate the results in an appropriate manner to the user and healthcare professionals while being low-cost, user-friendly, unobtrusive, and having minimal power requirements. Abbott's FreeStyleLibre (Care 2016), a wearable, minimally invasive, continuous blood glucose system, illustrates how far wearable noninvasive solutions have progressed recently and the potential for more comprehensive noninvasive monitoring of other bodily fluids. Miller and colleagues (Miller et al. 2014) describe a minimally invasive microneedle-based transdermal sensor that provides on-chip potentiometric determination of K+ (Figure 2.3). This K+ microneedle sensor includes a solid-state ion selective electrode that is integrated into a microfluidic channel. Another minimally invasive biosensor for monitoring glucose and lactate is described by Gowers et al. (2015). This 3D printed microfluidic analysis system integrates with clinical microdialysis probes and biosensors housed in 3D printed electrode holders (Figure 2.4).

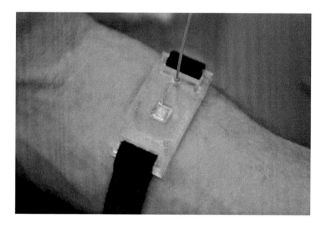

FIGURE 2.3
Shown is a prototype microneedle fluidic device placed on a human forearm. Plastic laminate technology was used to create a fluidic pathway between transdermal microneedle sampler, integrated electrode transducer, and exterior pump (with tube shown on back end). (Photo courtesy of Phillip Miller and Ronen Polsky.)

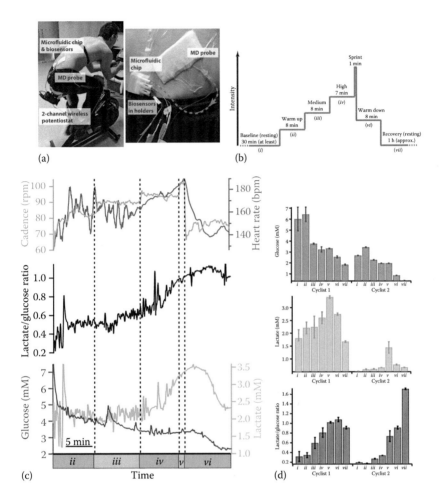

FIGURE 2.4

(a) Photograph of microfluidic device to measure tissue glucose and lactate levels in dialysate during the cycling protocol. Dialysate flowed into the microfluidic chip, housing the glucose and lactate biosensors, which were connected to wireless potentiostats, secured onto the bike. (b) Experimental protocol. Tissue levels were monitored during an initial resting period (i), followed by cycling at four levels of increasing rpm (ii–v), a level of warming down (vi), and a final period of resting (vii). (c) Dialysate glucose and lactate levels during the exercise phase of the cycling protocol. The bottom graph shows the glucose (red) and lactate (green) levels, the middle graph (black) shows the lactate/glucose ratio, and the top graph shows the rotations per minute (blue) and heart rate (purple) throughout the cycling protocol. Glucose and lactate traces have been despiked. The dotted lines indicate the stages of varying cycling intensity: (ii) 55 rpm, (iii) 65 rpm, (iv) 75 rpm, (v) sprint, and (vi) 55 rpm. Data have been time aligned, taking into account the time delay of the system. (d) Histograms showing mean dialysate levels for two different cyclists during key points in cycling protocol. Labels correspond to stages described in the experimental protocol: (i) baseline (ii) midway through warm up, (iii) midway through medium intensity, (iv) midway through high intensity, (v) end of sprint, (vi) end of warm down, and (vii) after 50 min of recovery. (Reprinted from Gowers, S.A. et al., *Anal. Chem.*, 87(15), 7763, 2015. With permission; Feuerstein, D. et al., *Anal. Chem.*, 81, 4987, 2009.)

The design of microfluidic devices for sampling biofluids is inherently more complex than sealed systems. In addition to material, signal detection, and electronic considerations, the device also needs to be capable of cleaning, self-diagnostics, and sample preparation and processing that may include separation, concentration, preservation, or amplification. The sensing of the presence of the biomarker is also complicated by variable concentration, the presence of confounding compounds, biological heterogeneity, nonspecific surface chemistry, and stability of signal readout. Additional challenges include calibration or inclusion of a reference detection component, the frequency of detection, switching between samples, having a lossless and fully reversible chemistry for capture and sensing, and being robust against environmental changes. The other consideration for these systems is that the biomarkers of interest need to have been identified and characterized in advance and the fluids that the device is sampling need to be within its operating parameters. Although much less common, devices that capture and store multiple samples for later off-chip analysis may provide a useful hybrid for cases where biofluids are not as well characterized, where the analytics would create a significant design burden, or when multiple complex biomarkers need to be tracked but without a high degree of urgency.

Electrochemical sensors meet many of the desirable criteria for integrated detection, including that they can be easily multiplexed, have a quantitative and specific readout for a chemical reaction in a controlled environment, and a relatively fast and sensitive response. For example, Puet al. (2016) have described a wearable, continuous glucose monitoring system that includes a microfluidic chip. The chip has an integrated three-electrode electrochemical sensor for continuous glucose monitoring in subcutaneous interstitial fluid, with a detection limit for glucose of 1.44 mg/mL and a linear range of 0–162 mg/mL.

Tattoo-based solid-contact ion-selective electrodes (ISEs) have also been developed for noninvasive potentiometric monitoring of epidermal pH levels. Bandodkar et al. (2013) combined polyaniline-based solid-contact ISEs, commercially available temporary transfer tattoo paper, and screen printing techniques using the hybrid fabrication protocol illustrated in the following. The tattoo sensors were printed on commercially available tattoo base paper using a combination of carbon, Ag/AgCl, and insulator inks. Testing on athletes showed that this approach yielded a highly flexible potentiometric sensor that was compliant with the skin, and its mechanical integrity and potentiometric behavior was minimally affected by repeated bending and stretching. However, the sensor functioned reliably only for 30 min, which was attributed to the combination of excessive sweating and the highly curvilinear morphology of the area being monitored (the neck of athletes).

By combining ionic liquids with polymer gels, so-called ionogels, it may be possible to retain some of the advantages of ionic liquids in a wearable system using a solid or semisolid gel-type structure. Curto et al. (2012) demonstrated a wearable and disposable optical barcode microfluidic device that incorporated ionogels. The microfluidic system was incorporated into an adhesive plaster to avoid direct contact of the ionogels with the skin. The authors used it to monitor pH of sweat in real time during an exercise period with the pH readout in the form of a barcode of color changing dyes over different pH ranges. They were able to demonstrate that the ionogel matrix was very robust even at harsh pH conditions, and there was no leaching of the dyes during the experiment. This suggested the potential for long durability of the device and accuracy on the pH measurement, making it useful for longitudinal studies.

Other sensing approaches have also been incorporated in wearable microfluidic devices. Optical sensors offer quite a few advantages over electrochemical sensors, primarily that physical contact is nonessential to monitor status, electrical noise can be minimized, and a wide range of approaches can be used to interrogate the output (Diamond 2004). Scaling is also simplified by spatial, temporal, and wavelength multiplexing of the measurements, though the positioning, power, and maintenance requirements for the emitters and sensors are more complicated. An integrated, miniaturized, wireless photometer that can be charged by electromagnetic induction and included ion-sensitive thin film optrodes was recently demonstrated that could track potassium concentrations in the micromolar range (Steinberg et al. 2014). Although potentially capable of a greater range of analytics and multiplexing, the complexity of integrating optical sensing into robust, power-efficient and comfortable, wearable packages remains a significant engineering challenge.

2.3 Potential Applications of Wearable Microfluidic Devices for Monitoring Bodily Fluids

The human body produces more than 30 distinct biofluids that may contain potential biomarkers related to disease and wellness. Some of these fluids can only be sampled through invasive means such as bile, lymph, cerebrospinal fluid, and blood serum; however, the majority can be sampled through noninvasiveness approaches, including natural orifice fluids (e.g., sputum, mucus, cerumen, saliva, breath condensates), skin secretions (e.g., sebum and sweat), excretions from the genitourinary system (e.g., urine, feces, sperm, cervical mucus), breast fluids (e.g., colostrum and nipple aspirate) as well as fluids that are generally associated with disease-states (e.g., vomit and exudates such as pus). This great diversity of fluids, with varied composition, levels of production, and accessibility provides a complicated but potentially rich source of both local and systemic responses to acute and chronic conditions. Although this section focuses on the potential for collection and analysis of bodily fluids from living humans using wearable devices, there is a lot of relevant work that has been conducted on bodily fluids for forensics (Roeder and Haas 2016) and on volatiles that are emitted by the body (de Lacy Costello et al. 2014, Hu et al. 2006).

The most common human fluids have been extensively analyzed using mass spectrometry to analyze the proteome and metabolome (Hu et al. 2006, Iadarola et al. 2016). Once potential biomarkers have been identified, many of these can be implemented as point-of-care diagnostics on a chip (Issadore and Westervelt 2013); these diagnostics also have the potential to be reduced further to a wearable device when there is need for more than a point measurement. An improving knowledge base of the relationship between fluid production, secretion, and excretion, and disease states and the ability to quantitate a wide panel of heterogeneous biomarkers to understand absolute and relative imbalances is accelerating the development of interest in potential biomarkers to track and the demand for point-of-care and wearable sensors.

The body orifices are a natural opportunity to sample biofluids. In humans, the mucosal membrane lining surrounding these orifices and cavities secretes several liters of protective mucus each day that is a rich biofluid containing a diversity of compounds including enzymes, proteins, glycoproteins, antibodies, and minerals. The glands producing mucus in the respiratory, urogenital, visual, and auditory systems respond to changes in environment, infection, body cycle, age, and chronic disease, providing potential biomarkers for microfluidic analysis.

However, as indicated previously, the analysis of bodily fluids is not straightforward. There are many confounding variables that contribute to intraindividual variation, including diet, lifestyle, natural human cycles, and medications. There is also significant interindividual variability driven by factors including genomics, environmental history, lifestyle, gender, and diet. Thirdly, there are technical sources of variability that are introduced through differences in the collection, preparation, and preservation of fluids for investigation. A fourth factor is that the biomarker of interest may be found in several fluids, though at different concentrations due to differences in expression level or time constants. Often biomarkers of interest may exist at low concentrations in a background of highly abundant proteins, in a highly viscous liquid, or conditions that lead to rapid degradation of the biomarker. The highly personal nature of biofluids, the desire to understand temporal changes, and the volatile and sensitive nature of many of the biomolecules align well with the potential capabilities of a body-worn microfluidic device that can repeatedly sample biofluids and provide rapid, quantitative analysis of a range of biomarkers to build up a longitudinal, personalized profile.

This section of the chapter will focus on the potential to collect and analyze human biofluids by noninvasive methods. Examples of recent work analyzing the three most common categories of fluids will be discussed, with comments on their analysis using wearable and microfluidic devices.

2.3.1 Aural, Ocular, Oral, and Respiratory Fluids

The respiratory system has several fluids that can be noninvasively sampled: saliva, phlegm, nasal mucus, and breath condensate. These fluids have been extensively studied and the quantity, color, and composition are routinely used for diagnosis purposes, so here we focus on approaches that are amenable to development as body-worn microfluidic devices. The assumption in this section is that the user can introduce samples of these fluids into the microfluidic system in a controlled and reproducible way. In each case, there is a risk of cross-contamination that would need to be considered in the design and a decision made on whether to simply use the microfluidic system for sample collection and preservation or to provide analysis as well. For sample collection and preservation, manual mechanical pumping may be sufficient. However, for analysis of samples, reliable power for a source and detector are required.

- *Saliva*—Saliva is a complex body fluid of proteins, nucleic acids, enzymes, electrolytes, and glycoproteins secreted primarily from the submandibular, sublingual, and parotid glands as well as oral debris that has the potential for early detection of many diseases (Lee and Wong 2009). Saliva has been extensively studied and developed for many point-of-care diagnostic applications (Chin et al. 2012, Hart et al. 2011, Kumar et al. 2013), with paper-based microfluidics becoming an attractive approach (Yetisen et al. 2013). Nearly a decade ago, a hands-free microfluidic system for detection of matrix metalloproteinase-8 (MMP-8) comprising a sample pretreatment step with a rapid (<10 min) immunoassay was demonstrated (Herr et al. 2007). More recently, microfluidic devices have been used to detect drug abuse using Raman spectroscopy (Andreou et al. 2013) and infrared spectroscopy (Wagli et al. 2013), the presence of low levels (~10 copies) of streptococcus bacterial DNA using real-time polymerase chain reaction (PCR) (Oblath et al. 2013), the level of nitrite that is associated with periodontal disease (Bhakta et al. 2014), and saliva urea nitrogen for monitoring kidney failure (Calice-Silva et al. 2014). The analysis of ejected, unstimulated whole saliva in a wearable system would provide some unique challenges in isolating, preserving, and potentially analyzing the biomarkers of interest from a highly proteolytic viscous fluid; however, on-chip separation and stabilization may provide a route for monitoring unpredictable dental or renal disease or tracking hormone levels such as cortisol.
- *Phlegm*—The visual study of sputum, coughed-up phlegm, from the trachea and bronchi is one of the oldest diagnostic point-of-care tests (phlegm was one of the four humors), providing rapid evaluation of a range of lung diseases including inflammation, tuberculosis, pneumonia, bronchitis, edema, and chronic obstructive pulmonary

disease (COPD). Phlegm is a complex mix of lipids, glycoproteins, and immunoglobulins as well as loose cells, infectious agents, and debris that have collected in the lungs. The mucosal base of phlegm is secreted in the airway, driven by disease and inflammatory processes, and its composition varies depending on many factors including state of the immune system, genetics, and environment. There is increasingly rapid development of point-of-care sputum tests for drug-resistant tuberculosis (TB) and other infectious agents, replacing more expert-dependent and subjective smear microscopy with molecular and PCR analysis (Lawn et al. 2013, Wang et al. 2013). With the development of upstream sample processing tools such as a microfluidic liquefier (Huang et al. 2015) and modular designs (Yafia et al. 2015), and downstream multiplexed (Luo et al. 2014) and all-on-chip (Meagher et al. 2008) methods, a fully integrated, wearable microfluidic sensor is potentially realizable.

- *Nasal mucus*—The secretions of the goblet cells in the nasal passage are primarily to prevent the airway drying out and a first-line defense for catching foreign particles such as dust, bacteria, and allergens. Mucus is composed of polypeptides, primarily the approximately 20 mucin genes, as well as cells and debris. Historically, several biomarkers have been studied in nasal secretions including eosinophil cationic protein (ECP) as an inflammatory response against parasites, bacteria, and viruses (Ruocco et al. 1998); however, the emergence of proteomic tools has now identified several hundred proteins, several of which have been linked to different diseases. In a number of recent studies, 12 proteins were found to correlate exclusively with allergic rhinitis compared to healthy controls (Tomazic et al. 2014), 124 proteins correlated exclusively with pollen exposure in healthy adults, and 68 proteins that exclusively correlated with pollen exposure in patients with allergic rhinitis (Tomazic et al. 2016). Other types of biomarkers have also been identified, including microRNA expression (Wu et al. 2015) and concentration of solids (Hill et al. 2014). Although there have been no significant demonstrations to date, body-worn microfluidic sensors could collect mucus with relative ease and track exposure to allergens and microbes.

- *Breath condensate*—Volatile and nonvolatile compounds can be easily condensed from exhaled breath (EBC) and are a potential source of biomarkers for lung disease, such as COPD, cystic fibrosis, pneumonia, or asthma. There are several reviews that highlight recent progress in this area (Ahmadzai et al. 2013, Beck et al. 2016, Davis et al. 2012) using mass spectrometry and chromatography for biomarker identification. Recently, an electrostatic precipitator has been shown to be an effective way of capturing aerosols from liters of air into a microfluidic device (Pardon et al. 2015) and a microfluidic device using a surface acoustic wave immunosensor for detecting carcinoembryonic antigen (CEA) from EBC was demonstrated with a detection limit of 1 ng/mL (Zhang et al. 2015). There is significant interest in developing point-of-care EBC analysis tools (Gubala et al. 2012) recognizing that collecting more basic biomarkers such as pH and ammonia levels(Hibbard et al. 2013) outside a controlled clinical environment may provide valuable insights into exacerbating environment situations.

- *Cerumen*—Cerumen, or earwax, is a complex mixture of keratins, long-chain fatty acids, cholesterol and alcohols, and debris secreted by the ceruminous and sebaceous glands to assist in cleaning and lubricating the ear canal. The texture and color of cerumen have been studied extensively; however, only recently has there been in-depth studies of the biomolecular composition (Feig et al. 2013). Earwax has a high degree of complexity with more than 2000 unique proteins identified supporting its role as an antimicrobial barrier and in local immune response. To date, there have not been any demonstrations of microfluidic systems to capture or analyze cerumen, though there are opportunities for microfluidic devices to monitor temperature, earwax buildup, biofilm formation, otitis media, and to use microfluidic channels for sound generation.

- *Tear fluid*—The lacrimal and meibomian glands and the conjunctival goblet cells secrete fluid to clean and lubricate the eye and provide a clearance mechanism for contaminants and irritants. The tear film separates into three layers: a lipid layer, an aqueous layer, and a mucous layer. Each of these layers contains a diverse array of biomolecules, with more than 1500 proteins present altogether (Aass et al. 2015). For example, the lipid layer, secreted from the meibomiam gland, is composed primarily of wax esters and cholesteryl esters, and the most common class of proteins are lipid binding proteins (Butovich 2013), though more than 90 different proteins have been identified (Tsai et al. 2006). Several putative biomarkers have been identified in tear fluid including ocular disorders, neurological disorders, and cancer (Aass et al. 2015, von Thun Und Hohenstein-Blaul et al. 2013). A microfluidic platform embedded in a contact lens for assessing lens care solution performance and type of bacterial infection has recently been demonstrated, which interrogates microliter volumes of tear fluid (Guan et al. 2016). A microfluidic design for a tear fluid immunoassay has also been demonstrated with a lower limit of detection of 3 nM and accurate to within 15% of a standard ELISA test (Karns and Herr 2011). One interesting approach that to date is relatively unexplored is whether biomarkers can be sensed in tear fluid from wearable devices such as eyeglasses, goggles, or an eye-mask.

2.3.2 Analysis of Skin Secretions

The outer covering of the human body serves many purposes, including acting as a low-permeability barrier to provide protection, regulating body temperature, sensing, absorption and excretion, and synthesis and storage of biomolecules. Human skin has a complex structure composed of several major cell types with sweat glands and sebaceous glands producing sweat and sebum, respectively, located in the reticular region of the dermal layer. Sebaceous glands are found all over the human body except on the palms and soles, while eccrine sweat glands are found all over the body. A second major class of sweat glands, apocrine glands, are found primarily in the armpits and perianal areas and active after puberty. The skin is also home to more than 1000 species of bacteria and is significantly influenced by aging, ultraviolet exposure, acute and chronic mechanical force, environmental conditions, diet, and hormonal areas.

Although the sebaceous and sweat glands are colocated in the dermis, the two main bodily fluids secreted by the skin are quite different in nature. Thus, the partitioning of biomolecules into sweat and sebum is quite different and allows identification and analysis of distinct and complementary biomarkers. These fluids can also be readily collected by a body-worn sensor, though isolating biomarkers of interest in a compact device may be challenging because of the significant amount of debris, bacteria, and cells present, in addition to the complex mixture of biomolecules. The variation of inter- and intrapersonal secretion is compounded by environmental conditions that increase evaporation, diseases that influence blood supply and gland secretion, and burns or other skin damage that impact skin integrity. More than one hundred volatile organic compounds are also emitted by the skin, and there is interest in analyzing these compounds as potential biomarkers (Gallagher et al. 2008). Several collection techniques have been studied, some of which would be compatible with a wearable microfluidic system.

- *Sweat*—Humans perspire up to 10 L of fluid every day (Godek et al. 2005). Sweat is slightly acidic (pH 4.5–7) and composed primarily of water (~99%), minerals, lactic acid, urea and small amounts of biomolecules, drugs, and other debris. Sweating is often induced in clinical studies, and the quantity and composition of sweat is influenced by environmental factors such as temperature and relative humidity, the hormonal and sympathetic nervous systems, diet, and sweat-inducing chemical compounds as well as inter- and intrapersonal variability. The use of hygiene products, hair and skin defects can act as confounding factors, though despite all these challenges, analysis of sweat has yielded biomarkers for diseases including cystic fibrosis, diabetes, kidney disease, and detection of drugs (Jadoon et al. 2015). Sampling sweat passively from people with a more sedentary lifestyle and measuring biomarkers in very low and variable concentrations are technically very challenging, but recently there have been several demonstrations of mechanically compliant sensors attached to the skin that can measure simple analytes with the potential for multiplexed measurements at lower concentrations (Heikenfeld 2016). A number of simple, potential biomarkers in sweat have been already been studied using wearable devices. Devices are available for measuring rate of perspiration (Salvo et al. 2010), for measuring lactate with a limited of detection in the range of 5–100 mM (Garcia et al. 2016), and for measuring sodium concentration using ion selective electrodes (Schazmann et al. 2010). Six years ago, a visually readable multiplexed approach using multiple colorimetric pH sensitive dyes and ionogels in an adhesive plaster design was demonstrated (Benito-Lopez et al. 2010). An alternative pump-free, flexible, disposable, wearable microfluidic design was also described with continuous pH readout of sweat during exercise using LEDs and a colorimetric pH indicator (Benito-Lopez et al. 2009). The microfluidic device was made using polymethylmethacrylate (PMMA) and pressure-sensitive adhesive (PSA) polymer sheets and lamination. The sensing area was a piece of textile (1 × 1 mm) embedded in the middle of the device with a pH-sensitive dye, which varied color according to the pH of the sweat.

- *Sebum*—Sebum is a waxy complex fluid composed of free fatty acids, waxy and cholesterol esters, squalenes, and fatty acids secreted by sebaceous glands in a number of regions including the skin, eyelids, nose, lips, gums, cheeks, surrounding female nipples, penis, and labia. Secretion is impacted by steroids, hormones, and has a number of constituents such as waxy esters, squalenes, and sapienic acid that are unique to sebum. Like other secreted bodily fluids, the thin layer of secretions provides a barrier against pathogens by providing an acidic environment and antimicrobial lipids. Imbalances in the composition of sebum are associated with a number of diseases and conditions. Sebum potentially has biomarkers for Parkinson's disease (Morgan 2016), inflammation (Lee et al. 2016), and environmental exposure (Boussouira and Pham 2016). The variability and low volume of sebum makes it more challenging to collect in a microfluidic device, though a large-area smart bandage approach embedded in clothing may be one solution.

2.3.3 Bodily Fluids from the Genitourinary System

The genital and urinary organs secrete and excrete a rich variety of bodily fluids that have been studied extensively throughout history. From the sweet smell of urine signaling potential diabetes to the changes in the consistency of cervical mucus indicating ovulation, all of the major schools of medicine have observed these fluids for centuries to gain prognostic insights. Urinalysis is one of the oldest clinical tests, and biomarkers in urine have been extensively reviewed (Albalat et al. 2011, An and Gao 2015, Rodriguez-Suarez et al. 2014, Zou and Sun 2015) and will not be discussed in detail here. However, it is worth noting that urine can be collected by absorbent structures embedded in clothing and analyzed using point-of-care tests such as a dipstick approach (Schultz 2013). There are several reasons why urine has been so extensively studied: from the practical perspective that it can be collected in large quantities at multiple time points noninvasively and by untrained personnel, and from the biological perspective that it is still relatively stable by the time it is voided because proteolytic degradation has essentially been completed in the bladder resulting in less need for sample preservation.

- *Urine*—Urine is a complex fluid of salts, metabolites, hormones, proteins, peptides, and volatile organic compounds secreted from the kidneys and excreted through the urethra along with some of the microbiome. Some simple, rapid, nonspecific biomarkers include color, pH, specific gravity, and volume. More than 1500 proteins have been identified in urine; approximately half are soluble, half as sediments, and approximately 3% in exosomes. Urine test strips and pregnancy test kits have been available for decades as point-of-care tools. Recently, a range of wearable pads particularly geared toward monitoring infants have been discussed and demonstrated (Fincher 2013, Nealon 2014, Ziai and Batchelor 2015), and there is significant interest in dipsticks (Higginbotham 2015) and films (Pathak et al. 2016) that can be analyzed with a cell phone. Over the coming decade, point-of-care and wearable urine sensors of increasing complexity are likely to become commercially available, spurred on by high-profile challenges such as the QualCommTricorder X-Prize (Foundation 2016).

- *Feces*—The excreted material from the digestive tract is a complex mixture of partially digested food, mucus, bile, bilirubin, gut flora, metabolic waste products, as well as many volatile compounds that are also often emitted as flatulence. There are many potential biomarkers to track, and recent work has looked at microbiome population biomarkers (Sung et al. 2016), colorectal cancer (Chen et al. 2016), inflammatory bowel disease (Soubieres and Poullis 2016), and the efficacy of intestinal transplants (Lauro et al. 2016) and fecal transplants (Choi and Cho 2016). Several stool point-of-care tests have been developed including for analysis of occult blood (Cho et al. 2016), amoebiasis (Korpe et al. 2012) and other pathogens (Phaneuf et al. 2016), and pancreatic function (Walkowiak et al. 2016). The demand for rapid detection of pathogens in a global health setting will continue to accelerate the development of point-of-care tools for analyzing stool samples, though there are also several potential monitoring applications for a sensor embedded in a wearable pad that could provide longer-term sampling of feces and flatulence.

- *Cervicovaginal fluid*—Secretions from Bartholin's gland and Skene's gland combine with other secretions from the reproductive ducts to produce a complex mix of several biofluids and the microbiota of the genital tract. For example, tubular mucous glands in the cervix produce the viscous, alkaline cervical mucus, which undergoes a series of changes during the menstrual cycle, while vaginal lubricant is acidic and composed of organic acids, complex alcohols, pyridine, glycols, and aldehydes (Owen and Katz 1999). There is extensive interest in cervicovaginal fluid biomarkers for monitoring pregnancy (Heng et al. 2015), changes in the microbiota that may indicate a dysbiotic state (van de Wijgert et al. 2014), and tracking exposure to sexually transmitted diseases (Keller and Herold 2009). Recently, a point-of-care test has been developed for detecting ruptured fetal membranes using an immunoassay (Rogers et al. 2016), highlighting the potential for extending this work to a wearable pad for continuous monitoring.

2.4 Conclusions and Future Directions

In this chapter, we have outlined two emerging use cases for wearable microfluidic systems: (1) the measurement of physical and physiological activity and (2) the collection and analysis of bodily fluids. Although the practical application of these technologies in large studies is at a nascent stage, the majority of challenges that remain are technical, social, or economic. Advances in rapid prototyping, soft lithography, and flexible hybrid electronics, combined with the consideration for power-efficient data collection strategies, user experience, and body area networks, are shaping our thinking about integrated systems for ubiquitous, unobtrusive, continuous monitoring of wellness. Microfluidics is the key underlying technology, because without accurate, reproducible, and predictable collection, manipulation, and sensing from small fluid volumes, results from these use cases will not have a significant impact on healthcare. One of the key challenges though is the specificity, sensitivity, and long-term reproducibility of sensor data from open systems for monitoring bodily fluids, suggesting that many of the near-term advances in the field will be on closed systems for monitoring activity and physiology.

Wearable microfluidic devices have been realized either as patches that stick to the skin like a temporary tattoo, or as close-body devices embedded in clothing. Both approaches have their advantages and disadvantages depending on the application. For physical measurement, conformal contact with the skin is not as critical, so devices embedded in clothing may provide a greater degree of comfort but would be more subject to operational uncertainty. For sampling bodily fluids, the primary design constraint is having access to that fluid, whether in the form of a contact lens, a sanitary towel, or skin patch, with each requiring some degree of obtrusiveness. A second consideration for bodily fluids is whether to provide analysis in addition to sample collection. A sampling-only approach could be achieved in a smaller, more passive device for fluids that can be easily stabilized and be made compatible with more complex, high-resource forms of fluid analysis, for example, to detect multiple, low-level biomarkers. Alternatively, if rapid feedback is required, relatively simple on-device analysis can be included using electrochemical, biochemical, or chromatographic approaches, though at the cost of higher power consumption. Emerging approaches for energy harvesting (Kim et al. 2016, Ostfeld et al. 2016, Reid et al. 2015), synthetic biology for creating whole-cell biosensors (Roda et al. 2013), and device networking (Ghamari et al. 2016) are rapidly building out a rich menu of options for future fully integrated, smart device designs.

The ability to capture and potentially analyze secreted bodily fluids in the natural environment will potentially be critical to developing diagnostic platforms and personalized treatments for a wide range of chronic diseases with an environmental or temporal component. Microfluidic approaches are attractive for these applications because of their small size, low manufacturing cost, ability to work with small fluid volumes, fast reaction times, modular and automated designs, and potential for biohazard containment. However, secreted bodily fluids are not well correlated with internal fluids such as plasma, so should be viewed as complementary to invasive sampling methods. Indeed, the composition, volume, and accessibility of secreted biofluids is a lot more variable than internal fluids and require more complex models of health and wellness to interpret. One of the long-term goals for these devices would be to provide minute-by-minute analysis of how the body is uptaking and reacting to drugs so that dosages could be more precisely determined or alternative treatment options considered. There are also many other bodily fluids that may be amenable to noninvasive analysis by microfluidic devices but that are relatively unexplored; for example, vomit and exudates offer access to unique biofluids associated directly with disease processes, while rheum and breast milk are not continuously produced, but may be sampled under relevant conditions and may open up new insights into specific biological process, comparative biology, the interaction between the microbiome and bodily fluids, and for real-time monitoring of therapy. For example, the burgeoning field of smart bandages for monitoring wound-healing (Farooqui and Shamim 2016, McLister et al. 2016, Mostafalu et al. 2015) has the potential to monitor ultrasound treatment of venous ulcers (Samuels et al. 2013).

Beyond the development of the microfluidic devices themselves, one important challenge in accelerating the field of wearable microfluidic sensors is the development of findable, accessible, interoperable, and reusable datasets that can help with establishing standards for quality assurance, providing data interpretation, and for comparison and interpretation of performance across devices. There have been several projects that have developed databases of the components of biofluids, most notably the Sys-BodyFluid database that contained details of more than 10,000 proteins in 11 kinds of body fluids including plasma/serum, urine, cerebrospinal fluid, saliva, bronchoalveolar lavage fluid, synovial fluid, nipple aspirate fluid, tear fluid, seminal fluid, human milk, and amniotic fluid (Li et al. 2009) and the Max-Planck Unified (MAPU) proteome database that has details on several bodily fluids including plasma, urine, and cerebrospinal fluid (Gnad et al. 2016).

The road to widely adopted wearable biosensors is littered with overpromised and underdelivered performance and usability. In addition to sensor reproducibility, power management, data management, and bodily fluid sample variability, some of the other challenges of wearable microfluidic devices include operator-dependent effects such as body shape or disabilities that may impact device placement and reproducibility, interpretation of data in the context of the wearer's daily life, and calibration standards that may limit accuracy and precise quantification. The development of smart contact lenses that will be acceptable by the general public has highlighted some of these challenges in designing a product that is both useful from a healthcare perspective and easily integrated into daily life.

There are also many exciting research directions in the development of smarter, connected microfluidic systems capable of more complex analyses. A natural challenge and point at which these devices will come of age is when their performance exceeds that of companion animals for sensing epileptic seizures, low blood sugar, or early-stage cancer over a fixed period of time of several weeks. The recent work suggesting a link between a distinct sweat odor and Parkinson's disease (Morgan 2016) highlights how much there is still to understand about the connection between body secretions and different health diseases and conditions. The development and application of wearable microfluidic devices is evolving rapidly and holds great promise for identifying and tracking activity and biomolecular and physiological biomarkers to realize personalized healthcare.

References

Aass, C., I. Norheim, E. F. Eriksen, P. M. Thorsby, and M. Pepaj. 2015. Single unit filter-aided method for fast proteomic analysis of tear fluid. *Anal Biochem* 480:1–5.

Ahmadzai, H., S. Huang, R. Hettiarachchi, J. L. Lin, P. S. Thomas, and Q. Zhang. 2013. Exhaled breath condensate: A comprehensive update. *Clin Chem Lab Med* 51 (7):1343–1361.

Albalat, A., H. Mischak, and W. Mullen. 2011. Clinical application of urinary proteomics/peptidomics. *Expert Rev Proteomics* 8 (5):615–629.

An, M. and Y. Gao. 2015. Urinary biomarkers of brain diseases. *Genomics Proteomics Bioinformatics* 13 (6):345–354.

Andreou, C., M. R. Hoonejani, M. R. Barmi, M. Moskovits, and C. D. Meinhart. 2013. Rapid detection of drugs of abuse in saliva using surface enhanced raman spectroscopy and microfluidics. *ACS Nano* 7 (8):7157–7164.

Bandodkar, A. J., V. W. Hung, W. Jia, G. Valdes-Ramirez, J. R. Windmiller, A. G. Martinez, J. Ramirez, G. Chan, K. Kerman, and J. Wang. 2013. Tattoo-based potentiometric ion-selective sensors for epidermal pH monitoring. *Analyst* 138 (1):123–128.

Beck, O., A. C. Olin, and E. Mirgorodskaya. 2016. Potential of mass spectrometry in developing clinical laboratory biomarkers of nonvolatiles in exhaled breath. *Clin Chem* 62 (1):84–91.

Benito-Lopez, F., S. Coyle, R. Byrne, and D. Diamond. 2010. Sensing sweat in real-time using wearable microfluidics. *Proceedings of the Seventh International Workshop on Wearable and Implantable Body Sensor Network*, Singapore.

Benito-Lopez, F., S. Coyle, R. Byrne, A. Smeaton, N. E. O'Connor, and D. Diamond. 2009. Pump less wearable microfluidic device for real time pH sweat monitoring. *Proceedings of the Eurosensors XXIII Conference*, Lausanne, Switzerland, 1 (1), pp. 1103–1106.

Bhakta, S. A., R. Borba, M. Taba, C. D. Garcia, and E. Carrilho. 2014. Determination of nitrite in saliva using microfluidic paper-based analytical devices. *Anal Chim Acta* 809:117–122.

Boussouira, B. and D. M. Pham. 2016. Squalene and skin barrier function: From molecular target to biomarker of environmental exposure. In *Skin Stress Response Pathways: Environmental Factors and Molecular Opportunities*, ed. T. G. Wondrak, pp. 29–48. Cham, Switzerland: Springer International Publishing.

Butovich, I. A. 2013. Tear film lipids. *Exp Eye Res* 117:4–27.

Calice-Silva, V., M. A. Vieira, J. G. Raimann, M. Carter, J. Callegari, N. W. Levin, P. Kotanko, and R. Pecoits-Filho. 2014. Saliva urea nitrogen dipstick—A novel bedside diagnostic tool for acute kidney injury. *Clin Nephrol* 82 (6):358–366.

Care, Abbott Diabetes. 2016. FreeStyle Libre. https://freestylediabetes.co.uk/, accessed October 19, 2016.

Chen, R., L. A. Lai, T. A. Brentnall, and S. Pan. 2016. Biomarkers for colitis-associated colorectal cancer. *World J Gastroenterol* 22 (35):7882–7891.

Chin, C. D., V. Linder, and S. K. Sia. 2012. Commercialization of microfluidic point-of-care diagnostic devices. *Lab Chip* 12 (12):2118–2134.

Cho, C. H., J. Kim, M. A. Jang, B. J. Lee, J. J. Park, and C. S. Lim. 2016. Evaluation of the performance of a fecal tumor M2-PK rapid kit using stool specimens for detection of colorectal tumors. *Ann Clin Lab Sci* 46 (2):154–160.

Choi, H. H. and Y. S. Cho. 2016. Fecal microbiota transplantation: Current applications, effectiveness, and future perspectives. *Clin Endosc* 49 (3):257–265.

Chossat, J.-B., H.-S. Shin, Y.-L. Park, and V. Duchaine. 2015. Soft tactile skin using an embedded ionic liquid and tomographic imaging. *J Mech Robot* 7 (2):021008.

Curto, V. F., C. Fay, S. Coyle, R. Byrne, C. O'Toole, C. Barry, S. Hughes, N. Moyna, D. Diamond, and F. Benito-Lopez. 2012. Real-time sweat pH monitoring based on a wearable chemical barcode micro-fluidic platform incorporating ionic liquids. *Sens Actuators B Chem* 171:1327–1334.

Davis, M. D., A. Montpetit, and J. Hunt. 2012. Exhaled breath condensate: An overview. *Immunol Allergy Clin North Am* 32 (3):363–375.

de Lacy Costello, B., A. Amann, H. Al-Kateb, C. Flynn, W. Filipiak, T. Khalid, D. Osborne, and N. M. Ratcliffe. 2014. A review of the volatiles from the healthy human body. *J Breath Res* 8 (1):014001.

Diamond, D. 2004. Internet-scale sensing. *Anal Chem* 76 (15):278A–286A.

Digiglio, P., R. Li, W. Wang, and T. Pan. 2014. Microflotronic arterial tonometry for continuous wearable non-invasive hemodynamic monitoring. *Ann Biomed Eng* 42 (11):2278–2288.

Farooqui, M. F. and A. Shamim. 2016. Low cost inkjet printed smart bandage for wireless monitoring of chronic wounds. *Sci Rep* 6:28949.

Feig, M. A., E. Hammer, U. Volker, and N. Jehmlich. 2013. In-depth proteomic analysis of the human cerumen—A potential novel diagnostically relevant biofluid. *J Proteomics* 83:119–129.

Feuerstein, D., K. H. Parker, and M. G. Boutelle. 2009. *Anal. Chem.* 81:4987–4994.

Fincher, J. 2013. Smart diapers test children's urine to monitor their health over time. http://newatlas.com/pixie-scientific-smart-diapers/28320/, accessed October 19, 2016.

Foundation, XPRIZE. 2016. QualComm Tricorder X PRIZE. http://tricorder.xprize. org/, accessed October 19, 2016.

Gallagher, M., C. J. Wysocki, J. J. Leyden, A. I. Spielman, X. Sun, and G. Preti. 2008. Analyses of volatile organic compounds from human skin. *Br J Dermatol* 159 (4):780–791.

Garcia, S. O., Y. V. Ulyanova, R. Figueroa-Teran, K. H. Bhatt, S. Singhal, and P. Atanassov. 2016. Wearable sensor system powered by a biofuel cell for detection of lactate levels in sweat. *ECS J Solid State Sci Technol* 5 (8):M3075–M3081.

Ghamari, M., B. Janko, R. S. Sherratt, W. Harwin, R. Piechockic, and C. Soltanpur. 2016. A survey on wireless body area networks for ehealthcare systems in residential environments. *Sensors (Basel)* 16 (6), 831–863.

Gnad, F., M. Oroshi, and M. Mann. 2016. Max-planck unified (MAPU) proteome database. http://www.mapuproteome.com/. Max Planck Institute of Biochemistry, Am Klopferspitz 18, 82152 Martinsried, Germany, accessed September 23, 2016.

Godek, S. F., A. R. Bartolozzi, and J. J. Godek. 2005. Sweat rate and fluid turnover in American football players compared with runners in a hot and humid environment. *Br J Sports Med* 39 (4):205–211; discussion 205–211.

Gowers, S. A. N., V. F. Curto, C. A. Seneci, C. Wang, S. Anastasova, P. Vadgama, G.-Z. Yang, and M. G. Boutelle. 2015. 3D printed microfluidic device with integrated biosensors for online analysis of subcutaneous human microdialysate. *Anal Chem* 87 (15):7763–7770.

Guan, A., Y. Wang, K. S. Phillips, and Z. Li. 2016. A contact-lens-on-a-chip companion diagnostic tool for personalized medicine. *Lab Chip* 16 (7):1152–1156.

Gubala, V., L. F. Harris, A. J. Ricco, M. X. Tan, and D. E. Williams. 2012. Point of care diagnostics: Status and future. *Anal Chem* 84 (2):487–515.

Hart, R. W., M. G. Mauk, C. Liu, X. Qiu, J. A. Thompson, D. Chen, D. Malamud, W. R. Abrams, and H. H. Bau. 2011. Point-of-care oral-based diagnostics. *Oral Dis* 17 (8):745–752.

Heikenfeld, J. 2016. Non-invasive analyte access and sensing through eccrine sweat: Challenges and outlook circa 2016. *Electroanalysis* 28 (6):1242–1249.

Heng, Y. J., S. Liong, M. Permezel, G. E. Rice, M. K. Di Quinzio, and H. M. Georgiou. 2015. Human cervicovaginal fluid biomarkers to predict term and preterm labor. *Front Physiol* 6:151.

Herr, A. E., A. V. Hatch, D. J. Throckmorton, H. M. Tran, J. S. Brennan, W. V. Giannobile, and A. K. Singh. 2007. Microfluidic immunoassays as rapid saliva-based clinical diagnostics. *Proc Natl Acad Sci USA* 104 (13):5268–5273.

Hibbard, T., K. Crowley, F. Kelly, F. Ward, J. Holian, A. Watson, and A. J. Killard. 2013. Point of care monitoring of hemodialysis patients with a breath ammonia measurement device based on printed polyaniline nanoparticle sensors. *Anal Chem* 85 (24):12158–12165.

Higginbotham, S. 2015. With $35 million, Scanadu seeks approval for its medical 'tricorder'. *Fortune*. April 27, 2015. http://fortune.com/2015/04/27/scanadu-35-million/.

Hill, D. B., P. A. Vasquez, J. Mellnik, S. A. McKinley, A. Vose, F. Mu, A. G. Henderson et al. 2014. A biophysical basis for mucus solids concentration as a candidate biomarker for airways disease. *PLoS One* 9 (2):e87681.

Hu, S., J. A. Loo, and D. T. Wong. 2006. Human body fluid proteome analysis. *Proteomics* 6 (23):6326–6353.

Huang, P. H., L. Ren, N. Nama, S. Li, P. Li, X. Yao, R. A. Cuento et al. 2015. An acoustofluidic sputum liquefier. *Lab Chip* 15 (15):3125–3131.

Iadarola, P., M. Fumagalli, A. M. Bardoni, R. Salvini, and S. Viglio. 2016. Recent applications of CE- and HPLC-MS in the analysis of human fluids. *Electrophoresis* 37 (1):212–230.

Issadore, D. and R. M. Westervelt. 2013. *Point-of-Care Diagnostics on a Chip*, Biological and Medical Physics, Biomedical Engineering. Heidelberg, Germany: Springer.

Jadoon, S., S. Karim, M. R. Akram, A.K. Khan, M. A. Zia, A. R. Siddiqi, and G. Murtaza. 2015. Recent developments in sweat analysis and its applications. *Int J Anal Chem* 2015:164974.

Karns, K. and A. E. Herr. 2011. Human tear protein analysis enabled by an alkaline microfluidic homogeneous immunoassay. *Anal Chem* 83 (21):8115–8122.

Keller, M. J. and B. C. Herold. 2009. Understanding basic mechanisms and optimizing assays to evaluate the efficacy of vaginal microbicides. *Sex Transm Dis* 36 (3 Suppl):S92–S95.

Kim, S., S. J. Choi, K. Zhao, H. Yang, G. Gobbi, S. Zhang, and J. Li. 2016. Electrochemically driven mechanical energy harvesting. *Nat Commun* 7:10146.

Korpe, P. S., B. R. Stott, F. Nazib, M. Kabir, R. Haque, J. F. Herbein, and W. A. Petri, Jr. 2012. Evaluation of a rapid point-of-care fecal antigen detection test for Entamoeba histolytica. *Am J Trop Med Hyg* 86 (6):980–981.

Kumar, S., S. Kumar, M. A. Ali, P. Anand, V. V. Agrawal, R. John, S. Maji, and B. D. Malhotra. 2013. Microfluidic-integrated biosensors: Prospects for point-of-care diagnostics. *Biotechnol J* 8 (11):1267–1279.

Lauro, A., I. R. Marino, and C. S. Matsumoto. 2016. Advances in allograft monitoring after intestinal transplantation. *Curr Opin Organ Transplant* 21 (2):165–170.

Lawn, S. D., P. Mwaba, M. Bates, A. Piatek, H. Alexander, B. J. Marais, L. E. Cuevas et al. 2013. Advances in tuberculosis diagnostics: The Xpert MTB/RIF assay and future prospects for a point-of-care test. *Lancet Infect Dis* 13 (4):349–361.

Lee, W. J., S. L. Kim, K. C. Lee, M. Y. Sohn, Y. H. Jang, S. J. Lee, and D. W. Kim. 2016. Effects of magnesium ascorbyl phosphate on the expression of inflammatory biomarkers after treatment of cultured sebocytes with propionibacterium acnes or ultraviolet B radiation. *Ann Dermatol* 28 (1):129–132.

Lee, Y. H. and D. T. Wong. 2009. Saliva: An emerging biofluid for early detection of diseases. *Am J Dent* 22 (4):241–248.

Li, S. J., M. Peng, H. Li, B. S. Liu, C. Wang, J. R. Wu, Y. X. Li, and R. Zeng. 2009. Sys-BodyFluid: A systematical database for human body fluid proteome research. *Nucleic Acids Res* 37 (Database issue):D907–D912.

Luo, J., X. Fang, D. Ye, H. Li, H. Chen, S. Zhang, and J. Kong. 2014. A real-time microfluidic multiplex electrochemical loop-mediated isothermal amplification chip for differentiating bacteria. *Biosens Bioelectron* 60:84–91.

McLister, A., J. McHugh, J. Cundell, and J. Davis. 2016. New developments in smart bandage technologies for wound diagnostics. *Adv Mater* 28 (27):5732–5737.

Meagher, R. J., A. V. Hatch, R. F. Renzi, and A. K. Singh. 2008. An integrated microfluidic platform for sensitive and rapid detection of biological toxins. *Lab Chip* 8 (12):2046–2053.

Miller, P. R., X. Xiao, I. Brener, D.B. Burckel, R. Narayan, and R. Polsky. 2014. Microneedle-based transdermal sensor for on-chip potentiometric determination of K+. *Adv Healthcare Mater* 3 (6):876–881.

Morgan, J. 2016. Joy of super smeller: Sebum clues for PD diagnostics. *Lancet Neurol* 15 (2):138–139.

Mostafalu, P., W. Lenk, M. R. Dokmeci, B. Ziaie, A. Khademhosseini, and S. R. Sonkusale. 2015. Wireless flexible smart bandage for continuous monitoring of wound oxygenation. *IEEE Trans Biomed Circuits Syst* 9 (5):670–677.

Nealon, S. 2014. Diaper pad to detect dehydration and bacterial infections in infants. http://phys.org/news/2014-09-diaper-pad-dehydration-bacterial-infections.html, accessed October 19, 2016.

Nie, B., R. Li, J. D. Brandt, and T. Pan. 2014. Microfluidic tactile sensors for three-dimensional contact force measurements. *Lab Chip* 14 (22):4344–4353.

Oblath, E. A., W. H. Henley, J. P. Alarie, and J. M. Ramsey. 2013. A microfluidic chip integrating DNA extraction and real-time PCR for the detection of bacteria in saliva. *Lab Chip* 13 (7):1325–1332.

Ostfeld, A. E., A. M. Gaikwad, Y. Khan, and A. C. Arias. 2016. High-performance flexible energy storage and harvesting system for wearable electronics. *Sci Rep* 6:26122.

Owen, D. H. and D. F. Katz. 1999. A vaginal fluid simulant. *Contraception* 59 (2):91–95.

Pardon, G., L. Ladhani, N. Sandstrom, M. Ettori, G. Lobov, and W. van der Wijngaart. 2015. Aerosol sampling using an electrostatic precipitator integrated with a microfluidic interface. *Sens Actuators B Chem* 212:344–352.

Pathak, A., J. Borana, J. V. Adhikari, and S. S. Gorthi. 2016. Indicator-impregnated agarose films for colorimetric measurement of pH. *SLAS TECHNOL: Transl Life Sci Innov.* 22 (1):81–88.

Phaneuf, C. R., B. Mangadu, M. E. Piccini, A. K. Singh, and C. Y. Koh. 2016. Rapid, portable, multiplexed detection of bacterial pathogens directly from clinical sample matrices. *Biosensors (Basel)* 6 (4):49–58.

Pu, Z., C. Zou, R. Wang, X. Lai, H. Yu, K. Xu, and D. Li. 2016. A continuous glucose monitoring device by graphene modified electrochemical sensor in microfluidic system. *Biomicrofluidics* 10 (1):011910.

Reid, R. C., S. D. Minteer, and B. K. Gale. 2015. Contact lens biofuel cell tested in a synthetic tear solution. *Biosens Bioelectron* 68:142–148.

Roda, A., L. Cevenini, S. Borg, E. Michelini, M. M. Calabretta, and D. Schuler. 2013. Bioengineered bioluminescent magnetotactic bacteria as a powerful tool for chip-based whole-cell biosensors. *Lab Chip* 13 (24):4881–4889.

Rodriguez-Suarez, E., J. Siwy, P. Zurbig, and H. Mischak. 2014. Urine as a source for clinical proteome analysis: From discovery to clinical application. *Biochim Biophys Acta* 1844 (5):884–898.

Roeder, A. D. and C. Haas. 2016. Body fluid identification using mRNA profiling. *Methods Mol Biol* 1420:13–31.

Rogers, L. C., L. Scott, and J. E. Block. 2016. Accurate point-of-care detection of ruptured fetal membranes: Improved diagnostic performance characteristics with a monoclonal/polyclonal immunoassay. *Clin Med Insights Reprod Health* 10:15–18.

Ruocco, L., B. Fattori, A. Romanelli, M. Martelloni, A. Casani, M. Samolewska, and R. Rezzonico. 1998. A new collection method for the evaluation of nasal mucus proteins. *Clin Exp Allergy* 28 (7):881–888.

Salvo, P., F. Di Francesco, D. Costanzo, C. Ferrari, M. G. Trivella, and D. De Rossi. 2010. A wearable sensor for measuring sweat rate. *IEEE Sens J* 10 (10):1557–1558.

Samuels, J. A., M. S. Weingarten, D. J. Margolis, L. Zubkov, Y. Sunny, C. R. Bawiec, D. Conover, and P. A. Lewin. 2013. Low-frequency (<100 kHz), low-intensity (<100 mW/cm(2)) ultrasound to treat venous ulcers: A human study and in vitro experiments. *J Acoust Soc Am* 134 (2):1541–1547.

Schazmann, B., D. Morris, C. Slater, S. Beirne, C. Fay, R. Reuveny, N. Moyna, and D. Diamond. 2010. A wearable electrochemical sensor for the real-time measurement of sweat sodium concentration. *Anal Methods* 2 (4):342–348.

Schultz, C. 2013. Diaper with pocket for an absorbent pad containing a test strip. Google Patents, US 20130296739 A1, https://www.google.com/patents/US20130296739.

Soubieres, A. A. and A. Poullis. 2016. Emerging role of novel biomarkers in the diagnosis of inflammatory bowel disease. *World J Gastrointest Pharmacol Ther* 7 (1):41–50.

Steinberg, M. D., P. Kassal, B. Tkalcec, and I.M. Steinberg. 2014. Miniaturised wireless smart tag for optical chemical analysis applications. *Talanta* 118:375–381.

Sung, J., V. Hale, A. C. Merkel, P. J. Kim, and N. Chia. 2016. Metabolic modeling with Big Data and the gut microbiome. *Appl Transl Genom* 10:10–15.

Tomazic, P. V., R. Birner-Gruenberger, A. Leitner, B. Obrist, S. Spoerk, and D. Lang-Loidolt. 2014. Nasal mucus proteomic changes reflect altered immune responses and epithelial permeability in patients with allergic rhinitis. *J Allergy Clin Immunol* 133 (3):741–750.

Tomazic, P. V., R. Birner-Gruenberger, A. Leitner, S. Spoerk, and D. Lang-Loidolt. 2016. Seasonal proteome changes of nasal mucus reflect perennial inflammatory response and reduced defence mechanisms and plasticity in allergic rhinitis. *J Proteomics* 133:153–160.

Tsai, P. S., J. E. Evans, K. M. Green, R. M. Sullivan, D. A. Schaumberg, S. M. Richards, M. R. Dana, and D. A. Sullivan. 2006. Proteomic analysis of human meibomian gland secretions. *Br J Ophthalmol* 90 (3):372–377.

van de Wijgert, J. H., H. Borgdorff, R. Verhelst, T. Crucitti, S. Francis, H. Verstraelen, and V. Jespers. 2014. The vaginal microbiota: What have we learned after a decade of molecular characterization?. *PLoS One* 9 (8):e105998.

von Thun Und Hohenstein-Blaul, N., S. Funke, and F. H. Grus. 2013. Tears as a source of biomarkers for ocular and systemic diseases. *Exp Eye Res* 117:126–137.

Wagli, P., Y. C. Chang, A. Homsy, L. Hvozdara, H. P. Herzig, and N. F. de Rooij. 2013. Microfluidic droplet-based liquid-liquid extraction and on-chip IR spectroscopy detection of cocaine in human saliva. *Anal Chem* 85 (15):7558–7565.

Walkowiak, J., A. Glapa, J. K. Nowak, L. Bober, N. Rohovyk, E. Wenska-Chyzy, P. Sobkowiak, and A. Lisowska. 2016. Pancreatic elastase-1 quick test for rapid assessment of pancreatic status in cystic fibrosis patients. *J Cyst Fibros* 15 (5):664–668.

Wang, S., F. Inci, G. De Libero, A. Singhal, and U. Demirci. 2013. Point-of-care assays for tuberculosis: Role of nanotechnology/microfluidics. *Biotechnol Adv* 31 (4):438–449.

Wu, G., G. Yang, R. Zhang, G. Xu, L. Zhang, W. Wen, J. Lu, J. Liu, and Y. Yu. 2015. Altered microRNA expression profiles of extracellular vesicles in nasal mucus from patients with allergic rhinitis. *Allergy Asthma Immunol Res* 7 (5):449–457.

Yafia, M., A. Ahmadi, M. Hoorfar, and H. Najjaran. 2015. Ultra-portable smartphone controlled integrated digital microfluidic system in a 3D-printed modular assembly. *Micromachines* 6 (9):1289–1305.

Yetisen, A. K., M. S. Akram, and C. R. Lowe. 2013. Paper-based microfluidic point-of-care diagnostic devices. *Lab Chip* 13 (12):2210–2251.

Zhang, X., Y. C. Zou, C. An, K. J. Ying, X. Chen, and P. Wang. 2015. Sensitive detection of carcinoembryonic antigen in exhaled breath condensate using surface acoustic wave immunosensor. *Sens Actuators B Chem* 217:100–106.

Ziai, M. A. and J. C. Batchelor. 2015. Smart radio-frequency identification tag for diaper moisture detection. *Healthc Technol Lett* 2 (1):18–21.

Zou, L. and W. Sun. 2015. Human urine proteome: A powerful source for clinical research. *Adv Exp Med Biol* 845:31–42.

3

Fabrication and Applications of Paper-Based Microfluidics

Xuan Mu and Yu Shrike Zhang

CONTENTS

3.1 Introduction

Microfluidics, or lab-on-a-chip, has been developed for nearly 30 years, providing a versatile toolbox with strong capability and huge potential to push forward the boundary of many disciplines, with particular applications in biomedical research (Whitesides 2006, Mu et al. 2013, Sackmann et al. 2014). In recent years, a new trend has emerged, which is to integrate microfluidic concepts and techniques into a form of paper-based devices, that is, paper-based microfluidics (Figure 3.1).

On the one hand, paper as a ubiquitous microfibrous material (Pelton 2009, Ren et al. 2013, 2014, Mahadeva et al. 2015), would offer unique structure-relevant merits in microfluidics other than conventional materials such as silicone, plastics, and glass. The advantages mainly include: (1) the cost of paper

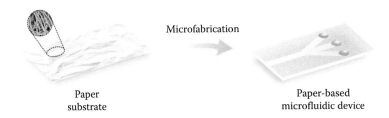

Paper
substrate

Microfabrication

Paper-based
microfluidic device

FIGURE 3.1
Paper-based microfluidic device is made of various paper substrates via a range of microfabrication strategies. The reconciliation of material advantages of paper and engineering advances of microfluidics shows huge benefits in developing novel clinical diagnostic techniques.

is much less expensive than others; (2) the fibrous nature of paper would lead to high surface-to-volume ratio and thus enhance a variety of size-relevant processes; and (3) the spontaneous wicking flow on paper is highly beneficial to the transport of liquid in the absence of external power sources. All of these advantages would render microfluidics a detection method much more accessible and affordable than conventional microfluidics.

On the other hand, the emerging paper-based microfluidics relies on the concept and techniques of microfluidics, especially surface patterning and vertical stacking (Webster and Kumar 2012, Cunningham et al. 2016). For example, by adopting microfluidic techniques, a colorimetric assay on paper not only allows for automated fluid distribution but also achieves as high as a throughput of 1024 reactions per test (Martinez et al. 2008). In another example, a four-step assay could be established on paper simply by a single activating procedure (Fu et al. 2012).

In fact, paper has for long been utilized in a myriad of commercial assays such as dot-immunoassay (Pappas et al. 1983, Coelho et al. 2007, Rodkvamtook et al. 2015), dried blood spotting (Spooner et al. 2009, Smit et al. 2014), Western/Northern blotting (Streit et al. 2008, MacPhee 2010), urine dipstick tests, and pregnant lateral flow tests (Wong and Tse 2009). Nevertheless, over these conventional diagnostic assays, the reconciliation of the unique characteristics of paper and the established microfluidic methods represents a great opportunity to forge new analytical and diagnostic strategies, demonstrating unprecedented and much more desired analytical functions. In our opinion, paper-based microfluidics is highly promising in developing functional analytical assays yet in a low-cost, less laborious, and easily accessible manner.

Although paper-based microfluidics is useful in a wide range of applications including environment monitoring (Ma et al. 2012), portable energy (Esquivel et al. 2014), screening of drugs (Weaver et al. 2013, Koesdjojo et al. 2014, He et al. 2016), and cell culture (Derda et al. 2009, Deiss et al. 2014, Kim et al. 2015b), its potential is fully demonstrated when it comes to the field of clinical diagnosis and point-of-care tests, especially in developing countries and resource-limited settings (Martinez et al. 2010, Mu et al. 2014, 2015).

The significance of clinical diagnosis doubtlessly soars in the landscape of globalization and population aging. It is a prerequisite to the downstream healthcare intervention and treatment. Although diagnosis itself only accounts for less than 5% of overall healthcare cost, it can influence as much as 60%–70% of healthcare decision-making (The Lewin Group 2005). However, most clinical diagnostic tests are instrument based, expensive, complicated, and thus limited in centralized medical centers and hospitals. This barrier, in fact, poses an elusive challenge of how to make these technically sophisticated diagnostic tests ultimately available to patients. Paper-based microfluidics, as mentioned earlier, is of great potential to address this challenge and may revolutionize the way of delivering diagnosis to patients.

The field has been developing rapidly, on the topic of which several extensive reviews have been previously published (Li et al. 2012b, Yetisen et al. 2013, Cate et al. 2014, Gomez 2014, Phillips and Lewis 2014, Chen et al. 2015, Su et al. 2015, Cheng et al. 2016). On the basis of these works, we further discuss up-to-date trends and recent achievements in this chapter. First, we will give a brief introduction regarding newly developed fabrication methods, and the choice of fabrication methods depends on specific contexts and paper used. Second, we will focus on the applications that are of the most clinical relevance, presenting the bottlenecks in current clinical diagnosis. We hope that this chapter would inspire more technological endeavors on continuously developing paper-based microfluidics devices.

3.2 Microfabrication Techniques

Microfabrication in paper-based microfluidics relies on the engineering techniques to pattern paper with hydrophobic areas, which are crucial features and prerequisites to achieve sophisticated analytical functions on paper. It also well distinguishes paper-based microfluidics from conventional paper-based tests. The microfabrication methods can be roughly divided into different categories from the technical perspective (Figure 3.2).

3.2.1 Photolithography

In the early stages, paper-based microfluidics is largely compliant with the conventional fabrication protocols in microfluidics. Photolithography is widely employed to pattern chromatographic paper and generate structures in a well-controlled and high-precision manner (Martinez et al. 2007, Carrilho et al. 2009b; Figure 3.2a). In a typical process, paper is first impregnated with the precursor of photoresist; upon the exposure of UV in a certain pattern, the photoresist can be selectively cross-linked in the paper and

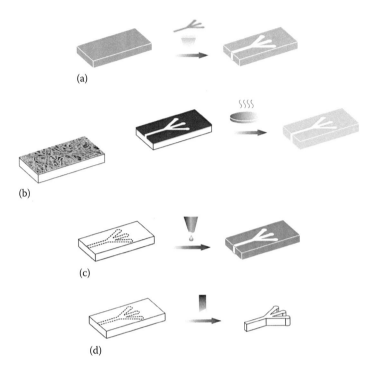

FIGURE 3.2
Microfabrication of paper-based microfluidics. (a) Photolithography. (b) Wax printing. (c) Inkjet
printing. (d) Mechanical cutting.

the uncured monomers will be subsequently washed away. As such, the
photoresist-occupied areas become hydrophobic, while the rest of the areas
still remain hydrophilic and allow for transport of liquids.

Besides two-dimensional (2D) patterning, multilayers of patterned paper
can be vertically aligned together to form a three-dimensional (3D) intercon-
nected network, leveraging analytical functions and throughput (Martinez et
al. 2008). Such a 3D network can be alternatively achieved by paper origami
(Liu and Crooks 2011, Kalish and Tsutsui 2014).

The photolithography-based fabrication proves the concept and the value
of paper-based microfluidics. However, the costly photoresist and instrument are hardly affordable to most research labs and, in particular, remote
regions, which seems incompatible with the original intention of using paper
to develop affordable analytical devices.

3.2.2 Wax Printing

Wax instead of photoresist has been employed to generate controlled hydrophobic areas (Carrilho et al. 2009a, Lu et al. 2009). Since both the wax and wax
printer are relatively inexpensive and can be easily adopted, wax printing has

soon become the most popular technique in fabricating paper-based micro-fluidics (Kurdekar et al. 2016, Li et al. 2016). The general process contains two steps: (1) printing the wax on the surface of paper; and (2) melting the wax on a heating device for it to penetrate the full thickness of the paper (Figure 3.2b). The second step inevitably reduces the fabricating resolution because of the wicking of the molten wax. Of note, even though the penetration of wax is troublesome in most cases, it can still be harnessed to achieve sophisticated functions, such as generating 3D and multilayer structures inside one single layer of paper (Li and Liu 2014, Renault et al. 2014).

3.2.3 Inkjet Printing

Inkjet printer, a common office instrument, is applicable to manufacturing paper-based microfluidics (Liao et al. 2014, Sun et al. 2015, Yamada et al. 2015b, Wang et al. 2016). To achieve this purpose, several hydrophobic materials in solutions with optimized viscosity have been developed to replace common printing ink, including alkyl ketene dimer (Li et al. 2010), resin (Xu et al. 2015), polystyrene (Abe et al. 2008), and polyacrylate (Apilux et al. 2013, Maejima et al. 2013). The printing or deposition of these hydrophobic materials on paper can form well-controlled hydrophobic patterns (Figure 3.2c). Besides printing the barriers for the channels, the printer may be equipped with a multicartridge system containing different inks, which is very useful to deposit chemical reagents necessary in the subsequent assay at the same time with the fabrication of the device.

More recently, the resistance to solutions containing surfactants is increasingly emphasized because of the potential of direct analysis of cell lysates using paper-based devices. To achieve this goal, improved hydrophobic barrier materials have been developed, including hydrophobic sol-gel-derived methylsilsesquioxane (Wang et al. 2014b), silicone resin (Rajendra et al. 2014), fluoropolymer (Chen et al. 2013), and Teflon (Deiss et al. 2014).

3.2.4 Cutting

The fabricating methods, mentioned earlier, always use hydrophobic materials to pattern papers. However, it is equally feasible to simply cut though the paper, allowing the geometric shape of the paper to guide the liquid flow (Figure 3.2d). Therefore, a myriad of cutting approaches have been developed and adopted on the basis of different cutting mechanisms and devices, including laser cutting (Nie et al. 2013, Spicar-Mihalic et al. 2013, Arrastia et al. 2015), plotter (Chen et al. 2016), mechanical cutting (Mu et al. 2014, 2015, Feng et al. 2015), and any combination of these techniques (Li et al. 2013b, Cai et al. 2014, Song et al. 2015).

Notably, some cutting methods provide an excellent alternative for patterning under room temperature. For example, nitrocellulose (NC) is a very useful paper substrate for constructing paper-based tests (Fridley et al. 2013, Arrastia et al. 2015). However, it is extremely vulnerable to high temperature over 100°C since it will decompose at 55°C and undergo autoignition at 130°C (Credou et al. 2013). Therefore, photolithography, wax printing, and even laser cutting is incompatible to pattern NC, while the mechanical cutting that avoids the generation of heat would be advantageous for this purpose. Furthermore, in some occasions, manual cutting, while seemingly less controlled, would provide necessary active intervention and maximally costumed flexibility (Fang et al. 2011, Nie et al. 2012).

3.3 Representative Applications of Paper-Based Microfluidics in Clinical Diagnosis

In this section, we will further discuss three specific applications of paper-based microfluidics in clinical diagnosis, that are, blood typing, ELISA, and sickle cell disease detection. A brief summary of broader applications of paper-based microfluidics is also provided in Table 3.1 but will not be discussed in details.

3.3.1 Blood Typing

Blood typing is of great clinical significance in blood transfusion and transplantation (Daniels and Bromilow 2014). The accurate and rapid detection of blood groups is imperative to prevent hemolytic transfusion reactions and other fatal consequences. Conventional tests heavily rely on laboratory-based instruments (e.g., centrifuges), requiring intensive and skilled manual operations, and thus limit the efficiency and accessibility of the assay. To develop an alternative blood grouping method, Gil, Shen, and colleagues harnessed the different transport behaviors on paper between agglutinated and non-agglutinated red blood cells (Khan et al. 2010; Figure 3.3a). The agglutinated red blood cells would form a spot with high optical density, allowing visual identification, while non-agglutinated ones would show nearly no visual trace of the spot. The paper-based assay not only enables streamlined operations with only one step of pipetting a drop of blood but also shows advantages on the aspects of assay time (several minutes) and cost (a few cents). It was further demonstrated that a step of elution could improve assay reliability (Al-Tamimi et al. 2012).

Shen and colleagues also made an effort to investigate the underlying mechanism of the agglutination of red blood cells on a piece of antibody-treated paper (Jarujamrus et al. 2012, Li et al. 2013a). It turns out that the antibodies desorbed from cellulose fibers, instead of the absorbed ones, played a more critical role in generating a large lump of agglutinated cells that are entangled in the network of paper fibers. The factors that may influence assay performance have been exploited, including paper structure (Su et al. 2012, Li et al. 2014a), papermaking additives (McLiesh et al. 2015,

TABLE 3.1

A Brief Summarization of Paper-Based Microfluidic Devices for Clinical Diagnosis

Clinical Samples	Disease	Detection Method	Analytical Target	Limit of Detection	References
Tear	Ocular disease and corneal epithelium disorders	Separation-based detection	Lactoferrin	0.1 mg/mL	Yamada et al. (2014), (2015a)
		Electrochemistry	Na^+ K^+	4.9 μM 6.8 μM	Chagas et al. (2015)
Sweat	Cystic fibrosis	Colorimetry	Anions	10 mM	Mu et al. (2015)
Saliva	Hemodialysis	Colorimetry	Nitrite	5 μM	Klasner et al. (2010)
	Tobacco smoke exposure	Distance-based detection	Thiocyanate	0.06 mM	Pena-Pereira et al. (2016)
Blood	Anemia	Colorimetry	Hemoglobin	1 g/L	Yang et al. (2013b)
Blister fluids	Bullous pemphigoid	Colorimetry	NC16A autoimmune antibody	NA	Hsu et al. (2014a)
Aqueous humor	Retinal ischemic condition	Colorimetry	Vascular endothelial growth factor (VEGF)	33.7 fg/mL	Hsu et al. (2014b)
Spiked Plasma	Phenylketonuria	Colorimetry	Phenylalanine	0.5 mg/L	Thiessen et al. (2015)
Semen	Infertility	Colorimetry	Live sperm Motile sperm	8.46 million/mL 15.18 million/mL	Nosrati et al. (2016)

Guan et al. 2016), and antibody stability (Guan et al. 2014a). The thin, porous, and lightweight paper is better to construct the blood group typing assay. Such paper could facilitate the elution of non-agglutinated red blood cells from the paper, and leads to a lower background and an improved signal-to-noise ratio. Papermaking additives have the potential to enhance the performance as well as accelerate the commercialization of the paper-based blood typing device.

Besides the agglutinated spot, other methods to enhance the visual detection has also been developed. Inspired by the magic paper in the movie of "Harry Potter," Shen and colleagues proposed a method to present the

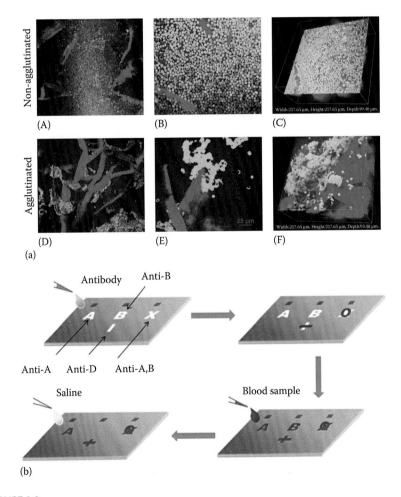

FIGURE 3.3
Clinical applications of paper-based microfluidics. (a) Blood typing based on agglutination of erythrocytes entangled in the fiber network of paper. (b) Display detection of blood types on paper.   (*Continued*)

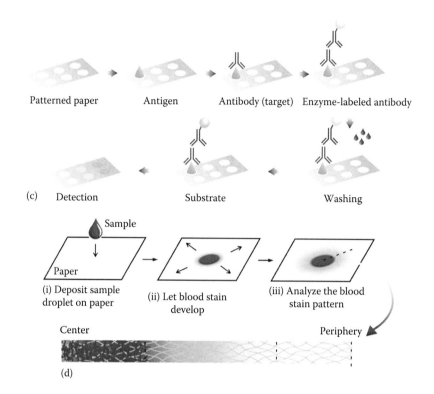

Patterned paper   Antigen   Antibody (target)   Enzyme-labeled antibody

(c)   Detection   Substrate   Washing

Sample

Paper

(i) Deposit sample droplet on paper

(ii) Let blood stain develop

(iii) Analyze the blood stain pattern

Center   Periphery

(d)

FIGURE 3.3 (*Continued*)
Clinical applications of paper-based microfluidics. (c) Paper-based ELISA procedure for the detection of autoimmune antibodies. (d) Paper-based diagnosis of sickle cell disease. ([a]: From Li, L.Z. et al., *Analyst*, 138(17), 4933, Copyright 2013a; [b]: From Li, M.S. et al., *Angew. Chem. Int. Ed.*, 51(22), 5497, Copyright 2012a; [d]: From Yang, X. et al., *Lab Chip*, 13(8), 1464, Copyright 2013a.)

detection results in written text (Li et al. 2012a). For example, a capital letter B, instead a red spot, would display on the paper when tested positive (Figure 3.3b), which is greatly beneficial for end users to interpret the assay results. In another case, a barcode-like format was proposed to take the advantages of smartphone readings (Guan et al. 2014b).

The utilization of paper-based assays has expanded to detect secondary blood groups (Li et al. 2014, Then et al. 2015), transform Indirect Antiglobulin Test (IAT) on paper (Yeow et al. 2015), and achieve reverse grouping (Noiphung et al. 2015). Although rare, minor, or secondary blood groups are of significant clinical importance.

3.3.2 ELISA

ELISA in the form of plastic well plate is one of the most ubiquitous assays performed in routine clinical laboratories. The transition of this assay into a form of patterned paper would improve its accessibility and efficiency, as well as expand the range of its potential applications (Figure 3.3c). Cheng, Whitesides, and colleagues developed a pioneering paper-based microfluidic ELISA (Cheng et al. 2010), which demonstrated significant advantages over conventional ones (Heller et al. 1998). The paper-based ELISA had the same layout as plastic 96-well plates, allowing high throughput. Each well was surrounded by hydrophobic SU-8 patterns that limited the spreading of liquid on paper. Therefore, each well of 5 mm in diameter only required 3 µL of solution to fill in, compared with 20–200 µL in plastic well-based ELISA. The high surface-to-volume ratio also contributed to the shorter assay time of 51 min, in comparison with the 213 min of conventional ELISA. This pioneering work set the tone for the following research on revolutionizing ELISA on patterned paper.

Currently, the role of paper-based ELISA has been widely expanded into detection of a variety of pathogenic and disease-relevant analytes, including Neuropeptide Y relative to cognitive performance (Murdock et al. 2013), Influenza H1N1 and H3N2 viruses (Lei et al. 2015), NC16A antibody of an autoimmune disease (Hsu et al. 2014a), *Escherichia coli* (Shih et al. 2015), hepatitis C virus (Mu et al. 2014), vascular endothelial growth factor (Hsu et al. 2014b), and Dengue virus serotype-2 envelope proteins (Wang et al. 2014a).

Several strategies have been developed to improve the sensitivity of paper-based ELISA, such as silicon dioxide beads to modify filter paper (Bai et al. 2013), polymerization-based amplification (Badu-Tawiah et al. 2015), poly(oligoethylene glycol methacrylate) (POEGMA)-based blocking agents (Deng et al. 2014), rolling circle amplification (Liu et al. 2016), modifications to monoclonal antibody (Hsu et al. 2014b), and Ring-Oven washing technique (Liu et al. 2015b).

3.3.3 Sickle Cell Disease

Sickle cell disease is a common recessively inherited blood disorder. It results in the altered conformation of hemoglobin and chronic anemia that is associated with life-long morbidity and significantly shortened life span (Yawn et al. 2014). Even though early diagnosis and intervention have been proven effective to control this disease, a rapid, reliable, and inexpensive method to diagnose sickle cell disease patients remains a huge challenge (Archer 2014).

The sick hemoglobin, due to the hydrophobic valine substitution, can be polymerized in a concentrated phosphate buffer solution. This phenomenon has been exploited to establish a liquid turbidity assay (SickleDex). Shevkoplyas and colleagues further developed an on-paper version of this assay mechanism (Yang et al. 2013a). The polymerized hemoglobin would entangle with the fiber network in the paper, and thus lead to differential patterns of blood stain (Figure 3.3d). They successfully employed this paper-based method to distinguish sickle cell trait carriers and sickle cell disease patients, and used it to quantify the ratio of sickle hemoglobin in blood that is beneficial to monitor the effectiveness of medical therapies (Piety et al. 2015).

3.4 Summary

Over the past several years, the field of paper-based microfluidics has developed rapidly and broadly. Paper-based microfluidics possesses a number of benefits such as reduced cost, speedy assay, increased portability, sensitivity, and multiplicity. Among them, we would like to emphasize the enhanced access for common patients to timely healthcare intervention, which may be the most influential aspect of paper-based microfluidics to clinical diagnosis.

The extraordinary material features of paper reconciled with microfluidic techniques are crucial to constructing a functional paper-based microfluidic device. The study on patterning and modifying paper, however, still requires continuous exploration and optimization.

The rapid growth of paper-based microfluidics has also inspired and echoed with the utilization of many other well-controlled and low-cost substrate materials, including eletrospun nanofibrous membrane (Yang et al. 2008), thread (Zhou et al. 2012, Nilghaz et al. 2014, Kim et al. 2015a), cotton (Lin et al. 2014), cloth (Liu et al. 2015a, Wu and Zhang 2015), and lignocellulose (from bamboo) (Kuan et al. 2015). We believe that the combination of these varieties of materials with paper will likely further enhance the functions of paper-based microfluidics and its applications in medicine.

Last but not least, the rational combination of paper-based microfluidics with other disciplines should not be overlooked. Several disciplines including chemometrics (Jalali-Heravi et al. 2015), nanotechnology (Sun et al. 2014, Warren et al. 2014), small molecular logic system (Ling et al. 2015), and synthetic biology/gene network (Pardee et al. 2014, Slomovic et al. 2015) have already demonstrated a glimpse of augmenting analytical functions on paper. Therefore, it is believed that the continual development of the paper-based microfluidics will ensure its translation into clinical diagnosis that spans across a much wider range of applications than currently available, hopefully in the near future.

Acknowledgments

YSZ acknowledges the National Cancer Institute of the National Institutes of Health Pathway to Independence Award (K99CA201603). XM acknowledges the support from National Natural Science Foundation of China (21305162 and 21375119) and the Chinese Scholarship Council Fund.

References

Abe, K., K. Suzuki, and D. Citterio. 2008. Inkjet-printed microfluidic multianalyte chemical sensing paper. *Analytical Chemistry* 80 (18):6928–6934.

Al-Tamimi, M., W. Shen, R. Zeineddine, H. Tran, and G. Garnier. 2012. Validation of paper-based assay for rapid blood typing. *Analytical Chemistry* 84 (3):1661–1668.

Apilux, A., Y. Ukita, M. Chikae, O. Chailapakul, and Y. Takamura. 2013. Development of automated paper-based devices for sequential multistep sandwich enzyme-linked immunosorbent assays using inkjet printing. *Lab on a Chip* 13 (1):126–135.

Archer, N.M. 2014. A diagnostic role for dense cells in sickle cell disease. *Proceedings of the National Academy of Sciences of the United States of America* 111 (41):14647–14648.

Arrastia, M., A. Avoundjian, P.S. Ehrlich, M. Eropkin, L. Levine, and F.A. Gomez. 2015. Development of a microfluidic-based assay on a novel nitrocellulose platform. *Electrophoresis* 36 (6):884–888.

Badu-Tawiah, A.K., S. Lathwal, K. Kaastrup, M. Al-Sayah, D.C. Christodouleas, B.S. Smith, G.M. Whitesides, and H.D. Sikes. 2015. Polymerization-based signal amplification for paper-based immunoassays. *Lab on a Chip* 15:655–659.

Bai, P., Y. Luo, Y. Li, X.D. Yu, and H.Y. Chen. 2013. Study on enzyme linked immunosorbent assay using paper-based micro-zone plates. *Chinese Journal of Analytical Chemistry* 41 (1):20–24.

Cai, L., Y. Wang, Y. Wu, C. Xu, M. Zhong, H. Lai, and J. Huang. 2014. Fabrication of a microfluidic paper-based analytical device by silanization of filter cellulose using a paper mask for glucose assay. *Analyst* 139 (18):4593–4598.

Carrilho, E., A.W. Martinez, and G.M. Whitesides. 2009a. Understanding wax printing: A simple micropatterning process for paper-based microfluidics. *Analytical Chemistry* 81 (16):7091–7095.

Carrilho, E., S.T. Phillips, S.J. Vella, A.W. Martinez, and G.M. Whitesides. 2009b. Paper microzone plates. *Analytical Chemistry* 81 (15):5990–5998.

Cate, D.M., J.A. Adkins, J. Mettakoonpitak, and C.S. Henry. 2014. Recent developments in paper-based microfluidic devices. *Analytical Chemistry* 87 (1):19–41.

Chagas, C.L.S., L. da Costa Duarte, E.O. Lobo, E. Piccin, N. Dossi, and W.K.T. Coltro. 2015. Hand drawing of pencil electrodes on paper platforms for contactless conductivity detection of inorganic cations in human tear samples using electrophoresis chips. *Electrophoresis* 36 (16):1837–1844.

Chen, B., P. Kwong, and M. Gupta. 2013. Patterned fluoropolymer barriers for containment of organic solvents within paper-based microfluidic devices. *ACS Applied Materials & Interfaces* 5 (23):12701–12707.

Chen, W., X. Fang, H. Li, H. Cao, and J. Kong. 2016. A simple paper-based colorimetric device for rapid mercury(II) assay. *Scientific Reports* 6:31948. http://www.nature.com/articles/srep31948#supplementary-information.

Chen, Y.-H., Z.-K. Kuo, and C.-M. Cheng. 2015. Paper—A potential platform in pharmaceutical development. *Trends in Biotechnology* 33 (1):4–9.

Cheng, C.-M., C.-M. Kuan, and C.-F. Chen. 2016. Low-cost in vitro diagnostic technologies. In *In-Vitro Diagnostic Devices*, pp. 59–91. Springer, Cham, Switzerland.

Cheng, C.M., A.W. Martinez, J.L. Gong, C.R. Mace, S.T. Phillips, E. Carrilho, K.A. Mirica, and G.M. Whitesides. 2010. Paper-based ELISA. *Angewandte Chemie-International Edition* 49 (28):4771–4774.

Coelho, J.S., I. da Silva Soares, E.A. de Lemos, M.C.S. Jimenez, M.E. Kudó, S. do Lago Moraes, A.W. Ferreira, and M.C.A. Sanchez. 2007. A multianalyte Dot-ELISA for simultaneous detection of malaria, chagas disease, and syphilis-specific IgG antibodies. *Diagnostic Microbiology and Infectious Disease* 58 (2):223–230.

Credou, J., H. Volland, J. Dano, and T. Berthelot. 2013. A one-step and biocompatible cellulose functionalization for covalent antibody immobilization on immunoassay membranes. *Journal of Materials Chemistry B* 1 (26):3277–3286.

Cunningham, J.C., P.R. DeGregory, and R.M. Crooks. 2016. New functionalities for paper-based sensors lead to simplified user operation, lower limits of detection, and new applications. *Annual Review of Analytical Chemistry* 9:183–202.

Daniels, G. and I. Bromilow. 2014. *Essential Guide to Blood Groups*, 3rd edn. Wiley-Blackwell, Chichester, U.K.

Deiss, F., W.L. Matochko, N. Govindasamy, E.Y. Lin, and R. Derda. 2014. Flow-through synthesis on teflon-patterned paper to produce peptide arrays for cell-based assays. *Angewandte Chemie-International Edition* 53 (25):6374–6377.

Deng, X., N.M.B. Smeets, C. Sicard, J. Wang, J.D. Brennan, C.D.M. Filipe, and T. Hoare. 2014. Poly (oligoethylene glycol methacrylate) dip-coating: Turning cellulose paper into a protein-repellent platform for biosensors. *Journal of the American Chemical Society* 136 (37):12852–12855.

Derda, R., A. Laromaine, A. Mammoto, S.K.Y. Tang, T. Mammoto, D.E. Ingber, and G.M. Whitesides. 2009. Paper-supported 3D cell culture for tissue-based bioassays. *Proceedings of the National Academy of Sciences of the United States of America* 106 (44):18457–18462.

Esquivel, J.P., F.J. Del Campo, J.L. Gomez de la Fuente, S. Rojas, and N. Sabate. 2014. Microfluidic fuel cells on paper: Meeting the power needs of next generation lateral flow devices. *Energy & Environmental Science* 7 (5):1744–1749.

Fang, X., H. Chen, X. Jiang, and J. Kong. 2011. Microfluidic devices constructed by a marker pen on a silica gel plate for multiplex assays. *Analytical Chemistry* 83 (9):3596–3599.

Feng, Q.M., M. Cai, C.G. Shi, N. Bao, and H.Y. Gu. 2015. Integrated paper-based electroanalytical devices for determination of dopamine extracted from striatum of rat. *Sensors and Actuators B: Chemical* 209:870–876.

Fridley, G. E., C.A. Holstein, S.B. Oza, and P. Yager. 2013. The evolution of nitrocellulose as a material for bioassays. *MRS Bulletin* 38 (4):326–330.

Fu, E., T. Liang, P. Spicar-Mihalic, J. Houghtaling, S. Ramachandran, and P. Yager. 2012. Two-dimensional paper network format that enables simple multistep assays for use in low-resource settings in the context of malaria antigen detection. *Analytical Chemistry* 84 (10):4574–4579.

Gomez, F.A. 2014. Paper microfluidics in bioanalysis. *Bioanalysis* 6 (21):2911–2914.

Guan, L., L. Li, X. Huang, J. Ji, J. Tian, A. Nilghaz, and W. Shen. 2016. REMOVED: Bioactive paper design for human blood analysis: Paper property suitable for large-scale sensor production. *Biochemical Engineering Journal* 105:473.

Guan, L.Y., R. Cao, J.F. Tian, H. McLiesh, G. Garnier, and W. Shen. 2014a. A preliminary study on the stabilization of blood typing antibodies sorbed into paper. *Cellulose* 21 (1):717–727.

Guan, L.Y., J.F. Tian, R. Cao, M.S. Li, Z.X. Cai, and W. Shen. 2014b. Barcode-like paper sensor for smartphone diagnostics: An application of blood typing. *Analytical Chemistry* 86 (22):11362–11367.

He, M., Z. Li, Y. Ge, and Z. Liu. 2016. Portable upconversion nanoparticles-based paper device for field testing of drug abuse. *Analytical Chemistry* 88 (3):1530–1534.

Heller, C., C. Stem, H. Wamwayi, and A. Grieve. 1998. Development of a filter paper-based ELISA for rinderpest antibodies. *Veterinary Record* 142 (26):729.

Hsu, C.-K., H.-Y. Huang, W.-R. Chen et al. 2014a. Paper-based ELISA for the detection of autoimmune antibodies in body fluid: The case of bullous pemphigoid. *Analytical Chemistry* 86 (9):4605–4610.

Hsu, M.-Y., C.-Y. Yang, W.-H. Hsu, K.-H. Lin, C.-Y. Wang, Y.-C. Shen, Y.-C. Chen, S.-F. Chau, H.-Y. Tsai, and C.-M. Cheng. 2014b. Monitoring the VEGF level in aqueous humor of patients with ophthalmologically relevant diseases via ultrahigh sensitive paper-based ELISA. *Biomaterials* 35 (12):3729–3735.

Jalali-Heravi, M., M. Arrastia, and F.A. Gomez. 2015. How can chemometrics improve microfluidic research? *Analytical Chemistry* 87 (7):3544–3555.

Jarujamrus, P., J.F. Tian, X. Li, A. Siripinyanond, J. Shiowatana, and W. Shen. 2012. Mechanisms of red blood cells agglutination in antibody-treated paper. *Analyst* 137 (9):2205–2210.

Kalish, B. and H. Tsutsui. 2014. Patterned adhesive enables construction of nonplanar three-dimensional paper microfluidic circuits. *Lab on a Chip* 14 (22):4354–4361.

Khan, M. S., G. Thouas, W. Shen, G. Whyte, and G. Garnier. 2010. Paper diagnostic for instantaneous blood typing. *Analytical Chemistry* 82 (10):4158–4164.

Kim, J., S. Bae, S. Song, K. Chung, and S. Kwon. 2015a. Fiber composite slices for multiplexed immunoassays. *Biomicrofluidics* 9 (4):044109.

Kim, S. H., H.R. Lee, S.J. Yu et al. 2015b. Hydrogel-laden paper scaffold system for origami-based tissue engineering. *Proceedings of the National Academy of Sciences of the United States of America* 112 (50):15426–15431.

Klasner, S.A., A.K. Price, K.W. Hoeman, R.S. Wilson, K.J. Bell, and C.T. Culbertson. 2010. Paper-based microfluidic devices for analysis of clinically relevant analytes present in urine and saliva. *Analytical and Bioanalytical Chemistry* 397 (5):1821–1829.

Koesdjojo, M.T., Y.Y. Wu, A. Boonloed, E.M. Dunfield, and V.T. Remcho. 2014. Low-cost, high-speed identification of counterfeit antimalarial drugs on paper. *Talanta* 130:122–127.

Kuan, C.-M., R.L. York, and C.-M. Cheng. 2015. Lignocellulose-based analytical devices: Bamboo as an analytical platform for chemical detection. *Scientific Reports* 5. Article ID 18570.

Kurdekar, A., L. Avinash A. Chunduri, E.P. Bulagonda, M.K. Haleyurgirisetty, V. Kamisetti, and I.K. Hewlett. 2016. Comparative performance evaluation of carbon dot-based paper immunoassay on Whatman filter paper and nitrocellulose paper in the detection of HIV infection. *Microfluidics and Nanofluidics* 20 (7):1–13.

Lei, K.F., C.-H. Huang, R.-L. Kuo, C.-K. Chang, K.-F. Chen, K.-C. Tsao, and N.-M. Tsang. 2015. Paper-based enzyme-free immunoassay for rapid detection and subtyping of influenza A H1N1 and H3N2 viruses. *Analytica Chimica Acta* 883:37–44.

Li, L.Z., X.L. Huang, W. Liu, and W. Shen. 2014a. Control performance of paper-based blood analysis devices through paper structure design. *ACS Applied Materials & Interfaces* 6 (23):21624–21631.

Li, L.Z., J.F. Tian, D. Ballerini, M.S. Li, and W. Shen. 2013a. A study of the transport and immobilisation mechanisms of human red blood cells in a paper-based blood typing device using confocal microscopy. *Analyst* 138 (17):4933–4940.

Li, M.S., W.L. Then, L.Z. Li, and W. Shen. 2014b. Paper-based device for rapid typing of secondary human blood groups. *Analytical and Bioanalytical Chemistry* 406 (3):669–677.

Li, M.S., J.F. Tian, M. Al-Tamimi, and W. Shen. 2012a. Paper-based blood typing device that reports patient's blood type "in writing". *Angewandte Chemie-International Edition* 51 (22):5497–5501.

Li, X., D.R. Ballerini, and W. Shen. 2012b. A perspective on paper-based microfluidics: Current status and future trends. *Biomicrofluidics* 6 (1):011301.

Li, X. and X. Liu. 2014. Fabrication of three-dimensional microfluidic channels in a single layer of cellulose paper. *Microfluidics and Nanofluidics* 16 (5):819–827.

Li, X., J. Tian, G. Garnier, and W. Shen. 2010. Fabrication of paper-based microfluidic sensors by printing. *Colloids and Surfaces B: Biointerfaces* 76 (2):564–570.

Li, X., P. Zwanenburg, and X.Y. Liu. 2013b. Magnetic timing valves for fluid control in paper-based microfluidics. *Lab on a Chip* 13 (13):2609–2614.

Li, Z., J. Yang, L. Zhu, and W. Tang. 2016. Fabrication of paper micro-devices with wax jetting. *RSC Advances* 6 (22):17921–17928.

Liao, W.-J., P.K. Roy, and S. Chattopadhyay. 2014. An ink-jet printed, surface enhanced Raman scattering paper for food screening. *RSC Advances* 4 (76):40487–40493.

Lin, S.-C., M.-Y. Hsu, C.-M. Kuan, H.-K. Wang, C.-L. Chang, F.-G. Tseng, and C.-M. Cheng. 2014. Cotton-based diagnostic devices. *Scientific Reports* 4:6976.

Ling, J., G. Naren, J. Kelly, T.S. Moody, and A. Prasanna de Silva. 2015. Building pH sensors into paper-based small-molecular logic systems for very simple detection of edges of objects. *Journal of the American Chemical Society* 137 (11):3763–3766.

Liu, H. and R.M. Crooks. 2011. Three-dimensional paper microfluidic devices assembled using the principles of origami. *Journal of the American Chemical Society* 133 (44):17564–17566.

Liu, M., C.Y. Hui, Q. Zhang, J. Gu, B. Kannan, S. Jahanshahi-Anbuhi, C.D.M. Filipe, J.D. Brennan, and Y. Li. 2016. Target-induced and equipment-free DNA amplification with a simple paper device. *Angewandte Chemie* 128 (8):2759–2763, International Edition.

Liu, M., C.S. Zhang, and F.F. Liu. 2015a. Understanding wax screen-printing: A novel patterning process for microfluidic cloth-based analytical devices. *Analytica Chimica Acta* 891:234–246.

Liu, W., Y. Guo, M. Zhao, H. Li, and Z. Zhang. 2015b. Ring-Oven washing technique integrated paper-based immunodevice for sensitive detection of cancer biomarker. *Analytical Chemistry* 87 (15):7951–7957.

Lu, Y., W.W. Shi, L. Jiang, J.H. Qin, and B.C. Lin. 2009. Rapid prototyping of paper-based microfluidics with wax for low-cost, portable bioassay. *Electrophoresis* 30 (9):1497–1500.

Ma, Y.X., H. Li, S. Peng, and L.Y. Wang. 2012. Highly selective and sensitive fluorescent paper sensor for nitroaromatic explosive detection. *Analytical Chemistry* 84 (19):8415–8421.

MacPhee, D. J. 2010. Methodological considerations for improving Western blot analysis. *Journal of Pharmacological and Toxicological Methods* 61 (2):171–177.

Maejima, K., S. Tomikawa, K. Suzuki, and D. Citterio. 2013. Inkjet printing: An integrated and green chemical approach to microfluidic paper-based analytical devices. *RSC Advances* 3 (24):9258–9263.

Mahadeva, S.K., K. Walus, and B. Stoeber. 2015. Paper as a platform for sensing applications and other devices: A review. *ACS Applied Materials & Interfaces* 7 (16): 8345–8362.

Martinez, A.W., S.T. Phillips, M.J. Butte, and G.M. Whitesides. 2007. Patterned paper as a platform for inexpensive, low-volume, portable bioassays. *Angewandte Chemie-International Edition* 46 (8):1318–1320.

Martinez, A.W., S.T. Phillips, and G.M. Whitesides. 2008. Three-dimensional microfluidic devices fabricated in layered paper and tape. *Proceedings of the National Academy of Sciences of the United States of America* 105 (50): 19606–19611.

Martinez, A.W., S.T. Phillips, G.M. Whitesides, and E. Carrilho. 2010. Diagnostics for the developing world: Microfluidic paper-based analytical devices. *Analytical Chemistry* 82 (1):3–10.

McLiesh, H., S. Sharman, and G. Garnier. 2015. Effect of cationic polyelectrolytes on the performance of paper diagnostics for blood typing. *Colloids and Surfaces B: Biointerfaces* 133:189–197.

Mu, X., X.L. Xin, C.Y. Fan, X. Li, X.L. Tian, K.F. Xu, and Z. Zheng. 2015. A paper-based skin patch for the diagnostic screening of cystic fibrosis. *Chemical Communications* 51 (29):6365–6368.

Mu, X., L. Zhang, S.Y. Chang, W. Cui, and Z. Zheng. 2014. Multiplex microfluidic paper-based immunoassay for the diagnosis of hepatitis C virus infection. *Analytical Chemistry* 86 (11):5338–5344.

Mu, X., W. Zheng, J. Sun, W. Zhang, and X. Jiang. 2013. Microfluidics for manipulating cells. *Small* 9 (1):9–21.

Murdock, R.C., L. Shen, D.K. Griffin, N. Kelley-Loughnane, I. Papautsky, and J.A. Hagen. 2013. Optimization of a paper-based ELISA for a human performance biomarker. *Analytical Chemistry* 85 (23):11634–11642.

Nie, J., Y. Liang, Y. Zhang, S. Le, D. Li, and S. Zhang. 2013. One-step patterning of hollow microstructures in paper by laser cutting to create microfluidic analytical devices. *Analyst* 138 (2):671–676.

Nie, J., Y. Zhang, L. Lin, C. Zhou, S. Li, L. Zhang, and J. Li. 2012. Low-cost fabrication of paper-based microfluidic devices by one-step plotting. *Analytical Chemistry* 84 (15):6331–6335.

Nilghaz, A., L.Y. Zhang, M.S. Li, D.R. Ballerini, and W. Shen. 2014. Understanding thread properties for red blood cell antigen assays: Weak ABO blood typing. *ACS Applied Materials & Interfaces* 6 (24):22209–22215.

Noiphung, J., K. Talalak, I. Hongwarittorrn, N. Pupinyo, P. Thirabowonkitphithan, and W. Laiwattanapaisal. 2015. A novel paper-based assay for the simultaneous determination of Rh typing and forward and reverse ABO blood groups. *Biosensors & Bioelectronics* 67:485–489.

Nosrati, R., M.M. Gong, M.C. San Gabriel, C.E. Pedraza, A. Zini, and D. Sinton. 2016. Paper-based quantification of male fertility potential. *Clinical Chemistry* 62 3:458–465.

Pappas, M.G., R. Hajkowski, and W.T. Hockmeyer. 1983. Dot enzyme-linked immunosorbent-assay (Dot-ELISA)—A micro technique for the rapid diagnosis of visceral leishmaniasis. *Journal of Immunological Methods* 64 (1–2):205–214.

Pardee, K., A.A. Green, T. Ferrante, D.E. Cameron, A.D. Keyser, P. Yin, and J.J. Collins. 2014. Paper-based synthetic gene networks. *Cell* 159 (4):940–954.

Pelton, R. 2009. Bioactive paper provides a low-cost platform for diagnostics. *TrAC: Trends in Analytical Chemistry* 28 (8):925–942.

Pena-Pereira, F., I. Lavilla, and C. Bendicho. 2016. Paper-based analytical device for instrumental-free detection of thiocyanate in saliva as a biomarker of tobacco smoke exposure. *Talanta* 147:390–396.

Phillips, S.T. and G.G. Lewis. 2014. The expanding role of paper in point-of-care diagnostics. *Expert review of Molecular Diagnostics* 14 (2):123–125.

Piety, N.Z., X. Yang, D. Lezzar, A. George, and S.S. Shevkoplyas. 2015. A rapid paper-based test for quantifying sickle hemoglobin in blood samples from patients with sickle cell disease. *American Journal of Hematology* 90 (6):478–482.

Rajendra, V., C. Sicard, J.D. Brennan, and M.A. Brook. 2014. Printing silicone-based hydrophobic barriers on paper for microfluidic assays using low-cost ink jet printers. *Analyst* 139 (24):6361–6365.

Ren, K., Y. Chen, and H. Wu. 2014. New materials for microfluidics in biology. *Current Opinion in Biotechnology* 25:78–85.

Ren, K., J. Zhou, and H. Wu. 2013. Materials for microfluidic chip fabrication. *Accounts of Chemical Research* 46 (11):2396–2406.

Renault, C., J. Koehne, A.J. Ricco, and R.M. Crooks. 2014. Three-dimensional wax patterning of paper fluidic devices. *Langmuir* 30 (23):7030–7036.

Rodkvamtook, W., Z.W. Zhang, C.C. Chao et al. 2015. Dot-ELISA rapid test using recombinant 56-kDa protein antigens for serodiagnosis of scrub typhus. *American Journal of Tropical Medicine and Hygiene* 92 (5):967–971.

Sackmann, E.K., A.L. Fulton, and D.J. Beebe. 2014. The present and future role of microfluidics in biomedical research. *Nature* 507 (7491):181–189.

Shih, C.-M., C.-L. Chang, M.-Y. Hsu, J.-Y. Lin, C.-M. Kuan, H.-K. Wang, C.-T. Huang, M.-C. Chung, K.-C. Huang, and C.-E. Hsu. 2015. Paper-based ELISA to rapidly detect *Escherichia coli*. *Talanta* 145:2–5.

Slomovic, S., K. Pardee, and J.J. Collins. 2015. Synthetic biology devices for in vitro and in vivo diagnostics. *Proceedings of the National Academy of Sciences of the United States of America* 112 (47):14429–14435.

Smit, P.W., I. Elliott, R.W. Peeling, D. Mabey, and P.N. Newton. 2014. An overview of the clinical use of filter paper in the diagnosis of tropical diseases. *The American Journal of Tropical Medicine and Hygiene* 90 (2):195–210.

Song, M.-B., H.-A. Joung, Y.K. Oh, K. Jung, Y.D. Ahn, and M.-G. Kim. 2015. Tear-off patterning: A simple method for patterning nitrocellulose membranes to improve the performance of point-of-care diagnostic biosensors. *Lab on a Chip* 15 (14):3006–3012.

Spicar-Mihalic, P., B. Toley, J. Houghtaling, T. Liang, P. Yager, and E. Fu. 2013. CO_2 laser cutting and ablative etching for the fabrication of paper-based devices. *Journal of Micromechanics and Microengineering* 23 (6):067003.

Spooner, N., R. Lad, and M. Barfield. 2009. Dried blood spots as a sample collection technique for the determination of pharmacokinetics in clinical studies: Considerations for the validation of a quantitative bioanalytical method. *Analytical Chemistry* 81 (4):1557–1563.

Streit, S., C.W. Michalski, M. Erkan, J. Kleeff, and H. Friess. 2008. Northern blot analysis for detection and quantification of RNA in pancreatic cancer cells and tissues. *Nature Protocols* 4 (1):37–43.

Su, J.L., M. Al-Tamimi, and G. Garnier. 2012. Engineering paper as a substrate for blood typing bio-diagnostics. *Cellulose* 19 (5):1749–1758.

Su, W., X. Gao, L. Jiang, and J. Qin. 2015. Microfluidic platform towards point-of-care diagnostics in infectious diseases. *Journal of Chromatography A* 1377:13–26.

Sun, J., B. Bao, M. He, H. Zhou, and Y. Song. 2015. Recent advances in controlling the depositing morphologies of inkjet droplets. *ACS Applied Materials & Interfaces* 7 (51):28086–28099.

Sun, J., Y. Xianyu, and X. Jiang. 2014. Point-of-care biochemical assays using gold nanoparticle-implemented microfluidics. *Chemical Society Reviews* 43 (17):6239–6253.

The Lewin Group. 2005. The value of diagnostics innovation, adoption and diffusion into health care Falls Church, VA.

Then, W.L., M. Li, H. McLiesh, W. Shen, and G. Garnier. 2015. The detection of blood group phenotypes using paper diagnostics. *Vox Sanguinis* 108 (2):186–196.

Thiessen, G., R. Robinson, K.D.L. Reyes, R.J. Monnat, and E. Fu. 2015. Conversion of a laboratory-based test for phenylalanine detection to a simple paper-based format and implications for PKU screening in low-resource settings. *Analyst* 140 (2):609–615.

Wang, H.-K., C.-H. Tsai, K.-H. Chen, C.-T. Tang, J.-S. Leou, P.-C. Li, Y.-L. Tang, H.-J. Hsieh, H.-C. Wu, and C.-M. Cheng. 2014a. Cellulose-based diagnostic devices for diagnosing serotype-2 dengue fever in human serum. *Advanced Healthcare Materials* 3 (2):187–196.

Wang, H.-L., C.-H. Chu, S.-J. Tsai, and R.-J. Yang. 2016. Aspartate aminotransferase and alanine aminotransferase detection on paper-based analytical devices with inkjet printer-sprayed reagents. *Micromachines* 7 (1):9.

Wang, J., M.R.N. Monton, X. Zhang, C.D.M. Filipe, R. Pelton, and J.D. Brennan. 2014b. Hydrophobic sol-gel channel patterning strategies for paper-based microfluidics. *Lab on a Chip* 14 (4):691–695.

Warren, A.D., G.A. Kwong, D.K. Wood, K.Y. Lin, and S.N. Bhatia. 2014. Point-of-care diagnostics for noncommunicable diseases using synthetic urinary biomarkers and paper microfluidics. *Proceedings of the National Academy of Sciences of the United States of America* 111 (10):3671–3676.

Weaver, A.A., H. Reiser, T. Barstis, M. Benvenuti, D. Ghosh, M. Hunckler, B. Joy, L. Koenig, K. Raddell, and M. Lieberman. 2013. Paper analytical devices for fast field screening of beta lactam antibiotics and antituberculosis pharmaceuticals. *Analytical Chemistry* 85 (13):6453–6460.

Webster, M. and V.S. Kumar. 2012. Lab on a stamp: Paper-based diagnostic tools. *Clinical Chemistry* 58 (5):956–958.

Whitesides, G.M. 2006. The origins and the future of microfluidics. *Nature* 442 (7101):368–373.

Wong, R. and H. Tse. 2009. *Lateral Flow Immunoassay*. Humana Press, New York.

Wu, P.J. and C.S. Zhang. 2015. Low-cost, high-throughput fabrication of cloth-based microfluidic devices using a photolithographical patterning technique. *Lab on a Chip* 15 (6):1598–1608.

Xu, C., L. Cai, M. Zhong, and S. Zheng. 2015. Low-cost and rapid prototyping of microfluidic paper-based analytical devices by inkjet printing of permanent marker ink. *RSC Advances* 5 (7):4770–4773.

Yamada, K., T.G. Henares, K. Suzuki, and D. Citterio. 2015a. Distance-based tear lactoferrin assay on microfluidic paper device using interfacial interactions on surface-modified cellulose. *ACS Applied Materials & Interfaces* 7 (44):24864–24875.

Yamada, K., T.G. Henares, K. Suzuki, and D. Citterio. 2015b. Paper-based inkjet-printed microfluidic analytical devices. *Angewandte Chemie International Edition* 54 (18):5294–5310.

Yamada, K., S. Takaki, N. Komuro, K. Suzuki, and D. Citterio. 2014. An antibody-free microfluidic paper-based analytical device for the determination of tear fluid lactoferrin by fluorescence sensitization of Tb3+. *Analyst* 139 (7):1637–1643.

Yang, D.Y., X. Niu, Y.Y. Liu, Y. Wang, X. Gu, L.S. Song, R. Zhao, L.Y. Ma, Y.M. Shao, and X.Y. Jiang. 2008. Electrospun nanofibrous membranes: A novel solid substrate for microfluidic immunoassays for HIV. *Advanced Materials* 20 (24):4770.

Yang, X., J. Kanter, N.Z. Piety, M.S. Benton, S.M. Vignes, and S.S. Shevkoplyas. 2013a. A simple, rapid, low-cost diagnostic test for sickle cell disease. *Lab on a Chip* 13 (8):1464–1467.

Yang, X.X., N.Z. Piety, S.M. Vignes, M.S. Benton, J. Kanter, and S.S. Shevkoplyas. 2013b. Simple paper-based test for measuring blood hemoglobin concentration in resource-limited settings. *Clinical Chemistry* 59 (10):1506–1513.

Yawn, B.P., G.R. Buchanan, A.N. Afenyi-Annan et al. 2014. Management of sickle cell disease: Summary of the 2014 evidence-based report by expert panel members. *JAMA* 312 (10):1033–1048.

Yeow, N., H. McLiesh, and G. Garnier. 2015. Indirect antiglobulin paper test for red blood cell antigen typing by flow-through method. *Analytical Methods* 7 (11):4645–4649.

Yetisen, A.K., M.S. Akram, and C.R. Lowe. 2013. Paper-based microfluidic point-of-care diagnostic devices. *Lab on a Chip* 13 (12):2210–2251.

Zhou, G., X. Mao, and D. Juncker. 2012. Immunochromatographic assay on thread. *Analytical Chemistry* 84 (18):7736–7743.

4

Printed Wax-Ink Valves for Multistep Assays in Paper Analytical Devices

Jacqueline C. Linnes and Elizabeth Phillips

CONTENTS

4.1 Introduction

Rapid environmental and point-of-care disease testing requires the translation of benchtop assays to portable and easy-to-use platforms in the field. The paper-based analytical device (PAD) is an easily fabricated platform lauded for their usability and disposal at extremely low costs compared to their plastic and glass microfluidic counterparts (Hu et al. 2014). Composed of porous membranes such as cellulose, nitrocellulose, and glass fibers, PADs are adaptable to a variety of sample types, chemical and biochemical assays, and detection output needs (Yager et al. 2008, Martinez et al. 2010b).

PADs leverage the inherent wicking ability of porous materials to transport fluid through multiple reagent zones. Traditional PADs, such as lateral flow immunoassays (LFIAs), operate without external pumping and offer a more affordable option than microfluidic chips for point-of-care diagnostics. Nevertheless, the limited fluidic control currently permitted in these porous membrane networks restricts the sophistication of assays that can be performed on paper (Byrnes et al. 2013).

Fluidic control in PADs can be categorized into three fundamental elements: pumps, routers, and valves, which facilitate the respective transport, mixing, splitting, and aliquoting of liquids. By automating these processes, PAD capabilities can be extended beyond single-step assays (Toley et al. 2015). Capillary flow, or pumping, is a fundamental property of the capillary networks themselves and is determined by porosity and tortuosity of the membranes (Smirnov 2010). Sophisticated flow direction can be routed through two- and three-dimensional channels defined by hydrophobic barriers made from PDMS, tape, and/or wax-ink (Bruzewicz et al. 2008, Martinez et al. 2010a, Renault et al. 2014). Valve mechanisms remain the most challenged elements to incorporate into paper-based devices (Byrnes et al. 2013, Toley et al. 2015). The simplest way to vary the flow rate and delivery time of reagents is to control the geometry of the channels such as their length and width (Fu et al. 2010, Fridley et al. 2014, Toley et al. 2015). Alternatively, fluid flow can be delayed by adding material to the channels, such as printer toner or paraffin wax (Noh and Phillips 2010, Ouyang et al. 2013). Similarly, pre-embedded surfactants have been used to accelerate the flow of liquid with delay and trigger valves but can potentially affect downstream assays (Chen et al. 2012, Jahanshahi-Anbuhi et al. 2014). However, these previously described methods to accelerate and decelerate the flow of liquid do not fully obstruct liquid flow and are thus incompatible with long assay incubation periods. Tunable valves that completely prevent and then release liquid flow through porous networks on demand will enable more sophisticated assays through controlled incubation and sequential liquid flow (LaFleur 2016).

We have developed a printed wax-ink valve mechanism that is low-cost, can be easily manufactured, can be tuned for various needs, can be actuated multiple times, and requires minimal user involvement (Phillips et al. 2016). In this chapter, we demonstrate how to prototype the tunable valve mechanism using wax-ink printing onto a nitrocellulose membrane. The wax-ink valve fully obstructs fluid flow and is actuated by heating to release a controlled amount of liquid past the valve. In this chapter, we show how the wax-ink valve can be integrated into an LFIA detecting bacterial contamination in water in order to increase the detection sensitivity with a gold enhancement step.

4.2 Materials

4.2.1 Patterning Wax Valve Strips

1. Vector design software (e.g., Adobe Illustrator) for designing the patterns for cutting and ink deposition

2. Vinyl cutter (e.g., Silver Bullet cutter plotter) and 45° blade with associated software (e.g., SCAL4) (see note Mat 1)
3. Nitrocellulose membranes (e.g., GE Healthcare FF120HP)
4. Copy paper (e.g., Boise multiuse copy paper)
5. Double-sided tape (e.g., 3M Scotch)
6. Transparency film (e.g., Staples multipurpose transparency film)
7. Tape (e.g., VWR general purpose laboratory labeling tape)
8. Wax printer (e.g., Xerox ColorCube 8580)
9. Solid wax-ink (e.g., Xerox Black ColorQube ink)
10. Filter forceps, blunt end (e.g., EMD Millipore XX6200006P)
11. Oven (e.g., VWR tabletop oven) or hotplate to hold the strips at a constant temperature to permeate strips with wax-ink

4.2.2 Fabrication/Assembly of Multistep Lateral Flow Immunoassay

1. Hot glue
2. Conjugate pad (e.g., GE Healthcare brand Fusion 5)
3. Thin-film heater (e.g., 28 Ω, 10 W/in.^{2} Omega) (see note Mat 2)
4. Power supply (e.g., 1550 B&K Precision Power Supply)
5. Gold enhancement solution (e.g., Nanoprobes GoldEnhance LM)
6. Tween-20 (Sigma-Aldrich)
7. Lateral flow immunoassay (e.g., Silver Lake Research Corporation Rapid Bacteria Pool water test strips)

4.2.3 Assay to Enhance LFIA Detection Signal

1. Test sample (e.g., *Escherichia coli* culture medium)
2. Glass dish (e.g., Pyrex 3140)
3. Vinyl electrical tape

4.3 Methods

4.3.1 Patterning

1. Use the vinyl cutter software to design a 50 mm by 20 mm rectangular path that will be used to cut the nitrocellulose.
2. Tape the nitrocellulose membrane facedown (plastic-backing facing up) onto the cutting mat with a transparency sheet sandwiched in

between by using general purpose lab tape to cover all four edges of the membrane. (See note Met 1.)

3. Using the Silver Bullet vinyl cutter set to a 45° blade offset and 0.65 mm overcut at 95 mm/s with a pressure set to 80, align the origin of the cutting knife with the corner of a nitrocellulose membrane sheet.

4. Cut the 50 mm by 20 mm strip from the nitrocellulose membrane.

5. Use Adobe Illustrator to create a single, 50 mm long horizontal black line (0.1 mm stroke) on an 8.5 in. by 11 in. artboard. Illustrator's Transform Panel function is helpful to specify the line's coordinate location (e.g., x = 40 mm, y = 40 mm will place the center point of the line 4 cm from the top and left side of the artboard). (See note Met 2.)

6. Adhere the nitrocellulose membrane strip faceup onto copy paper with 2 mm wide strips of double-sided tape on the leading and trailing edges of the nitrocellulose. The plastic backing of the nitrocellulose membrane should be against the copy paper and the nitrocellulose should be oriented such that its long side is parallel to the short side of the copy paper. Adhere the nitrocellulose membrane according to the coordinate that was set in 4.3.1.4. such that the line will print through the middle of the 50 mm by 20 mm strip. (See Figure 4.1.)

7. Print the 0.1 mm wide black line designed in step 4.3.1.4. onto the nitrocellulose membrane strip by feeding the copy paper into the manual tray, membrane facing down.

8. Gently peel the printed nitrocellulose membrane off the copy paper and tape using blunt end filter forceps to avoid crushing the membrane.

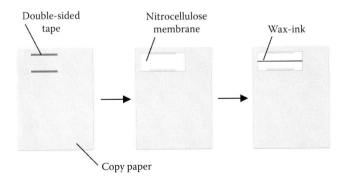

FIGURE 4.1
Nitrocellulose membrane alignment for wax ink printing.

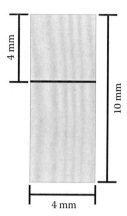

FIGURE 4.2
Final patterned wax valve.

9. Place printed nitrocellulose membrane (faceup) into an 85°C oven for 1 min so that the wax-ink band permeates into the nitrocellulose membrane. (See note Met 3.)

10. Cut 1 mm strips from the edges of the patterned membranes and discard these strips, as the wax does not melt evenly at the edges of the membrane. (See note Met 4.)

11. Cut the remaining patterned membrane into 4 mm by 10 mm strips, with the wax band about 4 mm from a short edge. (See Figure 4.2.)

4.3.2 Fabrication of Enhanced LFIA

1. The antibody–nanoparticle conjugate in the water test is provided from the manufacturer as a dried reagent in a tube. Rehydrate the conjugates with 40 µL of DI water for 10 min. Place 4 mm by 10 mm conjugate pad strips onto Parafilm and pipette the rehydrated conjugates onto the strips to dry overnight in ambient conditions. (See notes Met 5 and Met 6.)

2. Gently remove the sample pad from the lateral flow membrane and replace with the prepared conjugate pad.

3. Place the nitrocellulose membrane valve strip made in 4.3.1 facedown on lateral flow test membrane perpendicular to the test band. The valve strip should overlap the edge of the test membrane about 1 mm. Secure with a pea-sized drop of hot glue flattened with a spatula. A rounded glue drop can distort the test band and make it difficult to visualize later. (See note Met 7 and Figure 4.3 [front].)

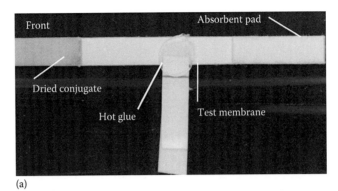

(a)

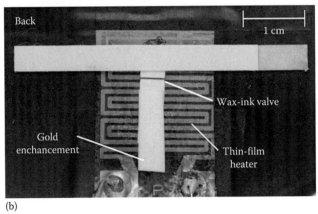

(b)

FIGURE 4.3
(a) Front and (b) back images of the assembled enhanced lateral flow immunoassay.

4. Adhere the modified lateral flow membrane assembly to a thin-film heater by sandwiching a strip of double-sided tape between the plastic backing of the valve strip and the thin-film heater. Ensure that the wax valve is located directly over a resistive metal element for optimal heating.

5. Complete the assembly by placing an untreated 4 mm by 10 mm strip of conjugate pad material (to deliver gold enhancement solution) on the valve strip. This second conjugate pad should overlap the valve strip by 5 mm. (See Figure 4.3 [back].)

4.3.3 Conducting a Multistep Assay

1. Connect the thin-film heater to a power supply. For maximum heating efficiency, adhere the thin-film heater and modified LFIA assembly to an upside-down glass dish with electrical tape along the edges of the thin-film heater to keep it in place.

2. Prepare GoldEnhance LM solution according to manufacturer instructions and add 0.015% Tween-20 solution.

3. Pipette 40 µL of liquid sample (e.g., *E. coli* culture) to the first conjugate pad. You should observe the sample rehydrating the conjugates and fluid wicking through the test membrane.

4. Pipette 40 µL of prepared GoldEnhance LM solution to the untreated conjugated pad. You should observe the GoldEnhance solution blocked by the wax-ink valve from flowing to the test membrane.

5. After 20 min room-temperature incubation, apply 0.21 amps of current to the thin-film heater for 50 s. (See note Met 8.)

6. After an additional 20 min incubation the test bands can be analyzed. Scanned images can be analyzed with MATLAB® or ImageJ to compare color intensity.

4.4 Notes

Mat 1: A laser engraver can also be used to cut valves.

Mat 2: A hotplate or other flat heating surface can also be used to actuate valves. However, care must be taken to prevent evaporation from the large heating surface.

Met 1: Taping all of the edges is important to prevent shredding the membrane during the cutting process. The transparency sheet prevents residual debris that may be on the cutting mat from damaging the nitrocellulose membrane.

Met 2: 0.1 mm is the smallest width that results in a solid wax line when melted on nitrocellulose membrane. Below this width, individual dots are printed that do not melt into a single line to block fluid wicking.

Met 3: A piece of aluminum foil is used to provide a clean surface in the oven for the membrane to lie on during heating.

Met 4: It is essential that thin strips be cut (step 4.3.2.2.) *after* melting the wax into the larger membrane strip.

Met 5: Strips of conjugate pad are placed on Parafilm (or other hydrophobic material) to prevent the conjugate solution from bleeding onto another surface while it is drying.

Met 6: Preparation of a conjugate pad and replacement of the sample pad are only necessary for some LFIAs, such as the Silver Lake Rapid Bacteria Pool test strips, in which the conjugate pad is not already a component of the lateral flow immunoassay. For LFIAs that already contain a conjugate pad upstream of the test membrane, the sample can be applied directly to the sample pad.

Met 7: Alternatively, secure with a 5 mm by 5 mm square of pressure-sensitive adhesive.

Met 8: Fifty seconds of 0.21 amps heats the 28 Ω, 10 W/in.^{2} thin-film heater to 48°C, the temperature at which the wax valve melts sufficiently for liquid to wick through. If using a different thin-film heater or wax-ink, the applied current and time may need to be adjusted to reach the appropriate melting temperature.

4.5 Conclusions

In this demonstration of the printed-wax valves, addition of the gold enhancement step in an LFIA for microbiological contamination in water samples improved the assay sensitivity by 10-fold. These printed-wax–ink valves can be applied to other multistep assays requiring sustained incubation and sequential reagent addition, such as isothermal DNA amplification and horseradish peroxidase-based enzymatic signal amplification reactions. Thermally actuated valves allow for additional sophistication in paper-based assays while maintaining low-cost fabrication and minimal user-steps, without obstructing downstream chemistries.

Acknowledgments

This work was supported in part by the Bill and Melinda Gates Foundation through the Grand Challenges Explorations Program (Grant No. OPP1150806), the National Science Foundation's Graduate Research Fellowship Program, the Purdue University Innovations in International Development Lab, and the Purdue Research Foundation.

References

Bruzewicz, D.A., M. Reches, and G.M. Whitesides. 2008. Low-cost printing of poly(dimethylsiloxane) barriers to define microchannels in paper. *Analytical Chemistry* 80(9):3387–3392.

Byrnes, S., G. Thiessen, and E. Fu. 2013. Progress in the development of paper-based diagnostics for low-resource point-of-care settings. *Bioanalysis* 5(22):2821–2836.

Chen, H., J. Cogswell, C. Anagnostopoulos, and M. Faghri. 2012. A fluidic diode, valves, and a sequential-loading circuit fabricated on layered paper. *Lab on a Chip* 12(16):2909–2913.

Fridley, G.E., H. Le, and P. Yager. 2014. Highly sensitive immunoassay based on controlled rehydration of patterned reagents in a 2-dimensional paper network. *Analytical Chemistry* 86(13):6447–6453.

Fu, E., P. Kauffman, B. Lutz, and P. Yager. 2010. Chemical signal amplification in two-dimensional paper networks. *Sensors and Actuators B, Chemical* 149(1):325–328.

Hu, J., S.Q. Wang, L. Wang, F. Li, B. Pingguan-Murphy, T.J. Lu, and F. Xu. 2014. Advances in paper-based point-of-care diagnostics. *Biosensors and Bioelectronics* 54:585–597.

Jahanshahi-Anbuhi, S., A. Henry, V. Leung, C. Sicard, K. Pennings, R. Pelton, J.D. Brennan, and C.D.M. Filipe. 2014. Paper-based microfluidics with an erodible polymeric bridge giving controlled release and timed flow shutoff. *Lab on a Chip* 14(1):229–236.

Lafleur, L., J.D. Bishop, E.K. Heiniger, R.P. Gallagher, M.D. Wheeler, P.C. Kauffman, X. Zhang, E. Kline, J. Buser, S. Ramachandran, S. Byrnes, N. Vermeulen, N. Scarr, Y. Belousov, W. Mahoney, B.J. Toley, P.D. Ladd, B. Lutz, and P. Yager. 2016. *Lab on a Chip* 16:3777–3787.

Martinez, A.W., S.T. Phillips, Z. Nie, C.-M. Cheng, E. Carrilho, B.J. Wiley, and G.M. Whitesides. 2010a. Programmable diagnostic devices made from paper and tape. *Lab on a Chip* 10(19):2499–2504.

Martinez, A.W., S.T. Phillips, G.M. Whitesides, and E. Carrilho. 2010b. Diagnostics for the developing world: Microfluidic paper-based analytical devices. *Analytical Chemistry* 82(1):3–10.

Noh, H. and S.T. Phillips. 2010. Fluidic timers for time-dependent, point-of-care assays on paper. *Analytical Chemistry* 82(19):8071–8078.

Ouyang, Y., S. Wang, J. Li, P.S. Riehl, M. Begley, and J.P. Landers. 2013. Rapid patterning of 'tunable' hydrophobic valves on disposable microchips by laser printer lithography. *Lab on a Chip* 13(9):1762–1771.

Phillips, E.A., S. Zhao, R. Shen, and J.C. Linnes. 2016. Thermally actuated wax valves for paper-fluidic diagnostics. *Lab on a Chip* 16(21):4230–4236.

Renault, C., J. Koehne, A.J. Ricco, and R.M. Crooks. 2014. Three-dimensional wax patterning of paper fluidic devices. *Langmuir* 30(23):7030–7036.

Smirnov, H.F. 2010. *Transport Phenomena in Capillary-Porous Structures and Heat Pipes.* CRC Press, Taylor & Francis, Boca Raton, FL.

Toley, B.J., J.A. Wang, M. Gupta, J.R. Buser, L.K. Lafleur, B.R. Lutz, E. Fu, and P. Yager. 2015. A versatile valving toolkit for automating fluidic operations in paper microfluidic devices. *Lab on a Chip* 15(6):1432–1444.

Yager, P., G.J. Domingo, and J. Gerdes. 2008. Point-of-care diagnostics for global health. *Annual Review of Biomedical Engineering* 10:107–144.

5

Mycofluidics: Miniaturization of Mycotoxin Analysis

Jonathan H. Loftus, Gregor S. Kijanka, and Richard O'Kennedy

CONTENTS

5.1 Introduction

5.1.1 Importance of Mycotoxins

Mycotoxins are toxic secondary metabolites produced by common fungal species such as *Aspergillus*, *Fusarium*, and *Penicillium*. They are important naturally occurring food adulterants with global occurrences and significant impact on food safety. Mycotoxins are ubiquitous, and it is estimated that 25% of the world's food supply is contaminated (CAST, 2003). Several hundred different mycotoxins have been identified and characterized. However, estimates suggest there are potentially hundreds of thousands of unique mycotoxin types. Mycotoxins of greatest agro-economic importance include aflatoxins (AFs), ochratoxin A (OTA), deoxynivalenol (DON), fumonisins (FB), zearalenone (ZEN), and patulin (Figure 5.1). The effects of these toxins can be both acute and chronic, and they are directly linked to hepatocellular carcinoma, immune suppression, inflammation, growth suppression, and many other diseases in humans and animals (Zain, 2011; Edite Bezerra da Rocha et al., 2014;

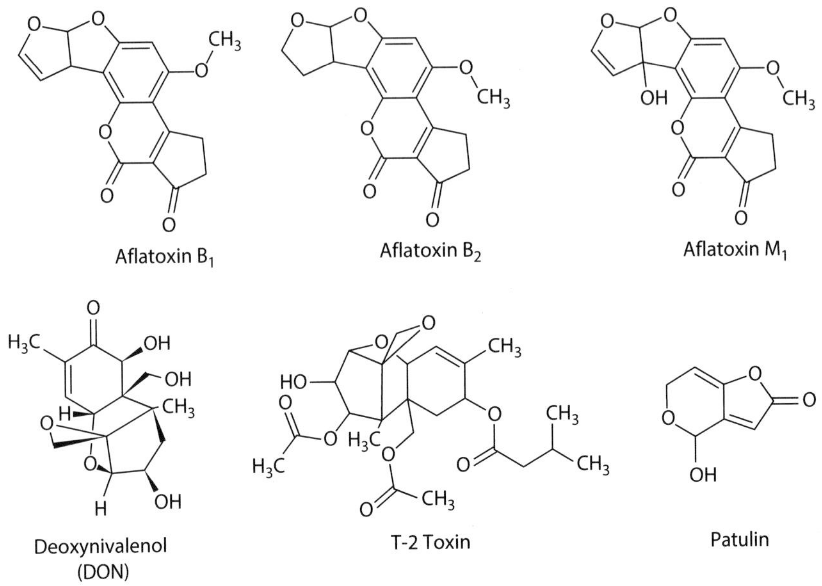

FIGURE 5.1
Chemical structures of important mycotoxins including aflatoxin B1, B2, M1, deoxynivalenol, T-2 toxin, and patulin.

Loftus et al., 2016). Aflatoxin B1 is classified as a Group 1 carcinogen, while aflatoxin M1, FB, and OTA are classified as Group 2B carcinogens by the International Agency for Research on Cancer (WHO IARC, 1993). Due to these severe effects, great efforts are being made to control and eliminate the risk of mycotoxin-contaminated foods by preventing exposure. Hence, mycotoxin analysis is regarded as one of the most important areas in food safety. The requirement for uncontaminated food sources is crucial to an ever-rising global population. It is estimated that 200,000 people are added to the global food demand daily and by the year 2050, the world population will surpass 9 billion (Marroquín-Cardona et al., 2014). Since the health of human populations is largely determined by the condition of food-producing ecosystems, pressures placed on supply may directly impact both the quantity and quality of available food. Increasing demand along with climate change underscores the importance of the role of mycotoxins in the changing environment. Governments and food safety authorities are now closely regulating and monitoring mycotoxin levels in foods for human and animal consumption. Detection, analysis, and monitoring of these adulterants at legislative limits are a worldwide priority (BIOMIN, 2016).

This chapter aims to briefly describe some of the established methods of mycotoxin analysis and highlight the limitations of these methods. The need to develop rapid, portable analytical platforms will be emphasized. These platforms must be able to compete with the gold standard techniques in areas such as sensitivity and specificity so that analysis can be moved from the laboratory to "on-site" monitoring. Current research on microfluidic-based devices will be examined and examples of devices utilizing microfluidic platforms to offer potential solutions for rapid analysis will be described throughout the chapter.

5.1.2 Current Methods of Mycotoxin Analysis

Many governments throughout the world have responded to the damaging health effects and economic impact of mycotoxins with the introduction of stringent regulatory and legislative limits (Zain, 2011). Countries are now implementing limits for a number of key mycotoxins. In order to monitor and enforce these limits, several methodologies are employed for food analysis. The variety in the structures and isoforms of mycotoxins (Figure 5.1) means that it is not currently possible to use one standard technique for their analysis. Turner et al. (2009) reviewed and compared some of the most commonly employed methods and found there was no one favorable method but that choice usually depended on: (1) the mycotoxin(s) being analyzed and (2) the matrix being used.

To quantitatively measure mycotoxin amounts, analytical approaches based on the chromatographic properties of the toxins have been established. Thin-layer chromatography (TLC) was historically the most commonly used separation technique in mycotoxin determination. TLC is still used as a preliminary screening technique for some mycotoxins; however, advances in the area of chromatography have led to a progression from TLC to more sophisticated methods based around liquid chromatographic (LC) separation coupled to detection methods such mass spectrometry (MS) (LC-MS), fluorometric detection (FD) (HPLC-FLD), or ultraviolet detection (UVD) (HPLC-UVD). Liquid-chromatography-based methods are the cornerstone of mycotoxin analysis, with the key methods established by the Association of Analytical Communities (AOAC) and centered on LC separation coupled with MS detection. It is accepted that LC-MS and LC-fluorescence are the gold standard against which all other methods are compared (Yeni et al., 2014).

The ability to generate highly specific antibodies is now well established and has proven hugely beneficial for mycotoxin analysis (Daly et al., 2000; Dunne et al., 2005; Edupuganti et al., 2013). Immunoassay is a widely utilized tool for the analysis of mycotoxins. It is based on molecular recognition for antigen by an antibody and provides detection with high sensitivity and specificity. Immunochemical detection platforms vary from simple lateral flow immunoassays and enzyme-linked immunosorbent assays (ELISAs) to highly sophisticated immunosensors. ELISA is one of the most commonly used immunoassay formats as it is an inexpensive, color-based test where the outputs may be assessed by simple absorbance determination. Many ELISA kits for mycotoxin detection have been successfully commercialized in the past two decades (Bahadır and Sezgintürk, 2015; Turner et al., 2015).

The portability of a test and opportunity for application in situations of minimal use (i.e., a customer requiring a single screening test instead of purchasing expensive analytical equipment) has meant that ELISA methodologies are still highly popular. The commercially available assays for the analysis of the most common mycotoxins have been validated by organizations such as the AOAC. These kits can be used in the field but do not offer the same levels of high-throughput sensitivity compared to lab-based methods. Chromatography-based analytical techniques and immunoassays have proven to offer suitable and sensitive solutions for determining mycotoxin contamination within a laboratory, but they have significant limitations, as outlined in the following section.

5.1.3 Limitations to Current Analysis Methods

Currently, chromatography remains the gold standard against which all other techniques are compared. The extreme sensitivity and flexibility of chromatography-based methods (Turner et al., 2015), as highlighted by the ability to detect multiple analytes (sometimes over 50) at ppb levels in complex samples, cannot be currently matched by other technologies. However, LC methods will always suffer practical issues. The lack of automation of TLC has generally made it a redundant technique, replaced by more sophisticated methods. The main issue with chromatography is that the analyses of mycotoxin levels are very time-consuming, costly, and require skilled personnel to operate. These techniques also require rigorous sample cleanup and pretreatment, and for GC analysis there is often a need for derivatization of nonvolatile mycotoxins. Often, mycotoxins can be lost or altered during these procedures, leading to inaccurate results (Selvaraj et al., 2015).

Immunoassay techniques lend themselves to being considerably more user-friendly and cost-effective when compared to chromatography, but ELISA may also require lengthy analysis times and so like chromatography methods they have significant limitations for implementation as rapid, "user-friendly" "on-site" testing platforms. It is also important to consider that due to their small size, mycotoxins must be coupled to large molecular weight carrier proteins to work in immunoassays. This conjugation process presents issues. Firstly, conjugations can be unstable and degrade over time. Secondly, variations in structures mean that mycotoxins have different functional groups, and as a result several different coupling chemistries need to be utilized. There is no universal technique. Finally, several problems have been encountered with the formation of cross-reacting, side-reaction products and interfering carrier toxin bridging groups. These interferences result in high background absorbances and reduced sensitivities in immunoassays (Xiao et al., 1995). ELISA formats are known to be reliable and excellent for screening; however, they also require multiple steps and plate readers. If information beyond simple screening is required, ELISA is not suitable for

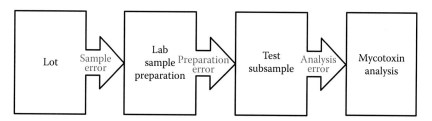

FIGURE 5.2
Overview of mycotoxin analysis procedure from lot-to-lab highlighting potential error areas of the procedure in red. Sampling error, preparation error, and analysis error together represent the total error in an analysis. The error found within the analytical method is low in comparison to that found in sampling and sample preparation.

field testing. Therefore, the integration of suitable molecular recognition elements, such as antibodies, directly with microfluidic systems is favored for portable, non-laboratory analysis.

Overall, the current analysis procedure for mycotoxin testing is flawed and faces the challenges of potential error introduction at all stages (Figure 5.2). It would be desirable to move this analysis away from the lab, into the field and thus to reduce some of the error while ultimately improving analysis.

5.2 Microfluidics for Mycotoxin Analysis

5.2.1 Advantages of Microfluidics for Mycotoxins Analysis

Mycotoxins provide excellent targets for microfluidic-based studies, from both the academic and commercial viewpoints. The development of microfluidic-based analytical methods is now beginning to outweigh chromatography applications (Marroquín-Cardona et al., 2014).

The physical properties of microfluidic systems have led to tools that can measure biological agents at a resolution that has not been possible with macroscale platforms. These systems can also be highly customized to suit a variety of target analytes. Most significantly, the emergence of fabrication methods that do not require highly specialized engineering facilities has allowed for rapid development of microfluidic systems and their adaptation to a broad range of biological applications (Alapan et al., 2015; Duncombe et al., 2015). Advancements in molecular biology research in conjunction with microfluidic approaches have the potential to transform mycotoxin analysis.

Microfluidic systems offer the ability to circumvent problems associated with traditional assay formats (Table 5.1). At these small scales, fluids exhibit

TABLE 5.1

Advantages and Disadvantages of Established and Emerging Methods of Mycotoxin Analysis

	Method	Advantages	Disadvantages
Chromatographic	TLC	Simple; "easy-to-use"; good screening technique	Time-consuming; requires organic solvents; does not allow for high-throughput
	HPLC	High sensitivity; good selectivity; reproducible; fully automated high-throughput; can be coupled to detector (MS); official methods available	Expensive equipment; specialist expertise required; may require derivatization; time-consuming; lab-based
	GC	High throughput; multiple mycotoxin analysis; good sensitivity; automated; official methods available	Expensive equipment; specialist expertise required; lab-based; derivatization required; matrix interference problems; issues with reproducibility and repeatability
	LC-MS	High throughput; multiple mycotoxin analysis; high sensitivity and selectivity; reproducible; provides confirmation; no derivatization required; recognized gold standard	Very expensive; specialist expertise required; lab-based; sensitivity relies on ionization technique; lack of internal standards
Immunoassay	ELISA Kits	Simple sample preparation; good screening technique; inexpensive equipment; good sensitivity; multiple mycotoxin analysis; limited use of organic solvents	Cross-reactivity with related mycotoxins; matrix interference; possible false positive/negative results; includes several steps; only semiquantitative without reader; often confirmatory LC analysis required.
Microfluidic	LFD	Rapid, no cleanup, no expensive equipment; simple; very "easy-to-use"; good sensitivity; reproducible; multiple mycotoxin analysis	Qualitative or semiquantitative; cross-reactivity with related mycotoxins; matrix interference
	Biosensors	Rapid; simple cleanup procedures; high throughput; multiple mycotoxin analysis; high sensitivity and selectivity; potential for full automation	Cross-reactivity with related mycotoxins; extract cleanup needed to improve sensitivity; variation in reproducibility and repeatability; no official methods available

Abbreviations: ELISA, enzyme-linked immunosorbent assay; GC, gas chromatography; HPLC, high performance liquid chromatography; LC-MS, liquid chromatography/mass spectrometry; LFD, lateral flow device; TLC, thin-layer chromatography.

Note: Shading shows the grouping of assay types and that microfluidic is sub group of immunoassay.

laminar flow, and mixing occurs by diffusion. Microfluidic immunoassays have several advantages over larger-scale formats, including increased surface area to volume ratios (speeding up antibody–antigen interactions) and smaller dimensions, which reduce reagent and sample volumes, and ultimately costs, and automated fluid handling, which can increase reproducibility and allow for higher-throughput analysis. These advantages allow for the improvement of operation, increase in speed, and reduction in cost of traditional immunoassays (Ng et al., 2010). Another major challenge for mycotoxin analysis is combining sample preparation and toxin detection into one integrated system. Microfluidics offers a possible solution to this problem through areas such as multilayer soft lithography, multiphase microfluidics, electrowetting-on-dielectric, electrokinetics, and centrifugal microfluidics (Sin et al., 2011). Preparation steps such as pre-concentrating, mixing, and separation can be utilized in microfluidic platforms to make complete system integration possible.

Microfluidic systems exhibit all the characteristics for a rapid mycotoxin analysis tool and there are now a plethora of examples available in the literature of these systems being utilized for this purpose.

5.2.2 Examples of Microfluidic Systems for Mycotoxins Analysis

A broad range of microfluidic platforms have been developed to detect key mycotoxins and are reported in the literature (Table 5.2). These systems utilize a variety of formats (Hervás et al., 2012; Guo et al., 2015). It is clear that immunoassay-based systems are a favored approach, evolving from ELISA-based methods and exploiting the potential of antibody affinity and specificity for reaching limits of detection (LODs) that are below legislative limits. Developments in DNA and RNA technology have resulted in aptamer-based biosensors with LODs similar to their antibody counterparts. Systems vary in complexity from simple lateral flow assays to sophisticated electrochemical systems. Overall, microfluidic-based systems are providing the foundation for fulfilling the requirements needed for a rapid "on-site" mycotoxin analysis tool, but they too have their challenges and limitations.

5.2.3 Challenges Associated with Microfluidic Systems

Microfluidics offers a powerful tool for mycotoxin analysis and development in this area has seen rapid advances in recent years (Atalay et al., 2011). There are, however, many challenges and obstacles to overcome in the design, optimization, and application of microfluidics platforms for analysis of biological contaminants such as mycotoxins. There is now an emphasis on overcoming these problems to ensure technologies can transition from research to commercial products.

TABLE 5.2

Summary of Recent Microfluidic Systems Used for Detection of Mycotoxins

Target	Matrix	System Type	LOD	Reference
AFB1	Peanut	LFTS	1 µg kg^{-1}	Zhang et al. (2011)
	Buffer	QCM	0.3 ng mL^{-1}	Wang and Gan (2009)
	Buffer	Multiplex microarray	4 pg mL^{-1}	Hu et al. (2013)
	Buffer	SPR	1 mg mL^{-1}	Park et al. (2014)
	Corn	Aptamer-based dipstick	0.3 ng g^{-1}	Shim et al. (2014)
AFB2	Almond extract	SPR	0.9 ng mL^{-1}	Edupuganti et al. (2013)
AFM1	Milk	LFTS	1 µg kg^{-1}	Wang et al. (2011)
	Milk	Electrochemical microsensor	0.008 µg L^{-1}	Parker et al. (2009)
DON	Buffer	REP	6.25 ng mL^{-1}	Olcer et al. (2014)
FB1	Maize	LFTS	199 µg kg^{-1}	Molinelli et al. (2009)
	Maize	Lateral flow	120 µg L^{-1}	Anfossi et al. (2010)
OTA	Green coffee	Chemiluminescence immunosensor	7 µg kg^{-1}	Sauceda-Friebe et al. (2011)
	Buffer	Chemiluminescence	0.85 ng mL^{-1}	Novo et al. (2013)
	Red wine		28 ng mL^{-1}	
	Buffer	Multiplex microarray	4 pg mL^{-1}	Hu et al. (2013)
ZEN	Corn silage	Electrochemical immunosensor	0.77 ng mL^{-1}	Panini et al. (2010)
	Feedstuff	Microbiochip immunosensor	0.41 µg kg^{-1}	Panini et al. (2011)
	Infant food	Electrochemical immunoassay	0.4 µg L^{-1}	Hervás et al. (2009)
	Sorghum	SPR	7.8 ng mL^{-1}	Edupuganti et al. (2013)
	Buffer	Multiplex microarray	4 pg mL^{-1}	Hu et al. (2013)

Abbreviations: AFB1, aflatoxin B1; AFB2, aflatoxin B2; AFM1, aflatoxin M1; DON, deoxynivalenol; FB1, fumonisin B1; LOD, limit of detection; LFTS, lateral flow test strip OTA, ochratoxin A; QCM, quartz crystal microbalance; REP, real-time electrochemical profiling; SPR, surface plasmon resonance; ZEN, zearalenone.

The main issues surrounding design and use of microfluidic systems are sample preparation and treatment, matrix effects, and complete system integration. Sample preparation and extraction are crucial steps in the detection of mycotoxins and are often a bottleneck in analyses. The technique employed is dependent on sample type and size. In some cases, multiplex detection of several targets in complex matrices is required, and this can result in interferences and cross-reactivity. In particular, extraction from complex food matrices is a major challenge to developing effective microfluidics platform for mycotoxins' detection. Extensive sample cleanup is often required prior to analysis. This does not allow for rapid detection, and the harsh conditions of extraction can have adverse effects on the assay (Wang et al., 2014). However, there is potential in the application of biological ligands such as antibodies and aptamers to isolate toxins from samples using bead-based techniques and immunoaffinity columns (Fitzgerald et al., 2010). Most systems will work optimally with buffers or spiked samples, but the translation to real-world samples is a major hurdle in the development process. "Label-free" assay formats tend to require less complex sample preparation and can allow "real-time" measurement, but these assays tend to still encounter matrix issues and nonspecific binding. Conversely, labeled assays are much less simplified and require several steps, but this can improve specificity and sensitivity of the assay. There is no ideal development strategy, and overcoming matrix effects in biological samples needs to be addressed with each system/analyte/matrix scenario (Sin et al., 2014).

Miniaturization can also cause adverse effects in microfluidic systems. Assays will always behave differently at microlevels due to the unique physical properties affecting liquid movement and binding events. Hence, it is crucial to ensure that the quality and performance of the assay remain unaffected by issues such as flux and signal-to-noise ratio during the miniaturization process (Dahlin, 2012).

Finally, system integration is possibly the greatest challenge in microfluidic systems development. It is this area that has proven the biggest obstacle in taking research to a commercial output. Great strides have been made in individual areas of development, but the amalgamation of these aspects into a single stand-alone platform remains elusive. A significant hurdle to the widespread adoption of microfluidic devices is the gap in expertise between engineers and biologists. Design and operation of microfluidic systems often need an understanding of the underlying fundamental physics of mass transport and fluid mechanics, thus limiting access. Also, where possible, biologists tend to use traditional macroscale systems rather than rely on emerging microscale techniques, even at the expense of convenience. Considering these obstacles, adoption and implementation of complete microfluidic systems will require time, maturation, and commercial availability of the underlying technologies.

5.3 Future Trends

Microfluidic platforms are particularly attractive for mycotoxin analysis because of the ease of integrating active forces, enhancing biological interactions and ultimately leading to faster analysis times, improved sensitivity, and lower costs. This area is growing at a rapid pace and new avenues of technology are appearing continually.

Multiplexing of several different mycotoxins in one system represents the latest and most exciting developments in this area. Systems incorporating microarrays and microbeads benefit from their flexibility and the capability to employ label-free detection.

Current techniques for enhancing antigen–antibody interaction will continue to improve, allowing for uniform multiplexed immunoassays (Ng et al., 2010). DNA and RNA aptamers also offer another avenue of detection (Iliuk et al., 2011). Fluid handling techniques are continually becoming more versatile and multiple modes can be incorporated onto a single platform. Improvements in surface immobilization will most likely provide ideal surfaces for ensuring high antibody binding activity with minimal nonspecific binding. Multiplexed immunoassays coupled with label-free detection strategies have the potential to produce devices capable of "on-site" multimycotoxin detection, ideal for developing countries and resource-poor areas. Reducing device complexity is also key in achieving this. Systems must be robust, cost-effective, and user-friendly. Lab-on-a-chip and Lab-in-a-trench systems (Dimov et al., 2010; Kijanka et al., 2015; Sharma et al., 2015) have shown progress toward miniaturized, total analysis assays. Some emerging platforms are providing sample cleanup along with quantification (Soares et al., 2014).

Mobile-phone-based diagnostics coupled with microfluidic systems offer another interesting approach to mycotoxin analysis. Currently, smartphones boast significant computational power and contain high-resolution cameras. It is considered that mobile-phone-based systems have excellent potential for allowing performance of analysis and interpreting results. Mobile phones are now so widespread and accessible that this technology could prove valuable for analysis and monitoring in developing countries and remote locations.

Additionally, the rapidly emerging area of nanotechnology and nanofluidics is now coming to the forefront of mycotoxin analysis. Systems incorporating nanomaterials have many advantages over other analysis methods and offer solutions to overcome the challenges posed. This technology is still in very early development stage but the progress toward the use of nanomaterials for mycotoxin analysis could be a significant step in food safety, and currently many investigations are ongoing into design and optimization of such platforms. Improvement in semiconductor technology has allowed production of electromechanical devices referred to as nanoelectromechanical systems (NEMS). A number of transducers have been developed using NEMS technologies, such as cantilevers, pillars, nanopores, carbon nanotubes (CNTs), nanoparticles, and nanowires. Performance of these nanotechnologies is highly dependent on biomolecules immobilized on the device as probes (Alapan et al., 2015). Transducers utilize different physical phenomena, including mechanical, electrical, or optical changes. As micro- and nanotechnologies allow for more accurate fabrication methods, the design and production of new systems will positively impact sensitivity, throughput, and specificity. These improvements will likely pave the way for the translation of micro/nanosystems from laboratories to the field.

Mycotoxins are a significant threat to human and animal health across the globe. Analysis of these adulterants is crucial to avoid their acute and chronic effects, and to maintain food integrity. This chapter has identified current and emerging technologies focusing on the development of rapid and sensitive microfluidic-based analysis platforms that will move mycotoxin analysis from the laboratory to the field. Research now must focus on producing commercial, complete microfluidic systems for total mycotoxin determination that will improve food safety worldwide. It is evident that in developing the next generation of microfluidic analysis systems, collaboration from an early stage between physical scientists, engineers, and molecular biologists is crucial. These collaborations offer the ability to address all engineering and analytical considerations. There are some excellent examples of these collaborations on research microfluidic platforms making the jump to commercial outputs, such as DCU's Biomedical Diagnostics Institute collaboration with industry partner Biosurfit to engineer a rapid centrifugal-based point-of-care test for C-reactive protein (CRP), a cardiac biomarker (http://biosurfit.com/). There are also ongoing projects such as the MARIne environmental *in situ* Assessment and monitoring tool BOX (MARIA BOX) and the MBio optical-planar waveguide platform utilizing centrifugal and lateral flow microfluidics respectively for the monitoring of marine toxins (Murphy et al., 2015). These highly promising research collaborations show the potential to be used for mycotoxin detection. Ultimately, it is clear that the continual expansion of biological investigations by microfluidics, and other emerging technologies, carried by interdisciplinary collaboration will produce significant progress in mycotoxin analyses.

Acknowledgments

The authors of this work are supported by the Irish Research Council (GOIPG/2013/380) and Science Foundation Ireland (14/1A/2646).

References

Alapan, Y., Icoz, K., and Gurkan, U.A. (2015) Micro- and nanodevices integrated with biomolecular probes, *Biotechnology Advances*, 33, 1727–1743.

Anfossi, L., Calderara, M., Baggiani, C., Giovannoli, C., Arletti, E., and Giraudi, G. (2010) Development and application of a quantitative lateral flow immunoassay for fumonisins in maize, *Analytica Chimica Acta*, 682(1–2), 104–109.

Atalay, Y.T., Vermeir, S., Witters, D., Vergauwe, N., Verbruggen, B., Verboven, P., Nicolaï, B.M., and Lammertyn, J. (2011) Microfluidic analytical systems for food analysis, *Trends in Food Science & Technology*, 22(7), 386–404.

Bahadır, E.B. and Sezgintürk, M.K. (2015) Applications of commercial biosensors in clinical, food, environmental, and biothreat/biowarfare analyses, *Analytical Biochemistry*, 478, 107–120.

BIOMIN. (2016) Mycotoxin report. 2015 BIOMIN mycotoxin survey. Available at: http://biomin.net/ (accessed May 25, 2016).

CAST (Council for Agricultural Science and Technology). (2003) Mycotoxins: Risks in plant, animal, and human systems. Task force report, Ames, IA, Vol. 139, pp. 1–199.

Dahlin, A.B. (2012) Size matters: Problems and advantages associated with highly miniaturized sensors, *Sensors*, 12(3), 3018–3036.

Daly, S.J., Keating, G.J., Dillon, P.P., Manning, B.M., O'Kennedy, R., Lee, H.A., and Morgan, M.R.A. (2000) Development of surface plasmon resonance-based immunoassay for aflatoxin B 1, *Journal of Agricultural and Food Chemistry*, 48(11), 5097–5104.

Dimov, I.K., Kijanka, G., and Ducree, J. (2010) Lab-in-a-trench platform for real-time monitoring of cell surface protein expression, *2010 IEEE 23rd International Conference on Micro Electro Mechanical Systems (MEMS)*, Hong Kong.

Duncombe, T.A., Tentori, A.M., and Herr, A.E. (2015) Microfluidics: Reframing biological enquiry, *Nature Reviews Molecular Cell Biology*, 16(9), 554–567.

Dunne, L., Daly, S., Baxter, A., Haughey, S., and O'Kennedy, R. (2005) Surface plasmon resonance-based immunoassay for the detection of aflatoxin B 1 using single-chain antibody fragments, *Spectroscopy Letters*, 38(3), 229–245.

Edite Bezerra da Rocha, M., Maia, F.E.F., Guedes, M.I.F., Rondina, D., and da Chagas Oliveira Freire, F. (2014) Mycotoxins and their effects on human and animal health, *Food Control*, 36(1), 159–165.

Edupuganti, S.R., Edupuganti, O.P., and O'Kennedy, R. (2013) Generation of anti-zearalenone scFv and its incorporation into surface plasmon resonance-based assay for the detection of zearalenone in sorghum, *Food Control*, 34(2), 668–674.

Fitzgerald, J., Leonard, P., Darcy, E., and O'Kennedy, R. (2010) Immunoaffinity chromatography, *Methods in Molecular Biology (Clifton, N.J.)*, 681, 35–59.

Guo, L., Feng, J., Fang, Z., Xu, J., and Lu, X. (2015) Application of microfluidic "lab-on-a-chip" for the detection of mycotoxins in foods, *Trends in Food Science & Technology*, 46(2), 252–263.

Hervás, M., López, M.Á., and Escarpa, A. (2009) Electrochemical immunoassay using magnetic beads for the determination of zearalenone in baby food: An anticipated analytical tool for food safety, *Analytica Chimica Acta*, 653(2), 167–172.

Hervás, M., López, M.A., and Escarpa, A. (2012) Electrochemical immunosensing on board microfluidic chip platforms, *TrAC Trends in Analytical Chemistry*, 31, 109–128.

Hu, W., Li, X., He, G., Zhang, Z., Zheng, X., Li, P., and Li, C.M. (2013) Sensitive competitive immunoassay of multiple mycotoxins with non-fouling antigen microarray, *Biosensors and Bioelectronics*, 50, 338–344.

Iliuk, A.B., Hu, L., and Tao, W.A. (2011) Aptamer in bioanalytical applications, *Analytical Chemistry*, 83(12), 4440–4452.

Kijanka, G.S., Dimov, I.K., Burger, R., and Ducrée, J. (2015) Real-time monitoring of cell migration, phagocytosis and cell surface receptor dynamics using a novel, live-cell opto-microfluidic technique, *Analytica Chimica Acta*, 872, 95–99.

Loftus, J.H., Kijanka, G.S., O'Kennedy, R., and Loscher, C.E. (2016) Patulin, Deoxynivalenol, Zearalenone and T-2 toxin affect viability and modulate cytokine secretion in J774A.1 Murine Macrophages, *International Journal of Chemistry*, 8(2), 22–32.

Marroquín-Cardona, A.G., Johnson, N.M., Phillips, T.D., and Hayes, A.W. (2014) Mycotoxins in a changing global environment—A review, *Food and Chemical Toxicology*, 69, 220–230.

Molinelli, A., Grossalber, K., and Krska, R. (2009) A rapid lateral flow test for the determination of total type B fumonisins in maize, *Analytical and Bioanalytical Chemistry*, 395(5), 1309–1316.

Murphy, C., Stack, E., Krivelo, S., McPartlin, D.A., Byrne, B., Greef, C., Lochhead, M.J. et al. (2015) Detection of the cyanobacterial toxin, microcystin-lR, using a novel recombinant antibody-based optical-planar waveguide platform, *Biosensors and Bioelectronics*, 67, 708–714.

Ng, A.H.C., Uddayasankar, U., and Wheeler, A.R. (2010) Immunoassays in microfluidic systems, *Analytical and Bioanalytical Chemistry*, 397(3), 991–1007.

Novo, P., Moulas, G., Prazeres, D.M.F., Chu, V., and Conde, J.P. (2013) Detection of ochratoxin A in wine and beer by chemiluminescence-based ELISA in microfluidics with integrated photodiodes, *Sensors and Actuators B: Chemical*, 176, 232–240.

Olcer, Z., Esen, E., Muhammad, T., Ersoy, A., Budak, S., and Uludag, Y. (2014) Fast and sensitive detection of mycotoxins in wheat using microfluidics based real-time Electrochemical profiling, *Biosensors and Bioelectronics*, 62, 163–169.

Panini, N.V., Bertolino, F.A., Salinas, E., Messina, G.A., Raba, J., and DeepDyve, I. (2010) Zearalenone determination in corn silage samples using an immunosensor in a continuous-flow/stopped-flow systems, *Biochemical Engineering Journal*, 51(1), 13–17.

Panini, N.V., Salinas, E., Messina, G.A., and Raba, J. (2011) Modified paramagnetic beads in a microfluidic system for the determination of zearalenone in feedstuffs samples, *Food Chemistry*, 125(2), 791–796.

Park, J.H., Kim, Y., Kim, I., and Ko, S. (2014) Rapid detection of aflatoxin B1 by a bifunctional protein crosslinker-based surface plasmon resonance biosensor, *Food Control*, 36(1), 183–190.

Parker, C.O., Lanyon, Y.H., Manning, M., Arrigan, D.W.M., and Tothill, I.E. (2009) Electrochemical Immunochip sensor for aflatoxin M 1 detection, *Analytical Chemistry*, 81(13), 5291–5298.

Sauceda-Friebe, J.C., Karsunke, X.Y.Z., Vazac, S., Biselli, S., Niessner, R., and Knopp, D. (2011) Regenerable immuno-biochip for screening ochratoxin A in green coffee extract using an automated microarray chip reader with chemiluminescence detection, *Analytica Chimica Acta*, 689(2), 234–242.

Selvaraj, J.N., Zhou, L., Wang, Y., Zhao, Y., Xing, F., Dai, X., and Liu, Y. (2015) Mycotoxin detection—Recent trends at global level, *Journal of Integrative Agriculture*, 14(11), 2265–2281.

Sharma, S., Zapatero-Rodríguez, J., Estrela, P., and O'Kennedy, R. (2015) Point-of-care diagnostics in low resource settings: Present status and future role of Microfluidics, *Biosensors*, 5(3), 577–601.

Shim, W.-B., Kim, M.J., and Mun, H. (2014) An aptamer-based dipstick assay for the rapid and simple detection of aflatoxin B1, *Biosensors and Bioelectronics*, 62, 288–294.

Sin, M.L., Gao, J., Liao, J.C., and Wong, P. (2011) System integration—A major step toward lab on a chip, *Journal of Biological Engineering*, 5(1), 6.

Sin, M.L., Mach, K.E., Wong, P.K., and Liao, J.C. (2014) Advances and challenges in biosensor-based diagnosis of infectious diseases, *Expert Review of Molecular Diagnostics*, 14(2), 225–244.

Soares, R., Novo, P., Azevedo, A., Fernandes, P., Aires-Barros, C.V., and Conde, J. (2014) On-chip sample preparation and analyte quantification using a microfluidic aqueous two-phase extraction coupled with an immunoassay, *Lab on a Chip*, 14(21), 4284–4294.

Turner, N.W., Bramhmbhatt, H., Szabo-Vezse, M., Poma, A., Coker, R., and Piletsky, S.A. (2015) Analytical methods for determination of mycotoxins: An update (2009–2014), *Analytica Chimica Acta*, 901, 12–33.

Turner, N.W., Subrahmanyam, S., and Piletsky, S.A. (2009) Analytical methods for determination of mycotoxins: A review, *Analytica Chimica Acta*, 632(2), 168–180.

Wang, J.-J., Liu, B.-H., Hsu, Y.-T., and Yu, F.-Y. (2011) Sensitive competitive direct enzyme-linked immunosorbent assay and gold nanoparticle immunochromatographic strip for detecting aflatoxin M1 in milk, *Food Control*, 22(6), 964–969.

Wang, L. and Gan, X.-X. (2009) Biomolecule-functionalized magnetic nanoparticles for flow-through quartz crystal microbalance immunoassay of aflatoxin B1, *Bioprocess and Biosystems Engineering*, 32(1), 109–116.

Wang, X., Lu, X., and Chen, J. (2014) Development of biosensor technologies for analysis of environmental contaminants, *Trends in Environmental Analytical Chemistry*, 2, 25–32.

World Health Organisation International Agency for Research and Cancer (WHO IARC). (1993) Toxins derived from *Fusarium moniliforme*: Fumonisins B1 and B2 and fusarin C. *IARC Monographs on the Evaluation of Carcinogenic Risks to Humans*, 56, 445–462.

Xiao, H., Clarke, J.R., Marquardt, R.R., and Frohlich, A.A. (1995) Improved methods for conjugating selected Mycotoxins to carrier proteins and Dextran for Immunoassays, *Journal of Agricultural and Food Chemistry*, 43(8), 2092–2097.

Yeni, F., Acar, S., Polat, Ö.G., Soyer, Y., and Alpas, H. (2014) Rapid and standardized methods for detection of foodborne pathogens and mycotoxins on fresh produce, *Food Control*, 40, 359–367.

Zain, M.E. (2011) Impact of mycotoxins on humans and animals, *Journal of Saudi Chemical Society*, 15(2), 129–144.

Zhang, D., Li, P., Yang, Y., Zhang, Q., Zhang, W., Xiao, Z., and Ding, X. (2011) A high selective immunochromatographic assay for rapid detection of aflatoxin B1, *Talanta*, 85(1), 736–742.

6

Planar Differential Mobility Spectrometry for Clinical Breath Diagnostics

Erkinjon G. Nazarov, Timothy Postlethwaite,
Kenneth Markoski, Sophia Koo, and Jeffrey T. Borenstein

CONTENTS

6.1 Introduction

Recent experience in emerging infectious diseases ranging from severe acute respiratory syndrome to avian influenza highlights a critical need for point-of-care diagnostics to immediately identify pulmonary infections. For decades, investigators have recognized that many diseases result in the production of distinctive volatiles or patterns of volatiles in human breath. Until recently, however, the technology to sample, identify, and classify these volatiles has been lacking. The result is that only certain diseases, such as *Helicobacter pylori* infection, are being clinically diagnosed through a breath test. The last several decades have brought advances in microsystems technology, computing power, and algorithms capable of rapid multivariate analysis. These new technologies enable inexpensive, portable, automated point-of-care systems capable of detecting biomarkers generated by specific infectious agents. A new era of clinical diagnosis could develop around technologies and techniques using noninvasive breath analysis. This advance could dramatically reduce the time spent by patients in clinical settings, increase the precision of differential diagnosis, shorten the response time for emerging epidemics, and reduce the cost burden for patient care.

Infectious diseases are the number one cause of mortality in the world and disproportionately ravage the developing world. Respiratory infectious diseases such as pneumonia and tuberculosis account for more than 10% of deaths in the world each year. In addition, many of the most common opportunistic infections that accompany AIDS in the developing world are also respiratory infections caused by bacteria or fungi. Together, respiratory infections cause millions of deaths each year and result in untold personal suffering and loss of productivity. In areas lacking robust diagnostic facilities (typical of a vast majority of health care facilities in the developing world), therapeutic approaches to respiratory illnesses are often empiric. Since many respiratory diseases have similar presentation, lack of diagnostic accuracy of specific pathogens often results in high rates of morbidity and mortality post-therapy, waste of scarce therapeutic resources, and, in cases such as cystic fibrosis, the risk of additional infection.

Most pulmonary infections are diagnosed and treated based on patient history and clinical findings rather than definitive lab-based tests. This can be problematic because in many cases this information is insufficient to narrow the etiology to a single pathogen, and the physician must treat with broader spectrum medications than necessary. In recent years, significant advances in the laboratory diagnostics available to detect respiratory viral infections have been achieved, including assays that use tissue culture, serology, and direct examination, as well as some rapid diagnostic techniques and molecular assays. Bacterial infections may also be confirmed via sputum and deep tracheal aspirates that are cultured and tested with standard microbiological techniques. In practice, however, these diagnostic tests have little impact on treatment decisions because patients are treated empirically based on clinical suspicion well before the studies are completed. If a point-of-care diagnostic tool were available, treatment could be immediately tailored to the relevant pathogen, improving the quality of care and reducing the spread of antibiotic resistance.

This chapter describes a device, and its technology underpinnings, which is capable of revolutionizing clinical breath diagnostics based on a combination of its small size and power requirements, ease of use, and applicability to a broad range of clinically relevant biomarker signatures. This technology, based upon the principle of ion mobility spectrometry, generates signature spectral patterns as distinctive as mass spectrometry, MS, but with far greater simplicity and adaptability. The differential mobility spectrometer (DMS) is a portable, handheld device that generates multidimensional biological spectra from volatile compounds found in exhaled breath. The current prototype model of the DMS fits in the palm of the hand, is highly durable, operates at atmospheric pressure, and can be operated with standard batteries. The technology is based upon the principles of ion mobility, where the specific mobility of a target species, rather than the molecular weight, is tracked as a function of electric field. The ion mobility spectra provide enhanced resolution because species with similar molecular weights can be distinguished, and further because the mobility of ions is a strong function of applied electric field. In contrast to existing time-of-flight ion mobility spectrometers (TOF-IMS), in which sensitivity is reduced as the instrument is miniaturized, the DMS sensitivity is enhanced as the device is made smaller, due to greater precision in the microscale device dimensions and control over local electric fields. A substantial body of data has been gathered using the DMS device in measurements of biomarkers of bacterial spores, human blood and urine, and chemical weapons simulants at parts-per-trillion levels. In the following, the technology for various implementations of the DMS will be described, along with applications in chemical sensing (to demonstrate the mechanisms involved in obtaining unique signature detection), biodefense, and in clinical breath diagnostics.

6.2 Ambient Pressure Ionization Instrument Classification: Gas-Phase Mobility Spectrometry

Ion-mobility-based spectrometers operating with one of a number of possible ionization means are capable of providing highly sensitive, lab-quality detection of trace targeted chemicals in field conditions. In this family of instruments, sample molecules are ionized directly at ambient pressure, and then the formed ions are identified according to their coefficient of mobility in a drift gas, typically N_2 or air. Because ionization and separation occur at ambient pressure, these instruments do not require cumbersome vacuum pumps, and therefore they are suitable for miniaturization and field use. Currently, there are a number of analyzers employing atmospheric pressure ionization, for example, conventional time-of-flight ion mobility spectrometry (IMS),[1] differential ion mobility spectrometry or field asymmetric ion mobility spectrometry (DMS/FAIMS),[2] aspirated IMS (AIMS),[3] and ambient pressure ionization mass spectrometer (API MS). In these instruments, ions are generated directly at ambient pressure, and then introduced into a vacuum for subsequent mass spectrometric (m/z) identification of ion species.[4] Many types of atmospheric pressure ionization analyzers have proven their effectiveness in addressing analytical needs when used in laboratory conditions. In a laboratory environment, users have access to functions enabling extensive sample preparation, including collection, pre-concentration, cleanup, and extraction. The advantage of incorporating these time-consuming pretreatment steps is that sample complexity is decreased, and the overall quality of the analysis is improved. In fielded applications, there are limited resources and time available for effective collection, pretreatment, and detection of targeted components. Therefore, for these applications, it is desirable to identify novel and rapid methods for sample collection and pretreatment. This need has served as a motivation for intensive efforts over the past two decades toward the development of instruments such as ion-mobility-based systems for ion pre-filtration and pre-separation. In this chapter, we will focus on relatively new differential mobility ion separation technology, which can be considered as a next step in the evolution of ion mobility spectrometry technology for applications in environmental detection, and, most importantly, to revolutionize point-of-care clinical diagnostics.

6.2.1 Technology Origins

The DMS/FAIMS method for ion species separation/identification in gases exploits the nonlinear dependence of an ion's coefficient of mobility under the effect of a strong electric field was first proposed in the Soviet Union during the 1980s by M. Gorshkov (Siberian Academy of Science, Novosibirsk).[5] The principle of operation for this new method involves separation of ions in a gas flow stream subjected to a superimposed electric field composed of a high-frequency, asymmetric waveform RF and DC field applied transverse to the direction to gas stream. Development efforts for this technology continued in the Soviet Union by researchers from laboratories at the Siberian and Uzbek Academies of sciences.[2,6–11] One of the principal motivations behind these efforts was the development of field-deployable instruments for the detection of explosives in the environment.

6.2.2 Chronological History of DMS and FAIMS Developments

During the late 1980s and early 1990s, the development process for DMS and FAIMS diverged with the efforts of two independently operated teams. The first group, Gorshkov's team at the Institute of Thermophysics of the Siberian Academy of Science, built curved geometry devices where ion separation occurs in analytical gap between two concentric cylindrical electrodes. In this design, the *nonhomogeneous electric field* is formed in the analytical gap when superimposed RF and DC voltages are applied to each of electrodes. This design was initially called field ion spectrometry and was eventually transferred to Mine Safety Appliances in Pittsburgh, Pennsylvania, to further develop and explore commercialization opportunities in this area.[12] A general advantage of the cylindrical device is that in the process of ion trajectory along analytical gap with inhomogeneous electric fields, the analyzed ions can be focused, which results in enhancing the efficiency of ion transmission through the sensor. In cylindrical designs, the ion's transmission can be changed from zero at low electric fields up to a maximum value at enhanced electric field conditions. In addition, the efficiency of focusing also depends on the relative difference between high field and low field ion mobility, defined by the ion's "alpha parameter." Therefore, different ion species with distinct alpha parameters display different level of focusing, which complicates quantitative analysis and system calibration. Over the next decade, the cylindrical design would become known as High Field Asymmetric Waveform Ion Mobility Spectrometry or FAIMS.[13] One motivation for this approach was to try to take advantage of the ion focusing properties of the inhomogeneous fields created with curved electrodes.[14,15]

A second scientific team, which included members from two research institutes, Novosibirsk and Tashkent, worked on a planar sensor design.[8,16] In this configuration, ion separation occurs in a *homogeneous electric field* in the gap between two planar electrodes. This sensor design was initially referred to as a drift spectrometer, which eventually changed to the more phenomenologically descriptive name Differential Mobility Spectrometer (DMS). The motivation for a planar approach was to create a device in which different ion species (independent of their polarity) would be transmitted through the sensor with the same efficiency, without being influenced by the value and sign of each ion's alpha parameters. Straightforward planar electrode designs provide the highest efficiency ion transmission even when separation voltages are turned off. This mode of operation is called the "transparent" regime of measurement, and enables the possibility of comparing the DMS output with and without ion separation. These characteristics were known to be lacking in the curved geometry cells.

6.2.3 DMS versus FAIMS

Both DMS and FAIMS share the same physical separation principle conceived by Gorshkov, fundamentally based on the difference between the high and low field mobility of a particular gas-phase ion. They both produce a continuous spatial separation of ion species, which takes place under superimposed effect of dispersion RF and compensation DC electric fields. It was also recognized that different geometries imparted different analytical properties, warranting distinguishing them with the separate terms FAIMS and DMS. For instance, Figure 6.1 provides a comparison between mobility spectra obtained for the same bradykinin samples (with formation of the same ion species $m/z = 531$ Da), which were obtained in two different designs: planar and cylindrical. This direct comparison shows that planar DMS provides higher resolution and sensitivity versus a cylindrical design. For example, the analysis presented in Figure 6.1 shows that when both systems are tuned to operate with comparable sensitivity, the resolving power of DMS is better by a factor of 2–4 times, and the operational speed is at least 20 times faster in the planar design.[17]

Table 6.1, which summarizes results reported from various scientific teams, compares the performance for these two approaches. A review of this information shows that the choice of geometry is particularly important, because the output and analytical performance of the DMS/FAIMS devices for the same samples can be significantly different.

6.2.4 Technology Transfer

During the 1990s, the DMS/FAIMS technologies were transferred from the East to the West. Figure 6.2 shows a chronological history of development and migration between institutions for both designs that started in the 1980s.

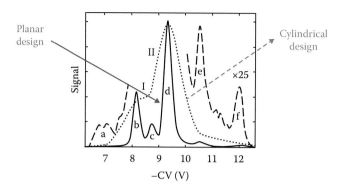

FIGURE 6.1
Comparison between the full spectra obtained by DMS and FAIMS for the same sample compounds (bradykinin): solid line corresponds to planar design and the dotted lines are for FAIMS design. The dashed line is fragment of DMS spectra (expanded ×25 for visualization) showing the separation power of a planar versus a cylindrical design.

It also provides a list of the companies and institutions that have played a major role in the growth of this technology from its starting points. The cylindrical version moved from the Siberian Academy of Sciences (Novosibirsk) to the Mine Safety Appliances (MSA) company in Pittsburgh (see bottom white color trajectory in Figure 6.2). The first commercial prototype of the cylindrical design was built and reported in 1995.[12] The Mine Safety Appliances cylindrical FAIMS device was utilized by the National Research Council in Ottawa to couple to a mass spectrometer.[14,15,18] This became the basis of Ionalytics Corp., which was subsequently bought by Thermo Fisher Scientific, Inc. in 2005 to commercialize this design as a FAIMS-MS system. Currently, Thermo Scientific's commercial product is called a FAIMS interface, which works in combination with a heated electrospray ionization source (HESI) and atmospheric pressure chemical ionization (APCI) of ion probes commercially available in combination with a triple-stage quadrupole mass spectrometer.

In 2004, Dr. Richard D. Smith's scientific team from Pacific Northwest National Laboratory (PNNL) began work with a cylindrical FAIMS system.[19] But later, after testing and comparison of performance of a new prototype planar version of DMS sensors versus cylindrical designs, the group transitioned to the flat design approach.[17]

Prof. Rick Yost's research team from the University of Florida also actively worked (from 2004) with the FAIMS system, as shown in the chronological map in Figure 6.2. In 2010, Yost's team offered a new three-dimensional (3D) geometry of the sensor with curved electrodes, which can be considered as derivative of two-dimensional (2D) cylindrical designs. These sensors are designed with hemispherical and spherical geometries.[20] They reported systematic experimental data for nine regular explosives. It conveyed that 3D designs provided enhanced sensitivity, resolution (up to twofold) and

TABLE 6.1

Comparison of Specific Features of Planar (DMS) and Cylindrical (FAIMS) Designs

	Ions' Residence Time	Focusing/Defocusing Ion Species	RF Dependence on Peak Width and Intensity	Selectivity (Relative to DMS)	Modes of Operation	Detection (+) or (−) ions	Time to Mount/Demount from MS	Cost
DMS	1–2 ms	None—this provides an option to generate dispersion plots	Moderate	1.0	Two modes operation: 1. Filtering (when RF on) 2. Transparent (when RF off)	Simultaneously detect both polarity ions	A few minutes	$
FAIMS	Significantly longer At least 100 ms	Some ions focused, some defocused	Strong	0.2–0.3	Single mode operation: Filtering only	Detect single polarity of ions [(+) or (−)]	A few hours	$$
DMS advantage over FAIMS	1. Reduced ion reaction losses due to diffusion 2. High-speed measurements possible	Coefficients of ion transmission for different species is similar, which make easy quantitative measurements	Operate with different values of RF voltage to turn sensor in optimal regimes for specific ion species	Ref. *Anal. Chem.* 2006, 78,3706	Fast comparison of filtered and unfiltered mass spectra	Simple to switch from one polarity to another	Rapid change from ESI-DMS-MS to any other configuration	Disposable sensor chips under development.

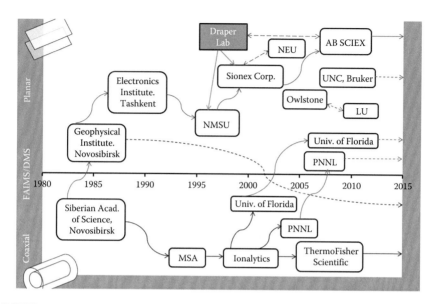

FIGURE 6.2

A chronological history of DMS (planar) and FAIMS (coaxial) developments, including the migration process of these two geometries between institutions. Trail for cylindrical is located below the horizontal axis and for planar is presented above the horizontal axis. This historical information was drawn from the literature and from personal communications with developers, which made contributions to this historical perspective. Used abbreviations: NMSU, New Mexico State University; NEU, Northeastern University; UNC, University of North Carolina; LU, Loughborough University; PNNL, Pacific Northwest Laboratory; MSA, Mine Safety Appliances.

resolving power (1.5-fold to twofold) for six different explosives. The best ion transmission was obtained in the spherical FAIMS cell, while a hemispherical FAIMS provided the best resolution and resolving power.[21]

A parallel trajectory related to the development of the DMS with planar electrodes started in 1996 from Tashkent (see upper green color trail in Figure 6.2). This technology was brought to Prof. Gary Eiceman's laboratory at New Mexico State University (NMSU), a leading center for new developments in ion-mobility-based technologies. The first tested prototype was a micromachined DMS sensor built by the Charles Stark Draper Laboratory in Cambridge, MA, as part of a Draper-funded collaboration with NMSU.[22] During this Draper-initiated and funded project (1998–2001), the planar geometry evolved further, in terms of a better understanding of the fundamentals of the DMS phenomena, miniaturization, and for providing new analytical applications of the technology. In addition to scientific investigations, the first prototypes of compact gas analyzers[23] and DMS detectors for use with gas chromatography (GC) were designed and built.[24] At that time, the technology began to be referred to in the literature as DMS, more closely reflecting the basic physical principles of operation.[25] Later, these prototypes were deployed as commercial prototypes at a Draper Laboratory spin-off company called Sionex Corporation. During the period 2001–2010, Sionex Corporation (following an OEM business model) provided numerous DMS sensors and electronics kits to companies specializing in the production of analytical systems for the detection and identification of traces of hazardous chemicals in complex mixtures.

In 2004, Owlstone Ltd was established. This company utilized a modernized planar multichannel design DMS sensor. The sensor design includes multiple (>15) parallel operated microchannels with an individual channel size height of 35 µm and length of 300 µm. Microscale analytical gaps enable a significant reduction in the residence time of ions, and can reach electric fields almost two times higher without breakdown. Decreasing the residence time of ions leads to increasing the speed of measurement and enhancing the magnitude of the electric field, leading to deeper fragmentation of analyte ions in the process of passing ions through the analytical gap. Fragmentation patterns can be used as a complementary piece of information about the ion species, which can improve identification accuracy. A consequence of using microscale channels is the necessity to increase the frequency of the RF generators, which imposed additional technical challenges.[26] The higher-frequency version of the analytical cell was called ultrahigh-frequency FAIMS. Based on this type of system, Owlstone produces several types of gas analyzers, including a stand-alone instrument (Lonestar™) and an OEM sensor module. Current micro- and macroscale gap (0.03–2 mm) DMS/FAIMS technologies have been adopted by various researchers, working in collaboration with instrumentation companies: Prof. Richard Yost (University of Florida) in collaboration with Agilent, and Prof. Gary Glish (University of North Carolina at Chapel Hill) with Bruker Daltonics Inc.

6.3 Comparison between Conventional IMS and DMS Operation

A primary focus of this chapter is to provide an overview of the different implementations of DMS analyzers (stand-alone and in combination with other technologies) that have been built and characterized on the basis of a planar DMS sensor. To clarify the advantages of this relatively new technology, a technical description of DMS operation is presented, along with a description of its features relative to conventional IMS.

6.3.1 Operational Principle of Conventional IMS

Classical time-of-flight ion mobility spectrometers (IMS) apply an instrumental approach, enabling characterization of ion species according to its absolute values of coefficient mobility.[1] This parameter can be considered as a unique "fingerprint" feature of individual ion species.[27] At moderate electric fields, the coefficient of mobility reflects structural information of ion species, including a reduced mass μ and cross-sectional area Ω (or size) of the analyzed ions, as described by Equation 6.1:

$$K(E) = \frac{e}{\mu v(E)} = \frac{3e}{16N}\left(\frac{2\pi}{\mu k T_{eff}}\right)^{\frac{1}{2}} \frac{1}{\Omega^{1.1}(T_{eff})} \tag{6.1}$$

The schematic and principle of operation of time-of-flight IMS is presented in Figure 6.3, in the left panel. An ion mobility spectrometer includes an ionization chamber, an ion injection shutter (or ion gate), and an ion drift tube with

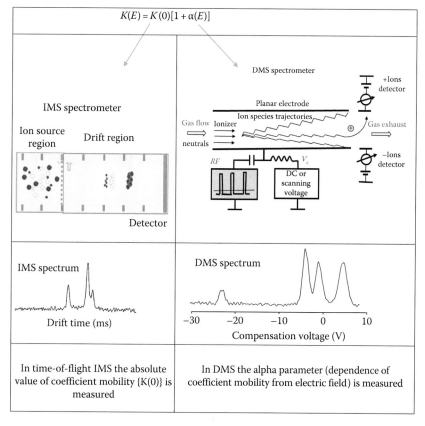

FIGURE 6.3

Comparison between principles of operation for conventional IMS and DMS. Left panel: Schematic and examples of output of IMS. Right panel: Operational schematic and examples of output for planar differential mobility spectrometer.

a homogeneously distributed low DC electric field (E = 100–200 V/cm) for pulling ion species in the direction of the detector (Faraday plate), the detector plate located at the end of drift tube. To inject ions from the ionization chamber into the drift tube area, periodic electric pulses are applied to the ion gate electrodes. After injection of a packet of ion cloud containing different ion species, all ions start to move through the drift area with distinct velocities, because the velocity of individual ion species is proportional to their coefficient mobility (K_i) and strength of electric field (E):

$$\vec{\vartheta}_i = K_i * \vec{E} \tag{6.2}$$

When the ion gate is operated in periodic mode, the detector records IMS mobility spectra, which include a series of ion pulses with different arrival time t_d. The value of t_d is used for calculation of coefficient mobility, and consequently for the identification of ion species. As can be seen, the principle of operation of an IMS is similar to the operation of the time-of-flight mass spectrometer (TOF MS), with the difference between IMS and MS occurring only in pressure conditions in analytical areas. Because MS operates in a vacuum, the arrival time of analyzed ions characterizes only the mass-to-charge ratio (m/z). Nevertheless, similar measurements in IMS operating at ambient pressure provide additional ion structural information.

6.3.2 Phenomenological Description of DMS Sensor Operation

A schematic and the operational principles of differential mobility spectrometer (DMS) are shown on the right panel of Figure 6.3. Construction of a DMS sensor is relatively simple in comparison with IMS. It contains the following three aligned segments: an ionization area, an analytical area between two electrodes for ion separation, and a pair of two detector electrodes for recording ions of each polarity (positive and negative). A formal description of the DMS shows that it operates in a manner similar to a quadrupole mass analyzer; ion separation occurs due to superimposed effect of dispersing RF and compensation DC electric fields in the analytical gap. When sample molecules are continuously introduced with transport gas flow into ionization area, the positive and negative resultant ions are formed and transported in analytical gap between two electrodes, where they then can be separated by adjusting specific combination of RF and DC electric fields. By regulation of the value of compensation voltage, it is possible to straighten trajectories for certain ion species. In this condition when values of V_c and RF are appropriately adjusted, only selected ion species can pass through the analytical gap and be continuously recorded on detector electrodes located in the exhaust of the analytical gap. Other ion species will have tilted trajectories; therefore, these ion species eventually reach one of the analytical electrodes (upper or bottom) and are neutralized. Instead of a constant compensation voltage, sweeping the voltage the output of DMS detectors can provide a sequence of peaks, as shown on DMS spectrum in Figure 6.3. The shape of the electrodes can be planar, as shown in the upper-left corner of Figure 6.2. This design is usually associated with the term DMS. Another cylindrical shape electrode design, shown in bottom-left corner of Figure 6.2, is associated with the term FAIMS. In any case, ion movement through the gap under the effect of gas stream along analytical gap and superimposed asymmetric waveform RF and DC electric fields applied across the two electrodes, causes ions to move in the analytical gap with a "zigzag" or up/down motion. Different ion species trajectories have different slopes. When the asymmetric waveform electric field is large enough ($E > 1000$ V/cm), the resulting trajectories of the different ion species diverge. The ion's alpha parameter characterizes the dependence of the coefficient of mobility of individual ion species on the strength of the RF electric field, E, as shown in Equation 6.3:

$$K_i(E) = K_i(0)\left[1 + \alpha_i(E)\right] \tag{6.3}$$

where $K_i(0)$ is the ion's low field coefficient of mobility. As ions travel in zigzag trajectories, their effective trajectories depend on their specific alpha parameters and can be shifted by either of the two electrodes. Ion species whose net movement under gas flow, the superimposed DC and asymmetric RF voltage adjusted to pass through the analytical gap, are subsequently detected at one of two Faraday plates placed on the exhaust of the analytical gap. Positive ions are detected at the bottom Faraday plate, which has a negative DC bias, and negative ions are detected at the upper detector plate, which has a positive bias. In order to "tune" the DMS sensor to pass the desired targeted ion species, a variable DC potential, known as the compensation voltage (V_c), is also applied across the two analytical electrodes. By varying either the RF or DC electric fields, it is possible to reach conditions where only specific ion species pass through the gap and are detected. Other ion species are neutralized on the top or bottom analytical electrodes. As such, DMS can be considered as a continuously operated ion species filter, when V_c is constant and tuned for filtering the targeted ions. So, in contrast to IMS, which provides ion separation in a pulsed regime according to the absolute value of ion coefficient mobility $K_i(0)$, the DMS separates ions continuously and provides ions filtration on the basis of the ion's alpha parameters. Equation 6.4, which is a derivative of Equation 6.3, shows that the alpha parameter of individual chemicals expresses the ratio of the differential mobility $\Delta K(E) = K(E) - K(0)$ to the low field ion mobility $K(0)$:

$$\alpha_i(E) = \frac{K_i(E) - K_i(0)}{K_i(0)} = \frac{\Delta K_i(E)}{K_i(0)} \tag{6.4}$$

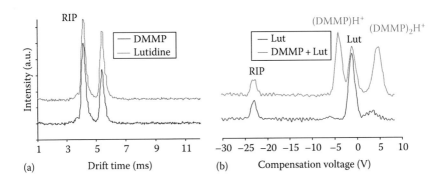

FIGURE 6.4
Comparison between IMS (a) and DMS (b) spectra for lutidine and DMMP samples.

The value of the alpha parameter, which characterizes the effect of a strong electric field on ion coefficient mobility $K_i(E)$, is specific for individual ions, and therefore can be used for the identification of an ion species. The sign of α_i can be positive, when ion coefficient mobility increases with increasing E, or can be negative, when mobility decreases with increasing values of E.

6.3.3 Comparison between the IMS and DMS Spectra

Figure 6.4 presents IMS and DMS spectra for DMMP (124 Da) and lutidine (107 Da) samples that were obtained separately in IMS (a) and DMS (b). As shown, the IMS spectra for both of these chemicals are fairly similar, and naturally include a reactant ion peak (RIP) with drift time $t_d = 4.2$ ms and analyte peaks in both spectra with same drift time $t_d = 5.4$ ms. In contrast, the DMS spectra of DMMP+Lutidine mixture probe (on Figure 6.4b) contain a combination of DMMP peaks (monomer $V_c = -4$ V and dimer $V_c = +4.5$ V) and a lutidine peak at $V_c = -1.5$ V. A control experiment of a solely lutidine sample unambiguously shows that the lutidine peak in fact has $V_c = -1.5$ V and is located between two DMMP peaks. So, for this particular component, we can see that while DMMP and lutidine are unresolved in IMS, they can be easily resolved in DMS. This was an expected result, because as already discussed, the IMS and DMS methods exploit different properties of ion species: IMS operation is based on measurement of the absolute value of coefficient mobility K_i; the DMS exploits the alpha parameter ($\alpha_i(E)$), which characterizes the ability of changing of ions conformation (cross section Ω) under the effect of strong electric field.

6.3.4 Use of DMS for Detection of Chemical Warfare Agents: GA, AC, and CK

Historically, ion mobility-based spectrometers were the most commonly deployed systems for chemical monitoring by the military for quantitative measurements and identifications. In this section, results are presented to

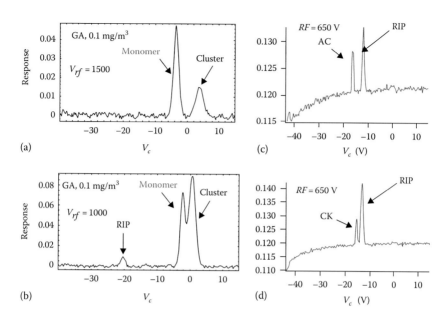

FIGURE 6.5
In the left column, DMS positive ions' linear spectra of GA agent are presented for two dispersion voltages: Panel (a) (1500 V) and (b) for (1000 V). In the right column—examples for negative ion spectra for two chemicals: panel (c) for AC agent and panel (d) for CK.

show the analytical potential and utility of DMS technology for homeland security applications. In Figure 6.5, in the left column, experimental positive ion spectra are presented for Tabun (GA—nerve class chemical agent with $MW = 162$ Da), and in the right column are two spectra of blood class agents: (d) CK—agent, which is cyanogen chloride (CNCl), $MW = 61$ Da; and (c) AC—agent, which is a very small hydrogen cyanide (HCN) ($MW = 27$ Da). GA spectra presented for two RF voltages: panel (a) for 1500 V and panel (b) for 1000 V. The transport gas was pure air with addition of 0.1 mg/m³ of GA vapors. GA spectra contain RIP and two analyte peaks, which were identified as monomer and cluster peaks. Comparison of both spectra shows that for this class of chemicals, increasing the RF voltage increases the separation power of a planar DMS sensor. Positions of each peak for a certain RF value are used for identification of the original ion species. The estimated LOD level for GA is ~0.007 mg/m³, which corresponds to a (V/V) concentration of 10 ppb.

Both AC and CK agent spectra are presented in Figure 6.5c and d, as obtained for same concentration of analyte vapors (~22 mg/m³). Each spectrum for these extremely volatile components contains two peaks: the leftmost peaks correspond to analyte ions that are detected at different compensation voltages. The rightmost peaks in each spectra are related to background (RIP) ions, and they naturally have the same peak position, $V_c = -11$ V in both measurements performed with $RF = 650$ V. These negative reactant peak ions that are formed in air correspond to oxygen/water molecules cluster ions, $(H_2O)_nO_2^-$. Comparison of the linear spectra for the two chemicals (in Figure 6.5c and d) shows that DMS is well matched for the identification of small molecular components, which is usually problematic for time-of-flight IMS. The estimated limit of detection (LOD) for both these blood class agents is ~4.1 mg/m^3.

6.3.5 Planar DMS Sensor Design Optimization for a Particular Application

Well-developed mathematical descriptions of the principle of DMS operation are available to explain the operation and predict DMS spectra for given planar designs. Calculation of peak position and width in DMS spectra involves several steps; a comprehensive description of the calculation can be found in a recent review article.[28] In the following, a common approach is used to get a final formula for calculation peak position V_c, peak width FWHM, which can be used for calculation resolution $R = V_c/FWHM$, and peak capacity (PC) used for characterizing resolving power for spectra of multicomponent DMS spectra $PC = (V_{c\,max} - V_{c\,min})/FWHM$.

6.3.6 Peak Position in Planar DMS Spectra

A mathematical formula for calculating a peak position in a DMS spectra was suggested in the first publication regarding DMS/FAIMS technology.[2] According to the DMS principle of operation, ion separation occurs when ions move under the superimposed effect of alternating strong RF (dispersion) and weak DC (compensation) electric fields acting in a direction perpendicular to the transport gas stream that transports ions through the analytical gap. The velocity of all ion species through a cell is determined solely by the linear velocity of the transport gas. Average dwelling time (τ) through a cell depends on geometric sizes (height, width, length) of the analytical gap and flow consumption gas rate $Q(cc/min)$. Usually, an ion's resident time in the analytical area $\tau = Q/(h * w * l)$ ranges from a few milliseconds to several hundred milliseconds, depending upon design geometry.

During flight time, ions experience the effect of an asymmetric waveform (alternating between low and very strong electric fields) encountered during each period of the RF waveform, roughly at least 10,000 times moving up and down perpendicular to the gas flow along to gap axis. Ion motion under effect of the electric field in gases can be described by simple equation $\vec{\vartheta} = K * \vec{E}$. In the case of superimposed very strong oscillated RF and weak DC fields, the equation is modified as follows:

$$\vec{\vartheta}_\perp(t) = K(\vec{E}) \times \vec{E}^{eff}(t) = K(\vec{E}) \times \frac{\vec{V}^{eff}(t)}{h} \qquad (6.5)$$

where

$V^{eff}(t) = SV(t) - V_c$ is the effect of superimposed alternating separating $SV(t)$ and constant V_c voltages

h is the distance between two DMS electrodes

Therefore, the effective electric field in the analytical gap is $\vec{E}^{eff}(t) = \vec{V}^{eff}(t)/h$.

To calculate the resulting drifting velocity of ions in the perpendicular direction $\langle \vartheta_\perp \rangle$, the integration of Equation 6.5 within one period (T) of RF voltage is needed:

$$\langle \vartheta_\perp \rangle = \langle \vartheta_\perp(t) \rangle = \frac{1}{T} \int_0^T \vartheta(t)dt \qquad (6.6)$$

For separating particular ions, the values of SV and V_c should be tuned to specific combinations, when the average velocity of targeted ions in the transfer direction should be zero$\langle \vartheta_\perp \rangle = 0$. In this case, the resulting ion zigzag movement along the analytical axis will have average zero tilt. For example, such trajectory is depicted as a medium ions' zigzag trajectory in the right column of Figure 6.3. This condition corresponds to the situation where an ion's shift under the effect of strong-pulsed asymmetric waveform $SV(t)$ electric field is compensated due to the continuous effect of the weak DC compensation voltage, and, therefore, ions move along the axis of the analytical gap.

Using this approach, Equation 6.7 may be defined and used for predicting the peak position for specific ion species (with given alpha functions) in DMS spectra:

$$V_c \approx \frac{\langle \alpha E_s f(t) \rangle h}{1 + \langle \alpha(E) \rangle} \qquad (6.7)$$

where

$f(t)$ is function describing the waveform of an alternating electric field

E_s is maximum magnitude of the alternating electric field

Equation 6.7 shows that ions with a high value of alpha have higher values of compensation voltage. The peak position of the DMS spectrum is increased by increasing the resulting product of the following three parameters $[\alpha * E_s * f(t)]$: alpha parameter $*$ strength of electric field $*$ RF pulse waveform. According to Equation 6.7, the value of the compensation voltage directly reflects the magnitude of the differential mobility of ion species connected with the alpha parameter.

6.3.7 Peak Width in Planar DMS Spectra

The mathematical procedure for calculating peak width is presented in a review[28] and shown in the following:

$$FWHM \approx \frac{h * Q}{w * l * K^{eff}} = \frac{1}{K^{eff}} \frac{h^2}{\tau_{min}} \tag{6.8}$$

where $K_{\perp}^{eff} = \frac{1}{T} \int K(E(t)) dt$ is the average (effective)value of the coefficient of mobility for a given ion species and RF waveform.

This equation predicts the peak width for arbitrary ion species in DMS spectra, if the ion's alpha function is known. In the process of the mathematical calculation, the planar design of the analytical gap was used. Calculated values of FWHM (full width half maximum) were then compared with experimentally measured values of FWHM in different sized DMS sensors (with different length, width, height). For confirmation, additional measurements of the FWHM for the same ion species were obtained in experiments with the same sensor design but with a variation of the gas consumption rates [Q]. Comparison between the experimental and calculated FWHM shows close agreement, within ~10% error.

Equation 6.8 expresses four fundamental properties of planar DMS sensors:

1. First, the ion residence time in the analytical gap is a universal parameter that provides comprehensive information about DMS sensor performance. Peak width inversely depends (hyperbolically: $Y = A/\tau$) upon ion residence time in the analytical gap of sensor.

2. Second, the peak width depends directly on the volumetric flow rate of transport gas and height of analytical gap.

3. Third, increasing the length and width of the gap helps to narrow peak width.

4. Finally, the effective coefficient of mobility for a given ion species can also affect observed peak widths: ions with higher effective coefficient of mobility have narrower FWHM.

6.3.8 Optimization of the DMS Design: Gap Dimension Effect

As shown at the beginning of this section, the performance of the planar DMS sensor depends upon: (1) design and size of the analytical gap, (2) alpha parameters $\alpha(E)$ of tested ion species, and (3) the strength and waveform of applied separating asymmetric waveform electric field $E_s * f(t)$. Variation of these parameters affects DMS sensor output, which can be manifested as changing of peak position, peak width, and peak intensity. For validation and demonstration of a relationship between DMS outputs and experimental parameters, a systematic investigation was conducted to explore the effect of each dimension of analytical gap on DMS performance. Protocol for the experimental investigation included the measurements of the same samples in 12 version of planar DMS sensors with the same gap height $h = 0.5$ mm but different gap widths w: 0.5,1,2,3 mm and lengths l: 5,10,15 mm. Transport gas was regulated for five flow rates (Q): 100, 200, 300, 400, 500 cc/min. The general conclusion from the obtained set of data in these experiments was *that the ion residence time in the analytical gap is a universal parameter that provides comprehensive information about its performance*. Equations 6.7 and 6.8, obtained on the bases of mathematical calculation, also support this fundamental conclusion. Equation 6.7 indicates that peak positions of ions in a planar design (with given gap height, h) depend only on the strength of electric fields and ion alpha parameters and do not contain Q.

To prove this important fundamental statement, results of direct experiments to measure the effect of ion residence times on DMS output signals were investigated. Figure 6.6 shows four experimental DMS spectra obtained for a 16-compound mixture acquired in same sensor with dimensions 1 × 10 × 30 mm, while applying the same separation RF field

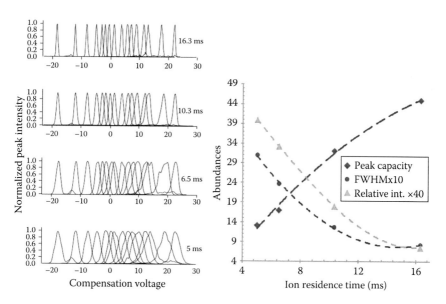

FIGURE 6.6
Demonstration of the effect of varying residence time on DMS output.

132 Townsends (Td). The only difference was flow rate, which provided the possibility of achieving different ion residence time in analytical gap ranging from 5 to 16.3 ms. A set of these experimental spectra are presented on the left panel.[29] In the right panel, the effect of changing residence time on peak width, peak intensity, and peak capacity is shown. Experiments explored 16 chemicals with masses ranging from 90.1 up to 649.1 Da: Alanine, Serine, Proline, Valine, Melamine, Methionine, Histidine, MDA, Minoxidil, Desipramine, Nordiazepam, Penbutolol, Propafenone, Angiotensin I (2+), Angiotensin II (2+), Angiotensin I (3+). For convenience, to compare the peak width and total spread of peak spectra, data are presented in normalized intensity view.

Following Equation 6.7 (which does not include term Q), the position of peaks V_c should be independent of changing flow rate (Q). According to Equation 6.8, reducing the residence time of ions in analytical gap (or increasing the flow rate) should strongly increase peak width, which clearly can be seen on experimental spectra. Calculated from experimental spectra, the effect of residence time on peak capacity (PC), FWHM, and intensity of peaks are presented in the right panel and show an expected result; increasing residence time of ions leads to increasing peak capacity of sensor. However, decreasing the residence time increases intensity and width of all peaks.

In summary, planar DMS sensor design optimization depends upon the particular application.

- The ion residence time in the analytical gap is a universal parameter that provides comprehensive information about the performance of the planar DMS sensor.
- The general relationship between sensor residence time and peak height shows that longer residence time reduces intensity but enhances selectivity, by narrowing peak width. Therefore, there is always a trade-off between peak height and peak width.
- Modifying analytical gap dimensions allows regulation of a DMS sensor performance to be optimized for specific applications. Examples of optimization toward this end include minimizing the flow consumption, enhancing selectivity, or optimizing system for maximum sensitivity, or minimizing the power consumption.

The general principles for the effect of sensor sizes on DMS sensor performance are as follows:

- Increasing the analytical gap length improves resolution of the DMS sensor due to increasing residence time, but also decreases the coefficient of transmission ions through the sensor.

- Increasing the analytical channel width reduces peak width but also requires higher-consumption gas flow rate to return to the same peak intensity.
- Decreasing the analytical gap height reduces gas consumption but requires a higher-frequency RF generator, and overall sensor resolution is also decreased.

6.4 Categorization of DMS Sensor Operation in Integrated Systems

6.4.1 Motivation for Integration of DMS with Other Analytical Instruments

The examples of operation of the DMS sensor presented earlier demonstrate the analytical potential of DMS system for detection and identification of individual chemicals. However, in applications where there is a need for fast screening of complex samples in the field, the resolving power of any stand-alone ionization-type instrument (including the powerful atmospheric pressure ionization mass spectrometric systems [API-MS]) becomes insufficient. This is primarily due to the presence of a high number of possible chemical interferents in environmental probes, which leads to additional complicating ions formation processes and, consequently, to changing of the sensor response. For example, the presence of traces of impurities in the ionization chamber or in the analytical channel can stimulate formation of (1) new ion-molecular complexes due to elastic interactions of targeted ion with impurity molecules, (2) initiation of fragmentation, and (3) neutralization due to charge exchange in gas-phase reactions with impurity molecules. Therefore, depending upon the nature of the targeted ion species and analysis conditions, the interaction of targeted ions with other gas-phase species can lead to undesirable consequences, resulting in the quenching or even loss of the response from the ion of interest or masking of the targeted ions response under enhanced intensity of chemical noise. One effective way to improve the quality of analysis of complex mixtures is the coupling of ionization-type instruments with other analytical techniques.

In analytical sciences, it is well known that integration of two or more chemical characterization methods can provide enhanced performance of chemical analysis. In integrated DMS systems, the analytical performance improvement is typically the result of the following factors[30,31]: (1) the analytical space of the combined system is increased due to the complementary chemical and physical characterization of the ion species, and (2) in hybrid systems, the total analytical burden can be distributed between the integrated methods, which helps to reduce the required level of performance of each of the integrated methods.

Hyphenated or hybrid design approaches provide additional flexibility to improve manufacturability and the cost of the total system. Due to the enhanced performance of the integrated system, design constraints and performance of the individual component subsystems can often be relaxed without a sacrifice in the performance of the overall system. In other words, integration of pre-separation and detection methods can help to enhance the ability of atmospheric pressure ionization-type analyzers, and make possible their use in more complex and harsh environments.

6.4.2 List of Products Where DMS Serves as System Engine

Once demonstration of the analytical potential of planar DMS systems was established, additional efforts started to commercialize DMS/FAIMS methodology. Currently, there are a number of DMS devices serving as highly sensitive analytical tools, which use the DMS sensor as an analytical system's engine, as presented in Figure 6.7. A goal of this chapter is to provide information about instrumentation and application developments for the planar geometry DMS system. In the following sections, we will focus only on systems that operate on the basis of planar DMS sensors with microscale dimensions. As was discussed in Table 6.1, the microchannel DMS design has a number advantages and greater potential to improve

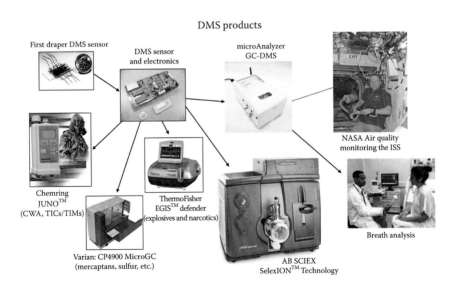

FIGURE 6.7
Illustration of developed systems around the DMS sensor with a microchannel analytical gap.

analytical performance of mobility-based instruments critically needed for biomedical applications.

Formally, all these systems can be categorized into three groups according to the function that the DMS sensor performs in each presented system:

1. *Simple gas analyzers*, where DMS operates as a single DMS spectral detector for analysis of simple samples.

2. *Hyphenated systems, where the DMS used as spectral detector* after any pre-fractioning techniques, for example, chromatography, temperature programming samples evaporating (or fractionating) systems, selective pre-concentrators with follow-on flash thermo-desorption.

3. *Tandem systems with a DMS interface* mounted in front of high-speed operated instruments (e.g., mass spectrometer or IMS). In this geometry, the DMS serves for selection and directs only targeted groups of ions in the analyzer. This approach has a special term: "Plasma chromatography."[32] In regular GC chromatography, the fractionation process of gaseous samples is time-consuming (usually 1–10 min), because molecule separation occurs due to multiple adsorption–desorption events on the internal surfaces of GC columns, and depends on the adsorption properties of analyte molecules. In plasma chromatography, analyte ion separation occurs in gas-phase media, where ion interaction with bulk gas molecules occurs with very high collision frequency ($>10^9$ s^{-1}); therefore, DMS version of plasma chromatography is capable of executing ultrafast separation of gaseous mixtures.

6.4.3 Operation of a Single DMS as a Spectral Detector in a Gas Analyzer

These type of analyzers provide fast measurements (second(s)) and can be used for analysis of simple gas mixtures. In this family of instruments, chemical identification occurs on the basis of peak position in DMS linear spectra (DMS response intensity = $f(V_c)$) obtained with fixed RF voltage). To achieve more reliable chemical identification, another multispectral method of chemical identification was suggested.[33] This advanced method for chemical identification offered simultaneously synchronized scans for strong asymmetric waveform dispersion voltage (SV) with weak DC voltage (V_c), and simultaneously recorded series of DMS spectra for different values of dispersion voltages. Integrated software helps to generate 2D dispersion plots from these data, which more thoroughly illustrates the process of shifting ion peak position as a function of separation voltage (SV). This method provides a panoramic view of the behavior of all ion species and reveals the specific nonlinear behavior for each individual ion species, facilitating enhanced chemical identification. In Figure 6.8, 2D traces for methyl salicylate (MSal)

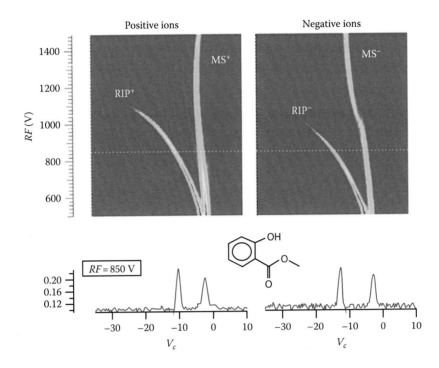

FIGURE 6.8
Dispersion plots and linear DMS spectra for both polarity methyl salicylate ions. In this particular case, placing the horizontal cursor in the position $RF = 850$ V therefore presented linear spectra correspond to 850 V.

ions are shown. To generate this particular 2D image, the V_c voltage is continuously scanned every second (between +10 up to −30 V), and the RF voltage is synchronized with V_c and scanned from 500 up to 1500 V with a step of 10 V. Analysis of these 2D traces tells us that this chemical is able to form simultaneously positive (left panel) and negative (right panel) ion species. Corresponding linear spectra (shown in the following) contain two peaks that correspond to RIP (background) and analyte (MSal) peaks. RIP ion traces show significantly stronger dependence from separation voltage, in contrast to MSI ions. The presented example shows that in dispersion plots, different behavior for individual ion species can be used as a source of additional information for ion species identification.

Figure 6.7 shows the Juno™ handheld analyzer, developed by Chemring Detection Systems (CDS) (2004). This device weighs ~2 lb, and has dimensions: 7.64 L × 3.95 W × 2.2 D (in.). It was designed for detection and identification of the traces of TIC and chemical warfare agents (CWA): VX, GA, GB, GD, GF, HD, L, HN3, AC, and CK in the field and in battlefield conditions, at levels less than IDLH (immediately dangerous to life or health).

6.4.4 DMS Operation as a Spectral Detector for Fractionating Systems

In particular geometries, the DMS sensor *can operate with separating techniques.* A typical example for such a combination is use of the DMS sensor as a chromatographic spectral detector. This geometry provides two advantages: pretreatment (fractionation) of complex sample probes, and simultaneous chromatographic characterization of each fraction of a mixture. Therefore, each fraction of a mixture is ionized and characterized independently in DMS. Such two-step characterization of chemicals of interest provides 2D characterization of analyte ions: the retention time of original molecules in the GC column and the ion's alpha parameter (which is connected with the position of the analyte peak in DMS spectrum). Such 2D characterization of individual chemicals enables more confident chemical identification and improves the accuracy of quantitative measurements. The following systems from Figure 6.6 belong to this category of instruments:

- The Varian CP-4900 analyzer was developed in 2004 for sensitive and precise monitoring of sulfur components (odorants) in gas samples.
- The ThermoFisher™ EGIS Defender was designed to operate with fast GC pre-separation and provide rapid (<20s) screening of passengers' bags for explosives and drugs in airports.
- The Draper Lab/Sionex microAnalyzer (2007) was developed for continuous, sensitive, and precise monitoring of the traces of individual volatile organic compounds (VOCs) and was targeted for many applications: breath samples analysis, monitoring environmental samples, petrochemical and pharmaceutical industry, and so on.
- Sionex Corporation built a version 1.0 of the microAnalyzer (2009) for NASA as a continuous air quality monitoring (AQM) and analyzer for the International Space Station. A version 2.0 of the microAnalyzer was built by Draper with deployment occurring in 2013. These systems have been successfully operating in the International Space Station since 2009.[34,35]

6.4.5 DMS Operation as an Ambient Pressure Ion Pre-Filter for Sophisticated Analytical Instruments

In this application, the DMS sensor operates as a tunable ion pre-filter for selection of the targeted ion species and exclusion of non-targeted ion species prior to mass spectrometry. Ion triaging prior to MS analysis helps to decrease the complexity of the ion population introduced into the mass analyzer and leads to improving the quality of MS measurements, resulting in: enhanced selectivity in MS measurements,[36–38] a reduction in the chemical noise in measured mass spectra,[39] extending the linear dynamic range in

MS measurements,[40] and at least a 10-fold improvement in the limit of MS detection. Examples of commercial planar DMS ion filters with ambient mass spectrometric systems are described in the following:

- AB SCIEX adopted the DMS technology and commercialized it in 2011 under the name AB Sciex SelexION™ Technology.[41] The system has been successfully used for challenging mass spectrometric applications related to monitoring and quantitative measurements of the chemical of interest in complex matrices. The technology was shown to be particularly useful for separating isobaric and isomeric ion species analysis in the pharmaceutical, food safety, environmental testing, proteomics, metabolomics, and other applications areas.

- Other groups have also combined commercial stand-alone DMS systems with potentially fieldable MS systems: Mini10[42] and NSTec Experimental.[43] These proof-of-concept experiments showed that DMS pre-filtering in front of compact/mobile ambient mass spectrometers provides significant value. It is typically the case that in the process of miniaturization the MS performance is reduced, and the analytical power of stand-alone MS systems can become insufficient to resolve quasi-isobaric components, such as those commonly encountered in background spectra or when mobile API MS devices operate in harsh environmental conditions. In several publications[42-44] it is shown that in applications when detection and quantitative measurement in field conditions are needed, even low-resolution portable mass spectrometers with DMS pre-filtering can provide a quality of analysis similar to stand-alone, high-performance desktop-type mass spectrometers. Therefore, adding DMS pre-filtering aids in restoring the analytical capability of compact mass spectrometers, which is lost during miniaturization. In addition to analytical advantages, long-term test results show that DMS pre-filtering improves the robustness of any API MS. Testing DMS-MS systems in harsh environment conditions[28] showed that the presence of a DMS interface in front of an API MS substantially increases the duration of service time before cleaning is required.

The foregoing presented a brief review of the chronology of a list of different prototypes, built in the last decade, and shows that DMS technology has significant analytical potential for detection and identification of traces of targeted chemicals in complex samples. One unquestioned advantage of this technology is its ability to operate with other analytical systems, when it is used for triage of ion species before analysis. This depends upon the particular application, condition of operation, and requirements that the DMS system can be optimized in various ways.

6.5 Advantages of Tandem Systems for Specific Applications

6.5.1 The GC-DMS System: Protecting Crew Health and Safety Aboard the International Space Station (ISS)

Crewmembers remain in the semiclosed environment of the International Space Station (ISS) for as long as 6 months, and during this time they rely on the ISS revitalization systems to keep the air and water safe for human consumption. It is vital to the health and safety of the crew that the air and water be periodically monitored and assessed.

The gas chromatograph-mass spectrometry (GC-MS) is the standard ground laboratory instrument for analysis of air contaminants. Unfortunately, it is too large, power hungry, and maintenance-intensive for use on the ISS. Replacing the MS with a DMS dramatically changes the resource issues of the GC-MS, thus allowing a small, low-power instrument that is relatively maintenance-free to monitor the contaminants onboard the ISS. The size and appearance of this system is presented in Figure 6.9, which was taken during a TV interview with an astronaut during a mission on the ISS. The reduction in size and maintenance resources is due to the fact that the DMS operates at atmospheric pressure as opposed to vacuum conditions required for MS. This was the motivation to develop a new air quality monitor for NASA

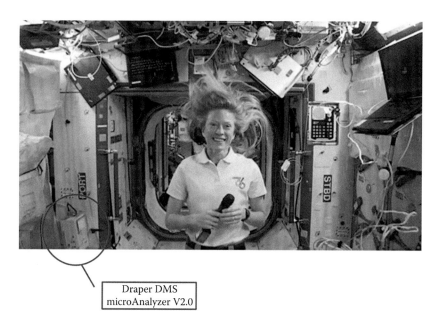

Draper DMS
microAnalyzer V2.0

FIGURE 6.9
Air Quality Monitor (AQM) aboard the International Space Station (ISS).

TABLE 6.2

List of Targeted Components for AQM

Target Compounds	
2-Butanone	Hexanal
2-Propanol	Hexane
Acetaldehyde	Hexamethylcyclotrisiloxane
Acetone	Methanol
Acrolein	m-p Xylenes
Benzene	n_Butanol
Dichloroethane	Octamethylcyclotetrasiloxane
Decamethylcyclopentasiloxane	Toluene
Ethanol	Trimethylsilanol
Ethyl acetate	Ammonia

needs on the basis of Sionex's existing GC-DMS system. Currently, the air quality onboard ISS is monitored every 73 h by the Draper microAnalyzer (referred to as the Air Quality Monitor—AQM), and the data are downlinked weekly for assessment by the NASA toxicologist. Numerous compounds have been detected on the ISS over its 15-year life, but only a handful of compounds meet the criteria to be monitored by real-time instrumentation. This list of compounds (Table 6.1) was developed by applying these simple criteria: (1) compounds frequently detected in spacecraft at concentrations above trace levels (e.g., ethanol, acetone), (2) compounds with significant toxicity at low concentrations, even though they are detected infrequently on spacecraft (e.g., benzene), and (3) compounds that can affect the response of continuously (autonomic) operating the environmental control systems (e.g., siloxanes, 2-propanol). The AQM monitors the list of compounds in Table 6.2, but more compounds could be targeted, if necessary, and the instrument is capable of detecting nontarget compounds as well. The NASA toxicologist sums the health effects for each compound, based upon the concentrations derived from the AQM and uses this number (total T-value) to determine the acceptability of the air quality on the ISS during missions. In nominal conditions, the main contributor to the T-value, not detected by AQM, is carbon dioxide. A health effects graph produced from AQM data is shown in Figure 6.10.

Additional value in having the technology present onboard the AQM was demonstrated in 2015, when an independently operated environmental control sensor system suddenly alarmed indicating a massive ammonia leak into the ISS. The crew was evacuated to a safe haven, sealed from the LAB module. It was thought that the alarm was false, but the options to confirm a false alarm were either to send the crew into the potentially contaminated LAB module to take samples or remotely activate the AQM from the ground and review the recorded data. The AQM was remotely activated, a method for detecting ammonia was uploaded from ISS ground control, and

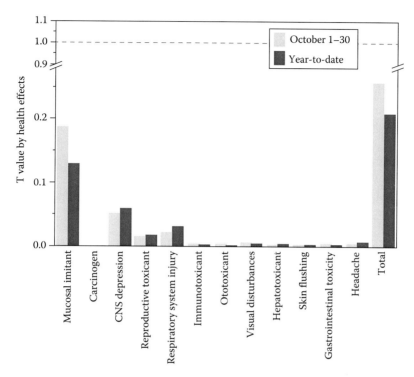

FIGURE 6.10
A health effects graph produced from AQM data.

the microAnalyzer confirmed that there was the normal amount of ammonia in the LAB atmosphere. This avoided the need to potentially put the crew in harm's way, which would have been required if they had to break the seal on the safe haven to enter the LAB.

A second important operational use of the AQM in 2015 was to help troubleshoot unusually high conductivity values in the water processing unit. Comparison of AQM response on headspace vapors with water processor data showed that higher than normal levels of ethanol were probably the cause of the high conductivity in the water processing unit.

6.5.2 DMS Operation as a GC Detector for Measurements in Harsh Environments

To demonstrate the enhanced analytical power of a GC-DMS system, experimental data related to the detection of trace amounts of CWA simulants in clean samples and in samples containing potential interferents are shown. Figure 6.11 shows the response of a microAnalyzer (GC-DMS) for an air mixture that contains traces of four phosphonates, which commonly serve

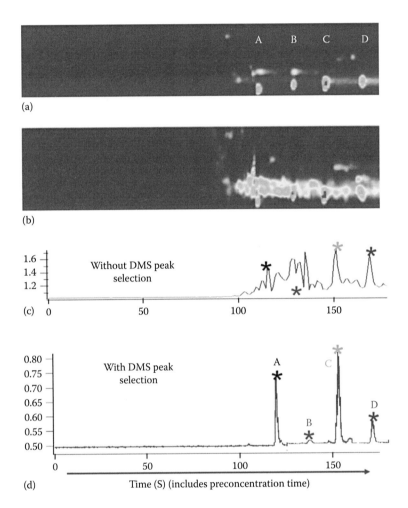

FIGURE 6.11
GC chromatograms obtained in a microAnalyzer (GC-DMS) for gas mixtures of four organophosphate chemicals commonly used as simulants of nerve agents. (a) 2D chromatogram for mixture sample with four chemicals (A,B,C,D). (b) 2D chromatogram for the same sample with adding interferents (AFFF and diesel). (c) Regular chromatograms extracted from raw 2D experimental data (experimental data (b)). (d) Extracted chromatogram from experimental data (b) by using DMS peak selection. (From Nazarov, E.G. et al., Planar differential mobility spectrometry as a powerful tool for gas phase ion separation and detection (Spectroscopy Solution: Premier Learning for Analytical Chemists.))

as simulants for nerve agents. Presented in the top panel (a) is a 2D chromatogram illustrating the DMS scanning response versus GC retention time for a clean sample. It contains four well-resolved spots related to each of the four simulants (A, B, C, D). Each spot is characterized as a specific combination of retention time (GC separation) and compensation voltage (DMS separation). This 2D chemical characterization in the GC-DMS system enhances the identification power of GC measurements in comparison with any regular total current measured detectors such as flame ionization, thermal conduction, and electron capture. The estimated values of LODs for each of the four chemicals were 65 ppt for A, 424 ppt for B, 20 ppt for C, and 107 ppt for D.

To model the challenging environmental conditions, additional vapors of interferents were added to the same analyte mixture. The interferents used were diesel fuel vapors and vapors of aqueous film forming foam (AFFF), a shipboard fire-fighting material known to cause interferences with IMS-based CWA sensor systems. A 2D GC-DMS chromatogram of this mixture is presented in panel (b) of Figure 6.11. As evidenced from the chromatogram, the addition of the interfering materials substantially increased the chemical noise, with the appearance of numerous new peaks that overlap with the analyte peaks. As a result, detection and identification of the target chemicals become problematic. A regular chromatographic view for total ion current measurements is presented in panel (c). Due to the high chemical noise, the peaks for A and B components cannot be resolved from interferences, and only identifiable peaks can be seen for C and D components. The final chromatogram presented in panel (d) was obtained using a regime of DMS operation with peak selection, wherein the RF and V_c parameters are optimized for the detection of each of the four individual components. As a result, the components A and B are now resolved from the interfering background signal and it is possible to detect, identify, and quantify all four targeted chemicals.

6.5.3 Example of Chemical Noise Reduction in DMS-MS

Experimental spectra that illustrate the advantages of integrating DMS to MS are discussed subsequently and shown in Figure 6.12a through c as reported in several publications.[38,39,46]

In Figure 6.12a, two mass spectra are presented for monitoring 2′-deoxycytidine (100 pg/μL) in mouse urine samples. 2′-Deoxycytidine (MW = 228 g/mol) is a radiation exposure biomarker and can be used in biodosimetry to determine the level of radiation exposure of individual live subjects.[39] The top spectrum was obtained without DMS ion pre-filtering (where RF voltage is turned off) and the bottom spectrum with DMS filtering (when RF = 3200 V). The first spectrum has significant chemical noise, which is typical for a complex sample such as urine. The spectrum contains a small peak (with an S/N of around 3–5) related to the targeted biomarker, 2′-deoxycytidine, which is the protonated molecular ions peak MH$^+$ with m/z = 229 Da. DMS pre-filtration becomes very simple. The recorded mass spectrum contains only one major peak with expected m/z of 229 Da. Most importantly, due to suppression of chemical noise, the S/N is now at least 50, which shows that DMS pre-filtration improved the value of the LOD for this assay by 10- to 15-fold.

6.5.4 Separation of Isobaric Ion Species in DMS-MS

Figure 6.12b shows DMS spectra[46] for five isobaric components with close molecular masses ($MW \sim 308$), but different structures: Benoxinate, $MW = 308.4158$; Phenylbutazone, $MW = 308.3743$; Bestatine $MW = 308.37$; Warfarin, $MW = 308.3278$, and Quinoxyfen, $MW = 308.135$. In mass spectrometric analysis with electrospray ionization, all of these chemicals form protonated ion species (MH^+) with close m/z ($\sim 309.25 \pm 0.15$ Da). Therefore, to resolve these components, one would need a mass spectrometer with enhanced resolution. At the same time, due to the fact that these chemicals have distinguishable structures, and hence ion mobilities, DMS is able to resolve these structures easily, as shown in Figure 6.12b. The additional parameter of DMS compensation voltage allows one to identify these isobaric components, even with

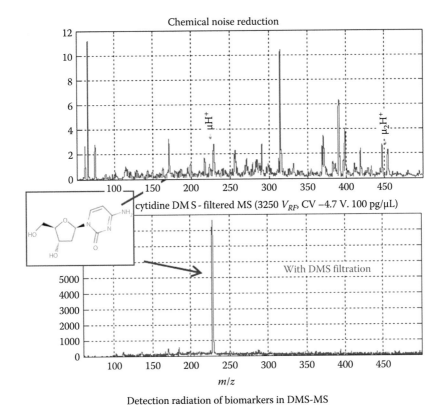

(a)

FIGURE 6.12

Sample spectra obtained with a DMS pre-filter in front of an API MS: (a) reducing chemical noise in mass spectra. *(Continued)*

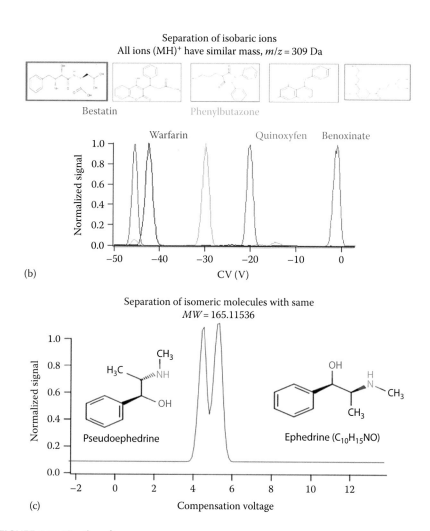

FIGURE 6.12 (*Continued*)
Examples that provide DMS pre-filter in front of an API MS: (b) separation of isobaric components, and (c) separation of isomeric components.

a low-resolution mass spectrometer (e.g., a field portable MS), which has resolving power of one mass unit, and possibly lower.

6.5.5 Selection and Identification of Isomeric Ion Species in DMS-MS

Figure 6.12c shows a DMS spectra obtained in a gas mixture that contains two stereoisomeric components: ephedrine and pseudoephedrine.[38] Both of these chemicals have the same molecular formula, $C_{10}H_5NO$, identical molecular weight, 165.11536, and similar molecular structures. The only difference between the two chemicals is the spatial arrangement of –OH groups in their molecular structures. Regardless of their similarities, these two chemicals have very different physiological effects: ephedrine is used in traditional medicine for the treatment of asthma and bronchitis, while pseudoephedrine is used for nasal congestion treatment. Therefore, it is important in the process of synthesis of these compounds to be capable of online control and identification of the desired final product. Even expensive, high-performance MS instruments cannot by themselves differentiate these compounds. But, as shown in Figure 6.12c, peak positions of ephedrine and pseudoephedrine ions are different and well resolved in DMS spectra. Therefore, by using a combination of DMS pre-filtration with MS, differentiation of these is isomeric compounds becomes possible.

6.5.6 DMS Operation as Interface in Front of IMS: DMS-IMS² System

Motivation for operating in the DMS-IMS² mode can be inferred from Figure 6.3, where a comparison between operating principles and outputs of both (IMS and DMS) ion-mobility-based sensors is given. Equation 6.3 shows that in general, the ion's comprehensive coefficient mobility $K(E) = K(0) [1 + \alpha(E)]$ is a function of electric field strength and consists of two terms: (1) $K(0)$, which is the absolute value of ion coefficient mobility at low electric field conditions, and (2) $\alpha(E)$, the alpha function that connects to the effect of a strong electric field on ion mobility (see Equation 6.4). A comparison between the operating principles of IMS and DMS reveals that these two systems operate in different regimes. In IMS, ion separation occurs in a low ($E \sim 200 \text{ V/cm}$) DC electric field, and values of $K(0)$ are obtained by measurement of ion arrival times. In DMS, ion spatial separation occurs in oscillating (between 1 and 35 kV/cm) asymmetric waveform electric field conditions. The resulting trajectories depend upon differences between analyzed ion's coefficient of mobility, which are different in high and low voltage portions of the separating RF voltage. Differences in methodologies of ion separation and experimental conditions lead to differences in IMS and DMS outputs:

- Output of an IMS contains solely information about low field coefficient mobility $K(0)$.
- Output of a DMS includes information about an ion's alpha coefficient $\alpha(E)$.

Therefore, integration of IMS and DMS spectra provides value in obtaining different portions of comprehensive coefficient mobility $K(E)$, which is described in Equations 6.3 and 6.4. Therefore, an integrated DMS-IMS system enables a 2D characterization of ion species, which contains enriched mobility-related information. This consequently has an enhanced level of ion species' identification in comparison to a stand-alone mobility instrument. This system was developed in collaboration with Hamilton Sundstrand

Corp. The objective was to develop a fast-operated tandem system, which minimizes the false alarm rate for detection and identification traces of targeted hazardous chemicals.

A schematic of T-tandem DMS-IMS^2 instrument consists of one planar DMS sensor and two independently operated cylindrical time-of-flight IMS(s) that are coupled to the output of the DMS. A block diagram and design of a tandem system are shown in Figure 6.13a. DMS itself can operate as a

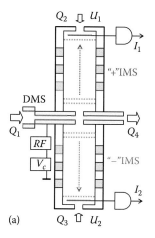

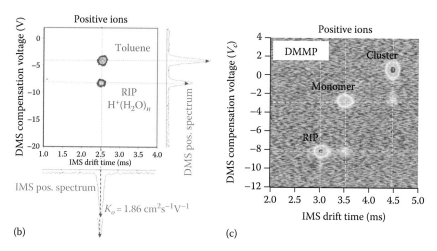

FIGURE 6.13
Tandem DMS-IMS^2 system and examples of its output. (a) Schematic of T-tandem (DMS-IMS^2) system. (b) Example of 2D pattern (V_c vs. t_d) recorded in T-tandem system for detection traces (45 ppb) of toluene vapors in nitrogen. (c) 2D pattern for positive dimethyl methyl phosphonate (DMMP) ions.

dual polarity DMS sensor, or as a filter for specific ion species, which after selection in DMS, are directed into the IMS cells. Drift time is measured and recorded on IMS detectors. This T-design configuration is capable of analyzing positive and negative ions in parallel.

Figure 6.13b and c presents 2D plots that were obtained in regime of operation "Compensation voltage vs. IMS Drift Time."In this regime, the DMS compensation voltage is periodically ($t \sim 1$ s) sweeping. At the same time, the IMS shutter runs continuously with a significantly faster period, which allows recording of IMS spectra every 0.01 s. Special software developed for DMS-IMS^2 system generates in real-time scale these 2D patterns (V_c vs. t_d) and displays for both polarity ions patterns on screen. In such a representation, any individual chemicals ions are revealed as specific spots in 2D surfaces with a particular V_c and t_d. Therefore, identification of a particular chemical can be realized by determining its response spot coordinates: t_d—drift time and V_c—compensation voltage. If need be, the software is able to separately display any IMS or DMS spectra too.

As expected, a 2D pattern shows the enhanced analytical space of a DMS-IMS system in comparison with a single sensor output. For example, in Figure 6.13b, the linear IMS spectrum (horizontal position) shows a single (with $t_d = 2.5$ ms) unresolved peak for RIP and toluene response, but an integrated 2D pattern shows two very-well resolved spots with the same $t_d = 2.5$ ms, but different $V_c. = 4$ and 8 V. This example shows the power of tandem measurements, which provide information about a comprehensive value of mobility; adding the DMS portion of mobility-related information (or alpha parameter) helps to solve the problem of chemical separation/identification. There are also possibilities for the opposite case, when IMS data introduce additional information *in comparison to DMS*.

Presented in Figure 6.13c is another example of a DMMP response in a T-tandem system. A 2D pattern for positive ions shows three spots corresponding to three ion species: RIP, monomer, and cluster peaks. In this case, both methods are certainly able to resolve all three peaks separately. But the 2D approach provides enhanced separation power in contrast to linear spectra. This is an expected result, and in this case we can explain this phenomenon on the basis of simple geometric considerations. In general, the resolving power of any type of spectral measurement can be presented as $R = l/FWHM_{av}$, where l is distance between two spots and $FWHM_{av}$ is average width of a response spot (or peak). In 2D cases, the distance between two spots can be determined as $l = \sqrt{a^2 + b^2}$, where a and b are distances between two peaks in linear spectra, which can be obtained from spectra obtained in DMS and IMS. This means that the value of l is longer than each of the segments of a or b. At the same time, the average value of $FWHM_{av}$ when a spot is symmetric (e.g., circle in this case) can be considered the same. Therefore, the resolving power R of a 2D system is in principle higher than can be obtained in a one-dimensional system. It means that for a DMS-IMS^2, there is a higher separation performance and an ability to operate with more complex samples.

So, based on the presented results and considerations, the following may be claimed.

The key benefits of the DMS-IMS^2 are as follows:

- High sensitivity for most TICs and TIMs. For instance, the typical sensitivity for CWAs and organophosphate compounds is in the low ppb-ppt range and comparable with stand-alone gas analyzers. This is achieved due to the high-efficiency (up to ~80%) transmission ion species between two sensors.
- High speed of operation. Overall speed for the detection of single targeted components may be ~1 s.
- Bipolar ion spectra. Both positive and negative ions are separated and measured simultaneously without instrumental switching.
- Enhanced separation power (peak capacity), small physical size, and moderate power consumption allow it to be used in the field or in handheld configurations.

6.6 Biodefense Applications: Aerosolized Pathogens as Potential Bioweapons

Many documented cases of intentional pathogen release have been recorded in modern history. Examples of agents used in chemical and bioterror attacks include *Salmonella*,[47] *Bacillus anthracis* spores,[48,49] and sarin nerve gas.[50] The biological toxin ricin was distributed in bioterror attacks on the U.S. Capitol.[51] Threats may not be limited to intentional release of aerosolized pathogens, with at least one confirmed accidental release to a community in the last several decades. In 1979, weapons-grade *B. anthracis* was released from a military facility in Sverdlovsk, former Soviet Union, resulting in the largest outbreak of inhalational anthrax in the twentieth century.[52]

The capability of *B. anthracis* to form highly resistant spores makes it a prime candidate for an easily released biological weapon. Anthrax spores are among the category A pathogens listed by the Centers for Disease Control and Prevention,[53] and can be aerosolized to target human inhalation. Early detection technologies are required for fast and reliable characterization of threat agents and for quickly exposing a hoax attack, if necessary. There remains a need for a robust multipurpose microanalyzer capable of both specific and sensitive environmental pathogen detection. Over the past several decades, scientists have adapted molecular biology techniques to detect

B. anthracis using DNA-based, antibody-based, and mass spectrometry analysis approaches. These tests vary greatly in sensitivity, response time, cost, availability, and complexity of use. With the identification of species-specific primers,[54] rapid polymerase chain reaction (PCR) has identified specific *Bacillus* species from both environmental[55] and clinical samples.[56] A novel detection method uses DNA-aptamers conjugated to magnetic electrochemiluminescent beads to bind and detect Sterne strain *B. anthracis* spores.[57] Sequencing on microchips containing gel-immobilized oligonucleotides has identified *B. anthracis* by single-nucleotide polymorphism (SNP) analysis,[58] and several commercial PCR kits/platforms are available that differ in sensitivity depending on sample type and preparation.[59] The most recent is based on rapid-cycle, real-time PCR, developed as a collaborative effort and dubbed the "Mayo-Roche Rapid Anthrax Test,"[60] which yields results in ~35 min, but may be difficult to deploy in the field.

Antibody-based methods traditionally use fluorescent-conjugated antibodies to spore-coat proteins to detect low levels of *Bacillus* spores. Phillips and Martin (1983) showed that it is possible to detect *Bacillus* spores with specificity using fluorescein-conjugated polyclonal antibodies directed toward the spore coat. However, it was found that multiple anthrax serotypes exist among *B. anthracis* strains, rendering specific detection with this method difficult.[61] More recently, monoclonal and polyclonal antibodies have been produced against *Bacillus* epitopes; these distinguish moderately well between *B. anthracis* and *B. subtilis*, but less effectively between *B. anthracis* and *B. cereus* spores. Additionally, variability exists in the specificity of antibodies between spore coat and vegetative cell epitopes.[62] Nevertheless, several novel antibody-based assays have been developed to identify *Bacillus* species. The electrochemiluminescent immunoassay (ECLIA) is based on a redox reaction between ruthenium (II)-trisbipyridyl $Ru[(bpy)_3]^{2+}$ labeled antibody and the excess of tripropylamine, which generates photons.[63] A magnetic particle fluorogenic immunoassay (MPFIA) technique employs antibody-coated magnetic beads as solid phase in suspension for bacterial capture and concentration in a 96-well microplate format.[16] Both the ECLIA and MPFIA are fast, but still require almost double the time of rapid PCR-based tests. Antibodies have also been immobilized onto silicon chips or membranes for higher-throughput screening of environmental samples. One significant limitation of these methods involves the specificity of the antibodies selected for use. However, fluorescent-labeled phage antibodies have recently been produced, and show promise as *Bacillus* species-specific markers[64]; antibody-based methods for *Bacillus* detection may further improve in the future.

Numerous large-scale benchtop chemical and analytical detectors have been explored to rapidly identify *Bacillus* spores. Most gas chromatograph (GC) detectors, such as the widely used flame ionization detector (FID), produce a signal indicating the presence of a compound eluted from the column; however, this signal lacks the information required for unambiguous compound identification. An expedient and simple method for identification of unknown analytes requires a detector to provide an orthogonal set of information for each chromatographic peak. The mass spectrometer (MS) is generally considered one of the most definitive detectors for compound identification, as it generates a fingerprint pattern of fragment ions for each GC eluent. Mass spectrometric information is often sufficient for sample identification through comparison to compound libraries, and has been used to identify species of bacteria.[65–69] Bacterial cell extracts themselves have been shown to produce reproducible spectra comprised mainly of phospholipids, glycolipids, and proteins.[70] As such, this is a very sensitive method for identifying *Bacillus* species, and even unique biomarkers have been identified between closely related *B. cereus* strains.[71] The so-called tandem MS method has yielded a wealth of specifically identified protein biomarkers for *B. cereus* using bioinformatic approaches.[72] Analysis by matrix-assisted laser desorption/ionization mass spectrometry (MALDI-MS) has also shown that very low mass biomarkers between 2 and 4 kDa distinguish *B. anthracis* from other closely related *Bacillus* species.[73] While this result was obtained using a very specific carrier matrix, it demonstrates that species-specific markers can exist if sample preparation is optimized. However, minor variations in sample/matrix preparations for MALDI-MS can produce significant changes in observed spectra.[74] Finally, MALDI-MS has been shown to distinguish bacteria in aerosolized samples, in a continuous fashion.[75]

While GCs are continuously being miniaturized and reduced in cost,[76] mass spectrometers are still very expensive, and their size remains relatively large, making them difficult to deploy in the field. The DMS produces spectra that can differentiate between compounds that co-elute in GC-MS, often yielding an improved ability to identify samples. For MALDI-MS, a statistical model has demonstrated the ability to distinguish between roughly 10 species similar to *B. subtilis* when the spectral masses are grouped in 1.5 Da ranges.[77] This is due to roughly the same number of proteins per unit-mass interval. Recent data also suggest a 75% correct identification rate using MALDI-MS with no false positives.[78] However, the DMS technology may easily distinguish between even larger numbers of species, as the spectra may be more easily deconvolved than those of MS due to differing ion mobilities.

Pyrolysis can be used to convert the spore sample into its component substances through the use of heat. Pyrolysis can be employed for identification and quantization of samples through the analysis of both the parent and the product ions. Detection of bacterial spore biomarkers by pyrolysis has been demonstrated using gas chromatography-ion mobility spectrometry and mass spectrometry,[49,50] and is a viable method of sample handling for DMS analysis.

Bacterial spore detection has been demonstrated utilizing a DMS system with a front-end pyrolysis experimental setup consisting of a CDS Pyroprobe 1000 (CDS Analytical, Inc., Oxford, PA) connected to the inlet of an HP 5890 gas chromatograph (GC) (Agilent Technologies, Palo Alto, CA). The GC was equipped with a 0.5 m deactivated fused silica column. A prototype DMS was connected to the detector outlet of the GC. The interface temperature of the pyrolyzer was set at 110°C, the GC inlet was set to 150°C, the GC oven was held constant at 200°C, and the GC detector heating block was set to 150°C. A slurry of *Bacillus* spores suspended in water was pyrolyzed by ramping the temperature up to 650°C at a rate of 0.01°C/ms, and then holding this temperature for 99.99 s. The spectra of the pyrolyzed spores corresponding to the detected positive and negative ions were recorded on a laptop computer connected to the DMS unit.

For each of the three species, *B. subtilis*, *B. cereus*, and *B. thuringiensis*, 100 experiments for each of three concentrations (900 experiments in total) were conducted. The concentrations used were 2×10^7 spores/mL (80,000 spores/experiment), 2.5×10^6 spores/mL (10,000 spores/experiment), and 1.25×10^6 spores/mL (5,000 spores/experiment). The data were then analyzed by ProteomeQuest® (Correlogic Systems Inc.), a proprietary pattern recognition software package that combines genetic algorithm elements first described by Holland[51] with cluster analysis elements described by Kohonen,[52] as previously described.[53–57]

The data from each species were randomly divided into three categories: a training set (50 spectra of each species), a testing set (150 spectra of each species), and a validation set (~100 spectra of each species). The training and testing sets consisted of files whose species' identities were known by the computer. The validation set, withheld from the modeling process, was then scored by the model to give an independent measure of the accuracy of the model on blinded data. The accuracy was calculated from the results of the independent validation set using the following equation: Accuracy = (True Positives + True Negatives)/(Total Number of Samples). The files were first compared in binary groups consisting of a single species at all three concentrations compared to a second species at all three concentrations, to create models that differentiated one species from another. The models giving the highest validation accuracies were as follows: *B. subtilis* versus *B. thuringiensis* 98.5%; *B. subtilis* versus *B. cereus* 92.0%; *B. cereus* versus *B. thuringiensis* 69.2%. The latter two species proved slightly more difficult to distinguish, which is not surprising as these two species are genetically very similar.

The biomarkers found across many models are displayed in Figure 6.14. Panel (a) shows the biomarkers found in 40 models that allowed discrimination of *B. subtilis* and *B. thuringiensis*. Note that there is one biomarker that was selected in many of the models, which indicates that it is important in the discrimination of these two species. Panel (b) shows a similar plot for *B. subtilis* and *B. cereus*, and again we see that the same biomarker appears in many of these models as well. When comparing the models of *B. cereus* and *B. thuringiensis* in panel (c), no biomarkers appear as frequently across all models, which is consistent with these two species being difficult to separate.

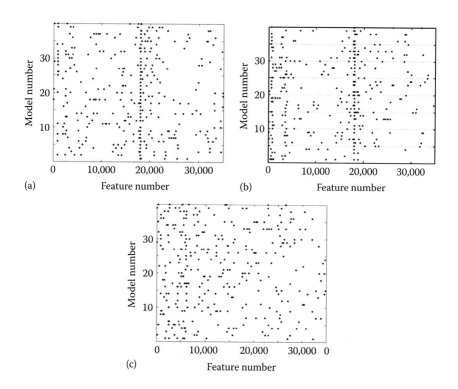

FIGURE 6.14
Distribution of features across 40 models. The models are: (a) *B. subtilis* versus *B. thuringiensis*, (b) *B. subtilis* versus *B. cereus*, (c) *B. cereus* versus *B. thuringiensis*.

To verify that *B. cereus* and *B. thuringiensis* tend to be more difficult to separate from each other than from *B. subtilis* due to their similarity, several binary models that distinguish *B. subtilis* from a pool of *B. cereus* and *B. thuringiensis* files were created. Again the 5 k, 10 k, and 80 k files for each species were combined and randomized prior to modeling. The model with the highest validation accuracy was 92.3%. The high classification obtained here shows that *B. cereus* and *B. thuringiensis* have biomarkers common to each other but different from *B. subtilis*.

As *B. cereus* and *B. thuringiensis* are the most difficult to classify, we modeled these two species at each concentration individually to determine if there is a concentration limit below which the species become indistinguishable. The models offering the highest accuracy were 60.8% at 5 k concentration, 64% at 10 k concentration, and 88% at 80 k concentration. Therefore, classification is more successful for these two closely related species when more spores are present.

A set of three-way comparisons were also performed to classify all three groups from one another in a single model. For these models only the 80 k data were used, since we determined that below that concentration *B. cereus* and *B. thuringiensis* are more difficult to distinguish. For each species, the spectra were randomly assigned to a training set of 25, a testing set of 50, and a validation set of 25. An overall accuracy of 77.3% was obtained in one model.

Representative spectra from the three species at 5000-spore concentration are shown in Figure 6.15. Biomarkers resulting from the three-way model are

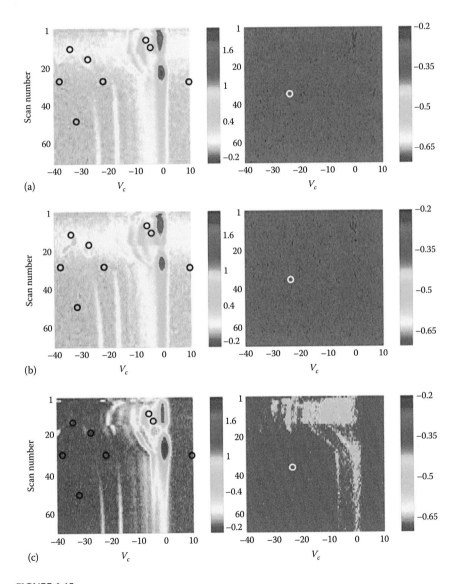

FIGURE 6.15
Representative DMS spectra of 80,000 spores undergoing pyrolysis at 650°C for 99.99 s. Positive ion spectrum (left), negative ion spectrum (right). (a) *B. subtilis*, (b) *B. cereus*, and (c) *B. thuringiensis*.

indicated with circles. The raw data are shown here, but the biomarkers were selected based on their relative ratio after normalization between zero and one. The data from these experiments look very similar by eye, yet the pattern recognition algorithms were able to find biomarkers present in sufficient quantities to reliably distinguish the species from one another.

A softer ionization technique, such as *Matrix-Assisted Laser Desorption/Ionization* (MALDI), may also be used as a sample introduction technique for DMS detection, as has been described earlier. In this method, spore samples are pretreated, such as with coronal plasma discharge or other chemical means, so that they will yield a high number of biomarkers. The pretreated spores are then complexed with a chemical matrix, usually an acid solution. The matrix–spore complex is excited by a laser using an energy level sufficient to excite the matrix but not the pretreated spore itself. The matrix and the spore then split apart, yielding electrostatic charged moieties that are introduced in the mass spectrometer to yield spectral biomarkers. Preliminary data taken with this front-end shows the ability to detect sample (Figure 6.16). There is no effect on the background spectra (panel a) due to the laser firing on a clean plate (panel b), which indicates that all signal detected in panel (c) results from the sample complexed with the matrix material.

Both, pyrolysis and MALDI introduction techniques should yield many useful biomarkers for spore samples, and it is possible that sample handling protocols may maximize the number of unique biomarkers produced.

6.7 Medical Applications

6.7.1 Breath Analysis

There are dozens of volatile organic compounds present in exhaled human breath, many of which show promise for diagnosis and management of diseases, but with little available technical or clinical research and development to date.[79–81] Many volatile gases are produced by disease conditions, and can often be smelled by physicians on the patient's breath. Examples include ketones in conditions such as starvation and ketoacidosis, feculent amines generated following bowel obstruction, and bacterial by-products related to anaerobic infections. Another example of breath analysis is the use of exhaled breath samples by police departments to measure blood alcohol levels of automobile drivers. Numerous diagnostic tests measure exhaled hydrogen after ingestion of a specific sugar or starch load to signal the presence of lactose deficiency, bacterial overgrowth of the small bowel, malabsorption, or deficits in pancreatic function resulting from cystic fibrosis.[82–84] One of the most common breath tests involves an office-based diagnostic for *H. pylori*, requiring the patient to first eat ^{14}C labeled urea, after which ^{14}C labeled CO_2

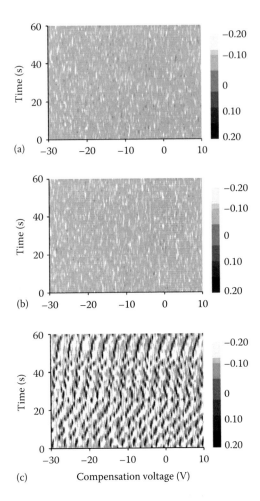

FIGURE 6.16
AP-MALDI-DMS spectra. (a) Background signal, equipment on, but laser not firing. (b) Laser firing on clean plate. (c) Laser firing on plate spotted with 100 fM desmosine in α-cyano-4-hydroxycinnamic acid matrix.

is detected in exhaled breath. There are other examples of radioactive labeled metabolites used in additional gastroenterology tests. Exhaled nitric oxide has been measured as a marker of inflammation in the lungs.[85–87] Analysis of exhaled breath is being explored as a rapid toxicology test for carbon monoxide and methanol.

6.7.2 Cardiovascular Applications

Cardiovascular applications of breath diagnostic testing are also emerging. For instance, two volatile hydrocarbons, ethane and pentane, are produced by the peroxidation of linoleic and linolenic acid, polyunsaturated fatty acids found in cellular membranes. These chemicals are oxidized during tissue ischemia and reperfusion injury.[88–94] Breath pentane has been found to be elevated in proportion to ischemia and inflammation in heart disease,[95–98] in cigarette smoking,[99] in ischemic bowel disease,[100] in cirrhosis,[101] in rheumatoid arthritis,[102] and even in schizophrenia.[103] Pentane may serve as a marker for reperfusion injury and could be used at the bedside to meter the rate of infusion of thrombolytic drugs or the percent of supplemental oxygen.

Phillips et al. demonstrated that the majority of 37 normal volunteers exhaled the same level of pentane as ambient air, some more and some less, with a normal distribution.[104] Cailleux established that a normal level of pentane is less than 10 pmol/L.[105]

Numerous literature reports have used gas chromatography or mass spectrometry, or both. Past breath analysis studies have been hampered by samples saturated with water vapor, variable ambient levels of gases being measured, ambient pentane dissolved in body fat, and co-elution of isoprene.[106] When exhaled gas is used to measure a process in the lung, exclusion of upper airway dead space gas may be necessary, but perhaps not when we are looking at diseases in other organs. Other measurement challenges have been related to earlier techniques of concentrating and detecting gases, using GC and MS, but may not remain problems with PFAIMS.

6.7.3 Diagnosis and Monitoring of Tuberculosis

Tuberculosis, one of the world's most prevalent killers, may be a diagnostic target particularly well suited for noninvasive diagnosis using DMS or IMS. Tuberculosis is caused by the obligate human pathogen, *Mycobacterium tuberculosis*. This bacterium currently infects~1 in 4 people worldwide. Each year, ~9 million cases of chronic TB infections become active, leading to both increased transmission and high morbidity. About 26% of those with active disease will die, making TB the eighth leading cause of death worldwide. The WHO lists TB as the fourth leading cause of disability adjusted life years (DALYs), a leading index for loss of per capita income and reduction in gross national product. Worldwide incidence of TB continues to increase dramatically, due in part to the rising prevalence of HIV/AIDS, which is associated with a negative catastrophic synergy with TB.

Treatment of TB is extensive and requires a minimum of three medications, each of which has important considerations and limitations to use. Inappropriate use of the medications has driven the emergence of multidrug-resistant isolates (MDR-TB) that have an extraordinarily poor prognosis and significantly increases the cost of therapy. Diagnosis and identification of chronic cases, which are then treated using a lower cost, more effective drug regimen is the most critical step in the management of TB. Unfortunately, definitive diagnosis requires laboratory culture of TB, a process that averages

15–19 days. For this reason, empiric use of anti-tuberculosis medications is widespread, resulting in further selection of MDR-TB isolates.

DMS technology can contribute to the control of the epidemic and the treatment of individual TB patients by capitalizing on the intersection between the instrumentation technology and modern bioinformatics. The respiratory form of TB produces a range of volatile organic compounds that are believed to be liberated into the exhaled breath of those with both chronic and active infections. Until very recently, ion separation technologies used on biomarkers lacked the sophistication to deconvolve these volatile organic signatures in a reproducible manner. Emerging proteomic algorithms coupled with DMS provide a method with which the fidelity and clarity of signatures may first be separated and subsequently identified by analyzing proteomic signatures.

6.7.4 Rapid Detection of Invasive Aspergillosis

Invasive aspergillosis (IA) is a leading cause of morbidity and death in patients with compromised immunity, particularly patients with hematologic malignancy and recipients of hematopoietic stem cell or solid organ transplantation. One of the major barriers to optimal care of these patients is the difficulty of identifying IA in its early stages—symptoms and radiologic findings are nonspecific, and existing microbiologic methods are insufficiently sensitive or specific to be reliable indicators of disease. Patients often require lung biopsies, which are technically difficult and risky in patients with compromised immunity and abnormal coagulation parameters.

In an immunocompromised host, IA can spread rapidly, with progressive pneumonia and even disseminated disease. Rapid, accurate, noninvasive identification of IA would improve clinical outcomes in these patients and guide efforts to prescribe antifungal therapy more precisely to patients who require treatment and spare those who do not—antifungal drugs are toxic, costly, and have numerous complicated interactions with other medications.

Aspergillus species are metabolically versatile, capable of producing secondary metabolites. It has been shown that *Aspergillus fumigatus* and other Aspergilli release unique sesquiterpene metabolite signatures unique to each species. In a proof-of-concept study analyzing breath samples from patients with suspected IA using thermal desorption GC-MS, a unique *A. fumigatus* sesquiterpene metabolite signature distinguished patients with IA from patients with other infections with 94% sensitivity and 93% specificity.[107] Detection of these metabolites has been translated onto a GC-DMS instrument, with identification of these metabolites within 30 min of breath sampling at the bedside (Figure 6.17).

Infections caused by other mold species are clinically similar to IA but are often optimally treated with other antifungal agents. There are no specific diagnostic modalities for these infections short of an invasive biopsy

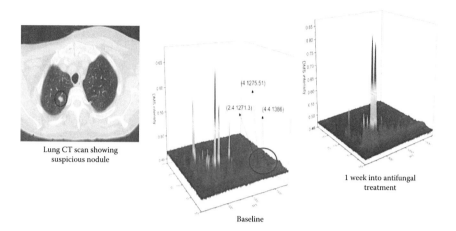

FIGURE 6.17
GC-DMS analysis of a breath sample from a patient with biopsy-proven invasive aspergillosis. Breath sample at baseline contains sesquiterpene secondary metabolites (circled in red), which disappeared after a week of effective antifungal therapy.

procedure. In *in vitro* studies, human pathogens such as the Mucorales, *Fusarium,* and *Scedosporium* have distinct secondary metabolite sesquiterpene signatures that distinguish them from *Aspergillus* species; these signatures may ultimately be harnessed for the noninvasive identification of infections caused by these fungal species and differentiation of these infections from IA.[108–110]

6.8 Conclusions

In the foregoing, DMS and FAIMS technologies have been described as a means to provide rapid, inexpensive, and unambiguous detection of analytes ranging from chemical species present in industrial processes or the environment to a host of biomarkers associated with various human diseases. The ability to obtain early detection of trace levels of signatures of human diseases in a noninvasive manner has the potential to revolutionize clinical diagnostics, and the data obtained for aspergillus detection and in a range of other applications show promise toward a novel approach to point-of-care diagnostics in settings far from advanced clinical care centers. As the technology continues to advance, its utilization as a clinical diagnostic is envisioned in doctor's offices and the home and in a wide range of developing world applications.

References

1. Eiceman G. and Z. Karpas. 2005. *Ion Mobility Spectrometry*, 2nd edn., CRC Press, Taylor & Francis LLC, Boca Raton, FL.
2. Buryakov I.A., E.V. Krylov et al. 1993. A new method of separation of multi-atomic ions by mobility at atmospheric pressure using a high-frequency amplitude-asymmetric strong electric field. *International Journal of Mass Spectrometry and Ion Processes* 128:143–148.
3. Makinen M., M. Nousiainen et al. 2011. Ion spectrometric detection technologies for ultra-traces of explosives: A review. *Mass Spectrometry Reviews* 30:940–973.
4. Bruins A.P. 1994. Atmospheric-pressure-ionization mass spectrometry: I. Instrumentation and ionization techniques. *TrAC: Trends in Analytical Chemistry* 13:37–43.
5. Gorshkov M.P. 1982. Inventor's certificate of USSR No. 966583, G01N27/62.
6. Avakov A.S., I.A. Buryakov et al. 1987. Mobility of multi-atomic ion species in air and new possibility of their separation. In: *Proceedings of the VII-th All-Union Conference on Low Temperature Plasma Physics*, Tashkent, Uzbek Republic.
7. Rasulev U.Kh., E.G. Nazarov et al. 1991. Identification of amine microimpurities in air-gas mixtures by means of surface ionization with a subsequent ion mobility separation of desorbing ions. In: *CIP 91 [Colloque international sur les procedes plasma] No8*, Antibes-Juanles-Pins, France, October 6, 1991, Vol. 47, pp. 409–411.
8. Buryakov I.A., E.V. Krylov et al. 1991. Analysis of ionic compositions of solutions using an ion gas analyzer. In: Malakhov V.V., ed. *Chemical Analysis of Environment*, Nauka, Novosibirsk, Russia, pp. 113–127.
9. Buryakov I.A., E.V. Krylov et al. 1991. Drift-spectrometer for trace amounts of amines in atmospheric air, Preprint #44. Arifov Institute of Electronics, Tashkent, Uzbekistan. Uzbek Academy of Sciences, p. 17.
10. Buryakov I.A., E.V. Krylov et al. 1991. Separation of ions according to mobility in a strong AC electric field. *Soviet Technical Physics Letters* 17:446–447.
11. Buryakov I.A., E.V. Krylov et al. 1993. Drift spectrometer for the control of amine traces in the atmosphere. *Journla of Analytical Chemistry* 48:156–165.
12. Carnahan B., S. Day et al. 1995. Development and applications of transverse field compensation ion mobility spectrometer. In: *Proceeding of Fourth International Workshop on IMS*, Cambridge, U.K.
13. Purves R.W. and R. Guevremont. 1999. Electrospray ionization high-field asymmetric waveform ion mobility spectrometry-mass spectrometry. *Analytical Chemistry* 71:2346–2357.
14. Guevremont R. and R.W. Purves. 1999. Atmospheric pressure ion focusing in a high-field asymmetric waveform ion mobility spectrometer. *Review of Scientific Instruments* 70:1370–1383.
15. Guevremont R. 2004. High-field asymmetric waveform ion mobility spectrometry: A new tool for mass spectrometry. *Journal of Chromatography A* 1058:3–19.
16. Nazarov E.G. and U.Kh. Rasulev. 1991. A surface ionization detector for amines, hydrazines, and their derivatives (SID). Science—Technical Advances. All-Union Institute of Scientific Information (VIMI), Moscow, Russia, Vol. 2, pp. 53–57.
17. Shvartsburg A.A., F. Li, K. Tang et al. 2006. High-resolution field asymmetric waveform ion mobility spectrometry using new planar geometry analyzers. *Analytical Chemistry* 78:3706–3714.

18. Guevremont R. 2001. High-field asymmetric waveform ion mobility spectrometry: A new tool for mass spectrometry. *Journal of Chromatography A* 1058:3–19.

19. Shvartsburg A.A., K. Tang et al. 2004. Understanding and designing field asymmetric waveform ion mobility spectrometry separations in gas mixtures. *Analytical Chemistry* 76:7366–7374.

20. Prieto M., T.A. Prox, and R.A. Yost. 2010. Design and evaluation of a novel hemispherical FAIMS cell. *International Journal of Mass Spectrometry* 298:41–44.

21. Marilyn P. and R.A. Yost. 2011. Spherical FAIMS: Comparison of curved electrode geometries. *International Journal for Ion Mobility Spectrometry* 14:61–69.

22. Miller R.A., G.A. Eiceman et al. 2000. A novel micromashined high-field asymmetric waveform-ion mobility spectrometer. *Sensors and Actuators B* 67:300–306.

23. Miller, R.A., E.G. Nazarov et al. 2001. A MEMS radio-frequency ion mobility spectrometer for chemical vapor detection. *Sensors and Actuators A* 91:301–312.

24. Eiceman G.A., E.G. Nazarov et al. 2002. A micro-machined planar field asymmetric IMS as a gas chromatographic detector. *Analyst* 127:466–471.

25. Nazarov E.G., R.A. Miller et al. 2002. Monitoring of trace amounts of sulfur compounds in air/hydrocarbon gas streams using a differential mobility spectrometer. *International Journal for IMS* 5(3):76–81.

26. Wilks A., M. Hart et al. 2012. Characterization of a miniature, ultra-high-field, ion mobility spectrometer. *International Journal for Ion Mobility Spectrometry* 15:199–222.

27. Mason E.A. and E.W. McDaniel. 1988. *Transport Properties of Ions in Gases*, Wiley, New York.

28. Schneider B.B., E.G. Nazarov et al. 2015. Differential mobility spectrometry/mass-spectrometry history, theory, design optimization, simulations, and applications. *Mass Spectrometry Reviews* 9999:1–51.

29. Schneider B.B., E.G. Nazarov et al. 2012. Peak capacity in differential mobility spectrometry: Effects of transport gas and gas modifiers. *International Journal for Ion Mobility Spectrometry* 15:141–150.

30. Anderson A.G., K.A. Markoski et al. 2008. DMS-IMS2, GC-DMS, DMS-MS: DMS hybrid devices combining orthogonal principles of separation for challenging applications. *Proceedings of SPIE* 6954:69540H (Apr.17).

31. Coy S.L., E.V. Krylov et al. 2008. DMS-prefiltered mass spectrometry for the detection of biomarkers. *Proceedings of SPIE* 6954:695411 (Apr.17).

32. Carr T.W., ed. 1984. *Plasma Chromatography*, Plenum Press, New York.

33. Petinarides J., M.T. Griffin et al. 2005. Implementation of a new technology for point detection. In: Gardner P.J., ed. *Chemical and Biological Sensing VI*, The International Society for Optical Engineering, Vol. 5, pp. 65–74, Bellingham, WA. Proceedings of SPIE: Volume 5795.

34. Limero Th., E. Reese et al. 2011. Preparation of a gas chromatograph-differential mobility spectrometer to measure target volatile organic compounds on the international space station. *International Journal for Ion Mobility Spectrometry* 14(2–3):81–91.

35. Limero Th., E. Reese et al. 2012. Results from the air quality monitor (gas-chromatograph-differential mobility spectrometer) experiment on board the international space station. *International Journal for Ion Mobility Spectrometry* 15:189–198.

36. Levin D.S., P.A. Vouros et al. 2006. Characterization of gas-phase molecular interactions on differential mobility ion behavior utilizing an electrospray ionization-differential mobility-mass spectrometer system. *Analytical Chemistry* 78(1):96–106.
37. Levin D.S., R.A. Miller et al. 2006. Rapid separation and quantitative analysis of peptides using a new nanoelectrospray-differential mobility spectrometer-mass spectrometer system. *Analytical Chemistry* 78(15):5443–5452.
38. Schneider B.B., T.R. Covey et al. Planar differential mobility spectrometer as a pre-filter for atmospheric pressure ionization mass spectrometry. *International Journal of Mass Spectrometry* 298:45–54.
39. Coy S.L., E.V. Krylov et al. 2010. Detection of radiation-exposure biomarkers by differential mobility pre-filtered mass spectrometry (DMS-MS). *International Journal of Mass Spectrometry* 291:108–117.
40. Hall A.B., S.L. Coy et al. 2013. Extending the dynamic range of the ion trap by differential mobility filtration. *Journal of the American Society for Mass Spectrometry* 24:1428–1436.
41. SCIEX. n.d. SelexION® ION Mobility Technology. https://sciex.com/products/ion-mobility-spectrometry/selexion-technology. Accessed March 20, 2017.
42. Tadjimukhamedov, F.Kh., A.U. Jackson et al. 2010. Evaluation of differential mobility spectrometer coupled to a miniature mass spectrometer. *Journal of the American Society for Mass Spectrometry* 21:1477–1481.
43. Manard M.J., R. Trainhama et al. 2010. Differential mobility spectrometry/mass spectrometry: The design of a new, field-portable mass spectrometer for real-time chemical analysis. *International Journal of Mass Spectrometry* 295:138–144.
44. Nazarov E.G. 2012. Differential ion mobility mass spectrometry—The next 5 years—Status and history of development. E-book *"Ion Mobility Mass Spectrometry—The Next 5 Years."* http://www.owlstonenanotech.com/ultrafaims/imsms-news/ebook-next-5-years. Accessed December 1, 2016.
45. Nazarov E.G., T.A. Postlethwaite et al. Planar differential mobility spectrometry as a powerful tool for gas phase ion separation and detection (Spectroscopy Solution: Premier Learning for Analytical Chemists). http://www.spectroscopy-solutions.org/Information/Archive/Featured-Articles/2220-/Planar-Differential-Mobility-Spectrometry-as-a-Powerful-Tool-for-Gas-Phase-Ion-Separation-and-Detection. Accessed December 1, 2016.
46. Schneider B.B., T.R. Covey et al. 2010. Control of chemical effects in the separation process of a differential mobility mass spectrometer system. *European Journal of Mass Spectrometry* 16(1):57–71.
47. Torok, T.J., R.V. Tauxe et al. 1997. A large community outbreak of salmonellosis caused by intentional contamination of restaurant salad bars. *JAMA* 278(5):389–395.
48. Keim, P., K.L. Smith et al. 2001. Molecular investigation of the Aum Shinrikyo anthrax release in Kameido, Japan. *Journal of Clinical Microbiology* 39(12):4566–4567.
49. Jernigan, J.A., D.S. Stephens et al. 2001. Bioterrorism-related inhalational anthrax: The first 10 cases reported in the United States. *Emerging Infectious Diseases* 7(6):933–944.
50. Okumura, T., N. Takasu et al. 1996. Report on 640 victims of the Tokyo subway sarin attack. *Annals of Emergency Medicine* 28(2):129–135.

51. Fernandez, M. and J. Weisman. 2004. Incident illustrates lapses in security net. Washington Post, February 4, 2004.

52. Meselson, M., J. Guillemin et al. 1994. The Sverdlovsk anthrax outbreak of 1979. *Science* 266(5188):1202–1208.

53. Darling, R.G., C.L. Catlett et al. 2002. Threats in bioterrorism. I: CDC category A agents. *Emergency Medicine Clinics of North America* 20(2):273–309.

54. Lee, M.A., G. Brightwell et al. 1999. Fluorescent detection techniques for real-time multiplex strand specific detection of Bacillus anthracis using rapid PCR. *Journal of Applied Microbiology* 87(2):218–223.

55. Makino, S.I., H.I. Cheun et al. 2001. Detection of anthrax spores from the air by real-time PCR. *Letters in Applied Microbiology* 33(3):237–240.

56. Turnbull, P.C., R.A. Hutson et al. 1992. Bacillus anthracis but not always anthrax. *Journal of Applied Bacteriology* 72(1):21–28.

57. Bruno, J.G. and J.L. Kiel. 1999. In vitro selection of DNA aptamers to anthrax spores with electrochemiluminescence detection. *Biosensors and Bioelectronics* 14(5):457–464.

58. Strizhkov, B.N., A.L. Drobyshev et al. 2000. PCR amplification on a microarray of gel-immobilized oligonucleotides: Detection of bacterial toxin- and drug-resistant genes and their mutations. *Biotechniques* 29(4):844–848, 850–842, 854 passim.

59. Higgins, J.A., M.S. Ibrahim et al. 1999. Sensitive and rapid identification of biological threat agents. *Annals of the New York Academy of Sciences* 894:130–148.

60. Uhl, J.R., C.A. Bell et al. 2002. Application of rapid-cycle real-time polymerase chain reaction for the detection of microbial pathogens: The Mayo-Roche Rapid Anthrax Test. *Mayo Clinic Proceedings* 77(7):673–680.

61. Phillips, A.P. and K.L. Martin. 1988. Investigation of spore surface antigens in the genus Bacillus by the use of polyclonal antibodies in immunofluorescence tests. *Journal of Applied Microbiology* 64(1):47–55.

62. Longchamp, P. and T. Leighton. 1999. Molecular recognition specificity of Bacillus anthracis spore antibodies. *Journal of Applied Microbiology* 87(2):246–249.

63. Yu, H. 1998. Comparative studies of magnetic particle-based solid phase fluorogenic and electrochemiluminescent immunoassay. *Journal of Immunological Methods* 218(1–2):1–8.

64. Zhou, B., P. Wirsching et al. 2002. Human antibodies against spores of the genus Bacillus: A model study for detection of and protection against anthrax and the bioterrorist threat. *Proceedings of the National Academy of Sciences USA* 99(8):5241–5246.

65. Shute, L.A., C.S. Gutteridge et al. 1984. Curie-point pyrolysis mass spectrometry applied to characterization and identification of selected Bacillus species. *Journal of General Microbiology* 130(2):343–355.

66. Wang, Z., K. Dunlop et al. 2002. Mass spectrometric methods for generation of protein mass database used for bacterial identification. *Analytical Chemistry* 74(13):3174–3182.

67. Demirev, P.A., Y.P. Ho et al. 1999. Microorganism identification by mass spectrometry and protein database searches. *Analytical Chemistry* 71(14):2732–2738.

68. Krishnamurthy, T., M.T. Davis et al. 1999. Liquid chromatography/microspray mass spectrometry for bacterial investigations. *Rapid Communications in Mass Spectrometry* 13(1):39–49.
69. Fox, A., G.E. Black et al. 1993. Determination of carbohydrate profiles of Bacillus anthracis and Bacillus cereus including identification of O-methyl methylpentoses by using gas chromatography-mass spectrometry. *Journal of Clinical Microbiology* 31(4):887–894.
70. Vaidyanathan, S., D.B. Kell et al. 2002. Flow-injection electrospray ionization mass spectrometry of crude cell extracts for high-throughput bacterial identification. *Journal of the American Society for Mass Spectrometry* 13(2):118–128.
71. Hathout, Y., P.A. Demirev et al. 1999. Identification of Bacillus spores by matrix-assisted laser desorption ionization-mass spectrometry. *Applied and Environmental Microbiology* 65(10):4313–4319.
72. Demirev, P.A., J. Ramirez et al. 2001. Tandem mass spectrometry of intact proteins for characterization of biomarkers from Bacillus cereus T spores. *Analytical Chemistry* 73(23):5725–5731.
73. Elhanany, E., R. Barak et al. 2001. Detection of specific Bacillus anthracis spore biomarkers by matrix-assisted laser desorption/ionization time-of-flight mass spectrometry. *Rapid Communications in Mass Spectrometry* 15(22):2110–2116.
74. Wang, Z., L. Russon et al. 1998. Investigation of spectral reproducibility in direct analysis of bacteria proteins by matrix-assisted laser desorption/ionization time-of-flight mass spectrometry. *Rapid Communications in Mass Spectrometry* 12(8):456–464.
75. Stowers, M.A., A.L. van Wuijckhuijse et al. 2000. Application of matrix-assisted laser desorption/ionization to on-line aerosol time-of-flight mass spectrometry. *Rapid Communications in Mass Spectrometry* 14(10):829–833.
76. Farquharson, S. and W.W. Smith. 2004. Differentiating bacterial spores from hoax materials by Raman spectroscopy, *Proceedings of SPIE*, 5269:9–15.
77. Pineda, F.J., J.S. Lin et al. 2000. Testing the significance of microorganism identification by mass spectrometry and proteome database search. *Analytical Chemistry* 72(16):3739–3744.
78. Jarman, K.H., S.T. Cebula et al. 2000. An algorithm for automated bacterial identification using matrix-assisted laser desorption/ionization mass spectrometry. *Analytical Chemistry* 72(6):1217–1223.
79. Phillips M. 1992. Breath tests in medicine. *Scientific American* July:74–79.
80. Zarling E.J. and M. Clapper. 1987. Technique for gas chromatographic measurement of volatile alkanes from single breath samples. *Clinical Chemistry* 33:140–141.
81. Phillips M. and J. Greenberg. 1992. Ion-trap detection of volatile organic compounds in alveolar breath. *Clinical Chemistry* 38:60–65.
82. Perman J.A., R.G. Barr et al. 1978. Sucrose malabsorption in children: Noninvasive diagnosis by interval breath hydrogen determination. *Journal of Pediatrics* 93:17–22.
83. Davidson G.P., T.A. Robb et al. 1984. Bacterial contamination of the small intestine as an important cause of chronic diarrhea and abdominal pain: Diagnosis by breath hydrogen test. *Pediatrics* 74:229–235.
84. Pauwels S., R. Fiasse et al. 1985. A simplified method of measuring breath hydrogen by end-expiratory sampling for diagnosis of lactose malabsorption. *Acta Clinica Belgica* 40:174–178.

85. Cheu H.W., D.R. Brown et al. 1989. Breath hydrogen excretion as a screening test for the early diagnosis of necrotizing enterocolitis. *American Journal of Diseases of Children* 143:156–159.

86. American Thoracic Society 1999. Recommendations for standardized procedures for the online and offline measurement of exhaled lower respiratory NO and nasal NO in adults and children. *American Journal of Respiratory and Critical Care Medicine* 160:2104–2117.

87. Djupesland P.G., W. Qian et al. 2001. A new method for the remote collection of nasal and exhaled NO. *Chest* 120:1645–1650.

88. Kharitonov P.P., D. Leak et al. 2000. Exhaled ethane, a marker of lipid peroxidation, is elevated in COPD. *American Journal of Respiratory and Critical Care Medicine* 162:369–373.

89. Morita S., M.T. Snider et al. 1986. Increased n-pentane excretion in humans: A consequence of pulmonary oxygen exposure. *Anesthesiology* 64:730–733.

90. Van Gossum A., R. Shariff et al. 1988. Increased lipid peroxidation after lipid infusion as measured by breath pentane output. *American Journal of Clinical Nutrition* 48:1394–1399.

91. Van Gossum A., J. De Cuyper et al. 1992. Assessment of lipid peroxidation in humans by breath pentane output measurement. *Acta Gastro-Enterologica Belgica* 55:245–248.

92. Jones M., N. Shiel et al. 1993. Application of breath pentane analysis to monitor age-related change in free radical activity. *Biochemical Society Transactions* 21:485S.

93. Kohlmuller D. and W. Kochen. 1993. Is n-pentane really an index of lipid peroxidation in humans and animals? A methodological reevaluation. *Analytical Biochemistry* 210:268–276.

94. Massias L., E. Postaire et al. 1993. Thermal desorption—Gas chromatographic determination of ethane and pentane in breath as potential markers of lipid peroxidation. *Biomedical Chromatography* 7:200–203.

95. Weitz Z.W., A.J. Birnbau et al. 1991. Skosey: High breath pentane concentrations during acute myocardial infarction. *Lancet* 337:933–935.

96. Mendis S., P.A. Sobotka et al. 1995. Breath pentane and plasma lipid peroxidases in ischemic heart disease. *Free Radical Biology and Medicine* 19:679–684.

97. Sobotka P.A., M.D. Brottman et al. 1993. Elevated breath pentane in heart failure reduced by free radical scavenger (captopril). *Free Radical Biology and Medicine* 14:643–647.

98. Sobotka P.A., D.K. Gupta et al. 1994. Breath pentane is a marker of acute cardiac allograft rejection. *Journal of Heart and Lung Transplantation* 13:224–229.

99. Euler D.E., S.J. Dave et al. 1996. Effect of cigarette smoking on pentane excretion in alveolar breath. *Clinical Chemistry* 42:303–308.

100. Kokoszka J., R.L. Nelson et al. 1993. Determination of inflammatory bowel disease activity by breath pentane analysis. *Diseases of the Colon & Rectum* 36:597–601.

101. Moscarella S., L. Caramelli et al. 1984. Effect of alcoholic cirrhosis on ethane and pentane levels in breath. *Bollettino della Società Italiana di Biologia Sperimentale* 60:529–533.

102. Humad S., E. Zarling et al. 1988. Breath pentane excretion as a marker of disease activity in rheumatoid arthritis. *Free Radical Research Communications* 5:101–106.

103. Phillips M., M. Sabas et al. 1993. Increased pentane and carbon disulfide in the breath of patients with schizophrenia. *Journal of Clinical Pathology* 46:861–864.
104. Phillips M., J. Greenberg et al. 1994. Alveolar gradient of pentane in normal human breath. *Free Radical Research* 20:333–337.
105. Cailleux A. and P. Allain. 1993. Is pentane a normal constituent of human breath? *Free Radical Research Communications* 18:323–327.
106. Springfield J.R. and M.D. Levitt. 1994. Pitfalls in the use of breath pentane measurements to assess lipid peroxidation. *Journal of Lipid Research* 35:1497–1504.
107. Koo S., H.R. Thomas et al. 2014. A breath fungal secondary metabolite signature to diagnose invasive aspergillosis. *Clinical Infectious Diseases* 59:1733–1740.
108. Yu X., M. Al-Kateb et al. 2016. *In Vitro Volatile Metabolite Signatures of Common Pathogenic Mucorales*, ASM Microbe, Boston, MA.
109. Yu X., S. Koshy et al. 2016. *In Vitro Volatile Metabolite Signatures of Common Pathogenic Fusarium Species*, IDWeek, New Orleans, LA.
110. Yu X., S. Koshy et al. 2016. *Examining the In Vitro Volatile Metabolite Profile of Pathogenic Scedosporium and Lomentospora Species*, IDWeek, New Orleans, LA.

Section II

Applications in Disease Detection

7

Rapid Diagnosis of Infectious Diseases Using Microfluidic Systems

Hardik Jeetendra Pandya, Mohamed Shehata Draz,
Majid Ebrahimi Warkiani, and Hadi Shafiee

CONTENTS

7.1 Introduction

Infectious diseases remain the primary public health challenge in many countries. Every year, infectious diseases account for more than 13 million deaths around the world, and for 30% of the total burden of disease. Developing countries are especially challenged with infectious diseases. According to world health organization (WHO), 50% of the total deaths in developing countries are attributed to various infections, including respiratory tract infections, diarrheal diseases, human immunodeficiency virus (HIV), tuberculosis, and malaria. In the healthcare system, a diagnostic cycle consists of several time-consuming steps besides sample transportation, pre- and post-analytical phases, result transmission, and batching practices augmenting the turnaround time from disease interpretation to results (Figure 7.1) [1–3]. The downside of experience-based empiric therapy management involves the choice of inappropriate antibiotherapy or late initiation of treatment often resulting in treatment failure [4–7].

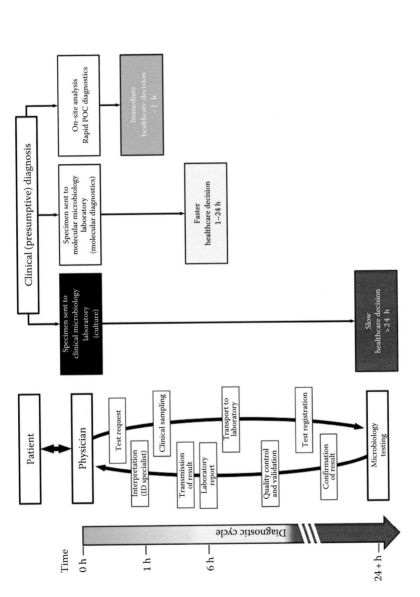

FIGURE 7.1
Personalized medicine in infectious disease management. The implementation of rapid point-of-care (POC) decreases the length of the diagnostic cycle in order to accelerate infectious disease management. (Reproduced from Bissonnette, L. and Bergeron, M.G., *J. Pers. Med.*, 2, 50, 2012. With permission.)

The development of efficient, rapid, and affordable diagnostic tests can have a major impact on the detection and control of infections, both in developed and developing countries. Recent technological advances have led to the emergence of new, rapid, and low-cost medical diagnostics, which are expected to revolutionize global healthcare systems and policies.

Microfluidics is one of the most important technologies that hold great promise for the management and control of infectious diseases. Microfluidics integrates multiple disciplines such as microfabrication, engineering, physics, and chemistry to enable the precise control and manipulation of fluids in the microscale environment. In combination with micro-electro-mechanical systems (MEMS) technology, advanced microfluidics platforms called lab-on-a-chip (LOC), point-of-care devices, or micro total analysis system (μTAS) were developed in which multiple preparations, analysis, and processing steps are integrated into one single chip. Microfluidic systems offer numerous advantages in medical diagnosis and bioanalytical applications, including minimal manual user intervention, lower sample consumption, shorter assay time, and enhanced data analysis and processing with full automation and portability [8–14]. Due to these numerous advantages, there is a great potential for this technology to be applied in the development of disposable, inexpensive, portable, and easy-to-use devices for detection of infectious diseases in a resource-limited setting [15–21]. In this chapter, we review the application of the microfluidics device and chips for detecting infectious diseases.

7.2 Microfluidic Devices and Chips for Infectious Diseases

Microfluidic platforms for infectious disease are divided into several categories based on their modalities. Here, we review (1) microfluidic devices based on optical detection: fluorescence [22–25], chemiluminescence [26,27], and absorbance [13,28–32]), (2) electrical sensing, and (3) centrifugal force-based sensing.

7.2.1 Microfluidics Based on Optical Detection

Optical detection is the most predominant method used in the microfluidic analyses due to the simplicity with which microfluidic devices can be coupled to various detection schemes, and their ability to detect low volume samples [33].

7.2.1.1 Fluorescence Microfluidics

A droplet-based device has dimensional scaling benefits which enable rapid and controlled mixing of fluids in the droplet reactors. This reduces the reaction time. A droplet-based microfluidic device for rapid detection of enzyme specific to *Mycobacterium tuberculosis* (Mtb) is shown in Figure 7.2.

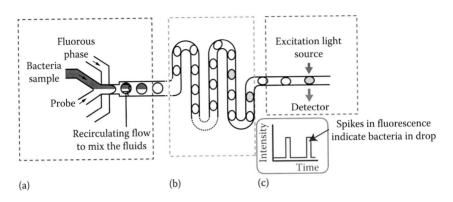

(a)   (b)   (c)

FIGURE 7.2

A schematic description of the droplet-based microfluidic device. The device consists of three parts: (a) Droplet generation and compartmentalization of the sample with probe. As droplets flow downstream in the microchannel, the content in the droplet is mixed rapidly. (b) Incubation for fluorescence to turn on. (c) Detection channel where the fluorescence from the drop is interrogated. (Reproduced from Moon, S. et al., *Biosens. Bioelectron*, 24, 3208–3214, 2009. With permission.)

The device works on the principle of isolation of bacteria from the picoliter droplets combined with a fluorescent probe by rapid detection of a reporter enzyme from Mtb. For Mtb detection, BlaC (an enzyme expressed/secreted by tubercle bacilli)-specific fluorogenic substrates as a probe are used [24]. The microfluidic channel facilitates the passing of the droplets formed by mixing fluorous phase, bacteria sample, and probe and fluorescence from the drop is interrogated in the detection zone for further analysis. The fluorescence from the drop is interrogated in the detection zone for further analysis. The device has the advantage of shortening the bacteria detection time by isolating the bacteria and the probe in a large number of picoliter droplets. Another advantage of the droplet-based microfluidic device for infectious diseases like Mtb is that due to a higher effective concentration of single bacterium in a smaller volume, the enzymatic reaction increases resulting in faster fluorescence signal in smaller drops.

Another example shows the capability of a fluorescent-based microchip to measure the CD4+ (a marker for HIV) percentage in real time from the microliter volume of blood (Figure 7.3). In this study, the microliter volume of blood is stained with fluorescent antibody without sample preparation. The device is connected to a computer via a charge-couple device (CCD) and the raw digital images are converted into absolute CD4+ counts and then into CD4 percentages [25]. A fluid delivery system is used to introduce the wash buffer and sample containing fluorescently stained lymphocytes in 0.9 μL of blood and to a capture flow cell. A fluorescence imaging station is used for capturing lymphocytes captured within the flow cell. The device was validated for its accuracy through testing in Botswana and the United States. The device was capable of discriminating clinically relevant CD4 thresholds with

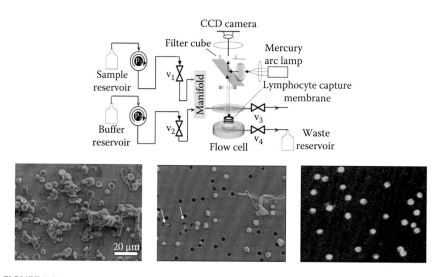

FIGURE 7.3

A fluorescent-based device for CD4+ T lymphocytes detection. The CD4+ lymphocytes were separated using a filter membrane in a microchip and counted using a CCD camera. Lymphocytes were selectively captured on the filter membrane in a microchip and stained for detection. Arrows show red blood cells passing through the filter membrane. (Reproduced from Rodriguez, W.R. et al., *PLOS Med.*, 2, e182, 2005. With permission.)

high specificity and sensitivity and showed close agreement with the standard flow cytometry (r = 0.95).

7.2.1.2 Colorimetric Microfluidics

Absorbance approaches like colorimetric detection are based on the color change of the detection system. The chemical/biochemical reactions between the colorimetric probes and target analytes result in the color change [28]. This facilitates the detection of analytes with the naked eye and eliminates the need of expensive camera for quantifying the results. This further eliminates the use of the bulky off-chip detection system [29]. Due to its unique advantages, the colorimetric has attracted interesting research for infectious disease detection [30–32]. A colorimetric microfluidic device developed by Sia et al. [13] demonstrates a low-cost POC with novel fluid handling, manufacturing, and signal processing techniques for detecting HIV for developing countries (Figure 7.4a). In this technique, the ELISA signals yielded by gold nanoparticle conjugated antibodies were amplified by silver-reduction amplification method. The results can be easily read by using a low-cost optical component such as LED even with the naked eye. The advantage of using this platform is threefold: (1) The device can be fabricated in a high-throughput manner at low cost as it uses injection molding compared to existing devices fabricated using silicon, glass, or Polydimethylsiloxane (PDMS). (2) Multistep reactions can be performed simultaneously by automatic delivery of multiple reagents using a bubble-based approach. This method does not require external instrumentation [34], electricity [34], or moving parts [35]. (3) A strong amplification of signals using minimum instrumentation was obtained using reduction of silver nanoparticles on to gold nanoparticles on a solid substrate in a continuous flow. The device could be integrated with the low-cost and robust optics as simpler to use as a cellular phone.

Figure 7.4b shows the technology for rapidly capturing and counting CD4 cells in an automated manner using magnetic bead and CD4 antibody. In this work, color intensity of the captured analytes was quantified using a smart phone showcasing the portability of this system [36].

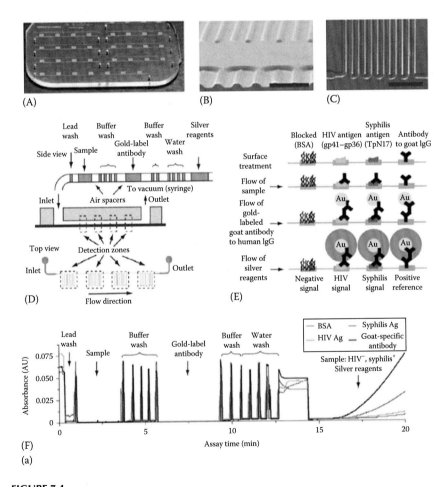

FIGURE 7.4

(a) ELISA-like-based HIV-1 detection on a microfluidic device. This method specifically detects anti-gp41 and anti-gp36 antibodies using an ELISA method. (a: Reproduced from Chin, C.D. et.al., *Lab Chip.*, 7, 41–57, 2007. With permission.) (*Continued*)

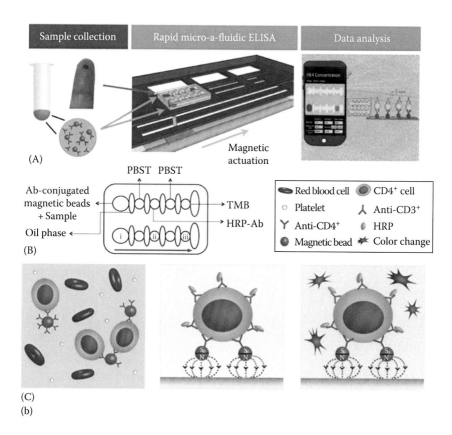

FIGURE 7.4 (*Continued*)
(b) Microfluidic ELISA assay (m-ELISA) to automatically isolate and quantify CD4 T lymphocytes in unprocessed whole blood samples. (b: Reproduced from Wang, S. et al., *Sci. Rep.*, 4, 3796, 2014. With permission.)

The advantage of this system is that unlike traditional techniques like flow-based ELISA, it does not require sample processing (i.e., cell fixing) to detect and capture the cells from whole blood. In addition, the micro-a-fluidic ELISA was capable of measuring CD4 T cell counts with an accuracy of 97% tested on whole blood samples from 35 patients at the clinical cut off of 350 cells/μL. Thus, in resource-limited settings, to detect CD4 in patients suffering from HIV, the m-ELISA offers a "plug-and-play" solution.

Colorimetric-based microfluidic systems have also been utilized for the detection of malaria. The microfluidic device shown in Figure 7.5 uses a nitrocellulose strip and can be used to detect malaria by detecting proteins derived from the blood. Blood obtained from the finger prick (usually around 5–20 μL) is placed on the strip and lysed to release the antigens within the red blood cells. The serum obtained contains the parasites within the cells (variable

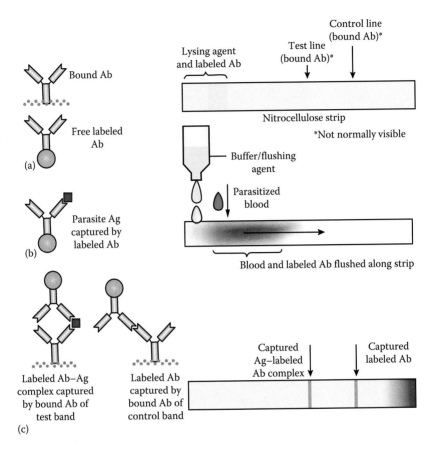

FIGURE 7.5
Schematic of the lateral flow strip chip to diagnose malaria. (Top) Device preparation with nitro-cellulose strip, (middle) operation principle of a lateral flow strip chip, and (bottom) expected results of a lateral flow strip. (Reprinted by permission from Macmillan Publishers Ltd. *Nat. Rev. Microbiol.*, Bell, D., Wongsrichanalai, C., and Barnwell, J.W., Ensuring quality and access for malaria diagnosis: How can it be achieved? 4, 682–695. Copyright 2006.)

amount of antibodies). As shown in the figure, the dye-labeled antibody specific for the target (antigen) is present at the lower end of the strip. The blood and buffer placed on the strip mix with the labeled antibody and are drawn up the strip. The labeled antibody is trapped on the test line if antigen is present and dye will be visible to the naked eye thus making it simple to use.

7.2.1.3 Chemiluminescence Microfluidics

Chemiluminescence-based microfluidic devices are based on using light emitted from the chemical reaction. A microfluidic chip with microfabricated pillars is developed to increase the contact area with the cells (Figure 7.6).

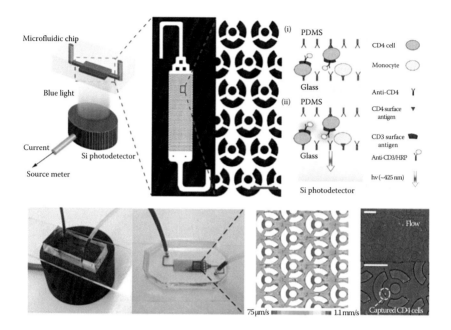

FIGURE 7.6
A microfluidic device for capturing and counting CD4$^+$ T lymphocytes using a chemilumi-nescence-based method. (Reproduced from Wang, Z. et al., *Anal. Chem.*, 82, 36–40, 2010. With permission.)

A small volume (3 µL) of human whole blood was passed on the chip to mea-sure the capture efficiency of CD4 T-cells. To eliminate the signal from cap-tured monocytes, anti-CD3 antibody was used for detection. After the CD4$^+$ cells are captured in the chamber, a luminol and H$_2$O$_2$ mixture was intro-duced into the chip and a silicon photodiode was used to monitor the mag-nitude of the light from the chemiluminescence. The difference in the current generated from the photodiode was used to generate a relation between the CD4 counts and measured photocurrent [27]. The results obtained at the end of the assay can be provided automatically and digitally.

7.2.1.4 Lens-Less Shadow Imaging

Lens-less shadow imaging is another approach of using a microfluidic device by leveraging the potential of CCD sensor and microfluidic device for point-of-care applications [38–40]. Using the lens-less imaging technique we can obtain aberration-free images, have large field of view and high-resolution imaging [38].

The microfluidic device shown in Figure 7.7 was used for capturing and counting CD4$^+$ from whole blood sample (<10 µL) without any pre-processing by emitting white light which passes through the glass slide

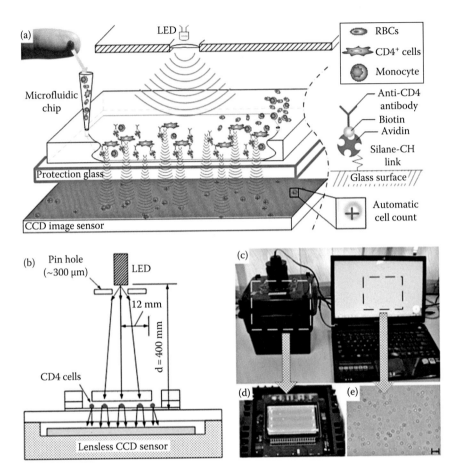

FIGURE 7.7
Lens-less ultra-wide-field cell monitoring array–based shadow imaging (LUCAS). (Reproduced from Moon, S. et al., *PLOS ONE*, 6, e21409, 2011. With permission.)

where CD4+ cells are captured and diffracted shadow signals of the cells fall on to the CCD image sensor. A ring diameter of the captured cells can be optimized by adjusting the distance between the CCD surface and captured cells. The preceding method does not require antibody-based fluorescent labeling and the results are produced within 10 min. The platform is inexpensive (<$1 materials costs) and contains a portable disposable microchip.

7.2.2 Electrical Sensing

Electrical sensing in microfluidic chips is insensitive to light intensity, cheaper, simpler, and a powerful modality to create sensitive portable biosensors [41–44]. Figure 7.8a shows a microfluidic device for counting CD4 cells using impedance spectroscopy. In this method, cells are immobilized inside

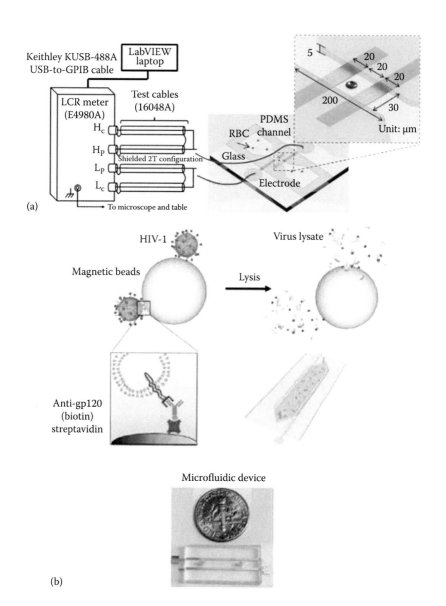

FIGURE 7.8
(a) Microfluidic device for differentiating *P. falciparum*-infected RBCs from uninfected RBCs.
(b) Electrical sensing of viral lysate on-chip for HIV-1 detection and viral load measurement
at the point of care. (a: Reproduced from Du, E. et.al., *Lab Chip*, 13 (19), 3903–3909, 2013. With
permission; b: Reproduced from Shafiee, H. et.al., *Small*, 9, 2553–2563, 2013. With permission.)

a microfluidic channel followed by lysing. A low-conductive, hypotonic media is used for lysing the cells causing the conductivity of the surrounding medium to change due to ions released from the lysed cells. The change in the impedance is measured by the interdigitated electrodes integrated within the microfluidic device. In point-of-care settings, this device can be used as a handheld instrument to provide affordable, fast, and simple cell counting.

Ducrée et al. [45] proposed a microfluidic device (Figure 7.8a) with integrated electrodes for studying the alterations during the multistage life of *Plasmodium falciparum* in red blood cells (RBCs) using electrical impedance measurement.

The device measured the change in impedance based on the capacitor formation upon cell crossing the electrodes integrated in the channel. The electrical properties (impedance) of the host RBCs change due to the biochemical alterations during the multi-stage life cycle of *P. falciparum*.

The microfluidic device could study the life of *P. falciparum* corresponding to the change in impedance of the host RBCs. The proposed platform can be potentially used as a non-invasive diagnostic tool for cell separation and a variety of diseases.

While, HIV-1 at early stage with a low concentration of antibody was not detectable with the current rapid POC HIV tests such as Unigold and OraQuick® Rapid HIV-1/2 Test, our recent work on label-free electronic biosensor showed a reliable and repeatable early-stage HIV-1 detection capability of the microchip by using viral lysate (Figure 7.8b). Streptavidin-coated magnetic beads conjugated with biotinylated anti-gp120 antibodies diluted in Dulbecco's phosphate-buffered saline (DPBS) without viruses were used as control samples. The magnetic beads with and without viruses were washed four times with 20% glycerol and were resuspended in 1% Triton X-100. The impedance magnitudes of the control samples and lysed HIV-1 was measured subsequently. Further, the presented technology could potentially be applied to measure other infectious diseases like malaria, tuberculosis, influenza, and hepatitis.

7.2.3 Centrifugal Force-Based Sensing

Centrifugal microfluidic technology includes rotating the microfluidic disc at various spinning rates generating Euler, centrifugal, and Coriolis forces that can be applied to various microfluidic device operations [16,45–51]. The centrifugal force-based sensing combines the benefits of both centrifugal forces and microfluidics in a single device. In addition, these devices are capable of pumping liquids in a wide range of flow and by alternating the direction of rotation, mixing can be easily accomplished [52]. For *in-vitro* diagnostics (IVD), centrifugal microfluidic technology has been identified as a strong candidate and has achieved significant commercial success [16,49]. Major multinationals such as 3M, and Roche among others, offer commercial products based on this technology.

Figure 7.9 shows a centrifugal-microfluidic "LabDisk" system as a point-of-care analyzer for rapid and highly sensitive pathogen detection. The

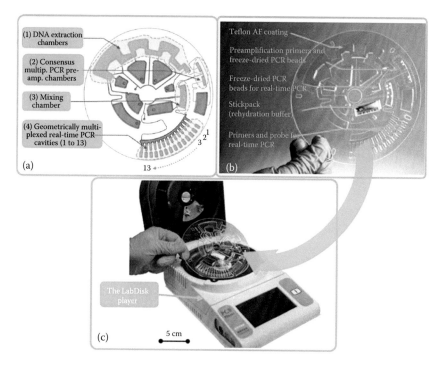

FIGURE 7.9

LabDisk design and LabDisk player. (a) LabDisk structure including DNA extraction chambers, consensus multiplex PCR preamplification chamber, mixing chamber, and 13 real-time PCR amplification chambers. (b) Structured LabDisk with prestored dry and liquid PCR reagents. (c) The portable LabDisk player for processing the LabDisk at the point-of-care. (Reproduced from Czilwik, G. et. al., *Lab Chip*, 15, 3749–3759, 2015. With permission.)

unit contains pre-stored reagents for performing automated multiplex PCR preamplification, geometrically multiplexed real-time PCR, and integrated DNA extraction.

The unit is capable of detecting low concentrations of various pathogens (5 colony-forming units [cfu] of *Escherichia coli*, 2 cfu of *Haemophilus influenza*, and 3 cfu of *Staphylococcus warneri*) in a 200 μL serum sample. The turnaround time from sample loading to analysis is around 3 h and 45 min.

Other examples of sensing methods are electrochemical [53], mass, or mechanical forces [54]. The drawback of the electrochemical sensing is that they are limited to only reagents and enzymes capable of producing the electrochemical reaction. However, with mechanical sensors there are still questions regarding its robustness necessary for POC diagnostic devices. Thus, we have not included the details about its mechanisms and application for infectious diseases in this chapter. While the research and feasibility of the microfluidic devices for infectious diseases have been rapid, the translation and commercialization is only the beginning of the reality.

In this chapter, we have focused on the recent microfluidic devices for the detection of infectious diseases. However, there are numerous micro/nano-technology-based devices used for point-of-a-care applications for infectious diseases. The impact of these devices is limitless, and in the near future it would potentially be available in every home like any other technology and would revolutionize the delivery of medical care. The question is how ready are we to get mesmerized by these amazing devices?

References

1. Faulstich K. and Haberstroh K., Handheld and portable test systems for decentralized testing: From lab to marketplace. *Proc. SPIE* 2009, 7306, 73060H1–73060H8.
2. Schimke I., Quality and timeliness in medical laboratory testing. *Anal. Bioanal. Chem.* 2009, 393, 1499–1504.
3. Bissonnette L. and Bergeron M.G., Infectious disease management through point-of-care personalized medicine molecular diagnostic technologies. *J. Pers. Med.* 2012, 2, 50–70.
4. Micek S.T., Welch E.C., Khan J., Pervez M., Doherty J.A., Reichley R.M., Hoppe-Bauer J., Dunne W.M., and Kollef M.H., Resistance to empiric antimicrobial treatment predicts outcome in severe sepsis associated with gram-negative bacteremia. *J. Hosp. Med.* 2011, 6, 405–410.
5. Nicolau D.P., Current challenges in the management of the infected patient. *Curr. Opin. Infect. Dis.* 2011, 24 (Suppl. 1), S1–S10.
6. Kumar A., Roberts D., Wood K.E. et al., Duration of hypotension before initiation of antimicrobial therapy is the critical determinant of survival in human septic shock. *Crit. Care Med.* 2006, 34, 1589–1596.
7. Lin J.-N., Lai C.-H., Chen Y.-H., Chang L.-L., Lu P.-L., Tsai S.-S., Lin H.-L., and Lin H.-H., Characteristics and outcomes of polymicrobial bloodstream infections in the emergency department: A matched case-control study. *Acad. Emerg. Med.* 2010, 17, 1072–1079.
8. Yetisen A.K., Akram M.S., and Christopher R. Lowe, paper-based microfluidic point-of-care diagnostic devices. *Lab Chip* 2013, 13, 2210–2251.
9. Huckle D., Point-of-care diagnostics: Will the hurdles be overcome this time? *Expert Rev. Med. Devices* 2006, 3, 421–426.
10. Petti C.A., Polage C.R., Quinn T.C., Ronald A.R., and Sande M.A., Laboratory medicine in Africa: A barrier to effective health care. *Clin. Infect. Dis.* 2006, 42, 377–382.
11. El-Ali J., Sorger P.K., and Jensen K.F., Cells on chips. *Nature* 2006, 442, 403–411.
12. Nge P.N., Rogers C.I., and Woolley A.T., Advances in microfluidic materials, functions, integration, and applications. *Chem. Rev.* 2013, 113, 2550–2583.
13. Chin C.D. et al., Microfluidics-based diagnostics of infectious diseases in the developing world. *Nat. Med.* 2011, 17, 1015–1019.
14. Myers F.B. and Lee L.P., Innovations in optical microfluidic technologies for point-of-care diagnostics. *Lab Chip* 2008, 8, 2015–2031.

15. Siegrist J., Peytavi R., Bergeron M.G., and Madou M., Microfluidics for IVD analysis: Triumphs and hurdles of centrifugal platforms—Part 1: Molecular fundamentals. *IVD Technol.* 2009, 15 (9), 27–33.

16. Gorkin R., Park J., Siegrist J., Amasia M., Lee B.S., Park J.-M., Kim J., Kim H., Madou M., and Cho Y.-K., Centrifugal microfluidics for biomedical applications. *Lab Chip* 2010, 10, 1758–1773.

17. Lien K.-Y. and Lee G.-B., Miniaturization of molecular biological techniques for gene assay. *Analyst* 2010, 135, 1499–1518.

18. Siegrist J., Peytavi R., Bergeron M.G., and Madou M., Microfluidics for IVD Analysis: Triumphs and hurdles of centrifugal platforms—Part 2: Centrifugal microfluidics. *IVD Technol.* 2010, 16 (1), 41–47.

19. Ferguson R.S., Buchsbaum S.F., Wu T.-T., Hsieh K., Xiao Y., Sun R., and Soh H.T., Genetic analysis of H1N1 influenza virus from throat swab samples in a microfluidic system for point-of-care diagnostics. *J. Am. Chem. Soc.* 2011, 133, 9129–9135.

20. Schumacher S., Nestler J., Otto T. et al., Highly-integrated lab-on-a-chip system for point-of-care multiparameter analysis. *Lab Chip* 2012, 12, 464–473.

21. Becker H. and Gärtner C., Polymer microfabrication technologies for microfluidic systems. *Anal. Bioanal. Chem.* 2008, 390, 89–111.

22. Moon S., Keles H.O., Ozcan A. et al., Integrating microfluidics and lensless imaging for point-of-care testing. *Biosens. Bioelectron.* 2009, 24, 3208–3214.

23. Rosenfeld L., Lyu F., Cheng Y., Rao J., and Tang S.K.Y., RAPID detection of tuberculosis using droplet based microfluidics, in *18th International Conference on Miniaturized Systems for Chemistry and Life Sciences*, San Antonio, TX, October 26–30, 2014.

24. Wealth Health Organization, Fluorescent light-emitting diode (LED) microscopy for diagnosis of tuberculosis: Policy statement, Geneva, Switzerland, 2011.

25. Rodriguez W.R., Christodoulides N., Floriano P.N. et al., A microchip CD4 counting method for HIV monitoring in resource-poor settings. *PLOS Med.* 2005, 2, e182.

26. Sia S.K. and Whitesides G.M., Microfluidic devices fabricated in poly (dimethylsiloxane) for biological studies. *Electrophoresis* 2003, 24, 3563–3576.

27. Wang Z., Chin S.Y., Chin C.D. et al., Microfluidic CD4+ T-cell counting device using chemiluminescence-based detection. *Anal. Chem.* 2010, 82, 36–40.

28. Vilela D., González M.C., and Escarpa A., Sensing colorimetric approaches based on gold and silver nanoparticles aggregation: Chemical creativity behind the assay. A review. *Anal. Chim. Acta* 2012, 751, 24–43.

29. Wu L. and Qu X., Cancer biomarker detection: Recent achievements and challenges. *Chem. Soc. Rev.* 2015, 44, 2963–2997.

30. Li X., Ballerini D.R., and Shen W., A perspective on paper-based microfluidics: Current status and future trends. *Biomicrofluidics* 2012, 6, 011301-1–011301-13.

31. Gao Z., Xu M., Lu M., Chen G., and Tang D., Urchin-like (gold core)@(platinum shell) nanohybrids: A highly efficient peroxidase-mimetic system for in situ amplified colorimetric immunoassay. *Biosens. Bioelectron.* 2015, 70, 194–201.

32. Fang W.-F., Chen W.-J., and Yang J.-T., Colorimetric determination of DNA concentration and mismatches using hybridization-mediated growth of gold nanoparticle probes. *Sens. Actuators B* 2014, 192, 77–82.

33. Baker C.A., Duong C.T., Grimley A., and Roper M.G., Recent advances in microfluidic detection systems. *Bioanalysis* 2009, 1 (5), 967–975.

34. Thorsen T., Maerkl S.J., and Quake S.R., Microfluidic large-scale integration. *Science* 2002, 298, 580–584.

35. Oh K.W. and Ahn C.H., A review of microvalves. *J. Micromech. Microeng.* 2006, 16, R13–R39.

36. Wang S., Tasoglu S., Chen P.Z. et al., Micro-a-fluidics ELISA for rapid CD4 cell count at the point-of-care. *Sci. Rep.* 2014, 4, 3796.

37. Bell D., Wongsrichanalai C., and Barnwell J.W., Ensuring quality and access for malaria diagnosis: How can it be achieved? *Nat. Rev. Microbiol.* 2006, 4, 682–695.

38. Moon S., Gurkan U.A., Blander J. et al., Enumeration of CD4$^+$ T-cells using a portable microchip count platform in Tanzanian HIV-infected patients. *PLOS ONE* 2011, 6, e21409.

39. Inci F., Tokel O., Wang S., Gurkan U.A., Tasoglu S., Kuritzkes D.R., and Demirci U., Nanoplasmonic quantitative detection of intact viruses from unprocessed whole blood. *ACS Nano* June 2013, 7 (6), 4733–4745.

40. Shafiee H., Lidstone E., Jahangir M., Inci F., Hanhauser E., Henrich T.J., Kuritzkes D.R., Cunningham B.T., and Demirci U., Nanostructured optical photonic crystal biosensor for HIV viral load measurement. *Sci. Rep.* January 2014, 4, 4116.

41. Cheng X., Liu Y.S., Irimia D. et al., Cell detection and counting through cell lysate impedance spectroscopy in microfluidic devices. *Lab Chip* 2007, 7, 746–755.

42. Holmes D. and Morgan H., Single cell impedance cytometry for identification and counting of CD4 T-cells in human blood using impedance labels. *Anal. Chem.* 2010, 82, 1455–1461.

43. Watkins N.N., Sridhar S., Cheng X. et al., A microfabricated electrical differential counter for the selective enumeration of CD4$^+$ T lymphocytes. *Lab Chip* 2011, 11, 1437–1447.

44. Shafiee H., Jahangir M., Inci F. et al., Acute on-chip HIV detection through label-free electrical sensing of viral nano-lysate. *Small* 2013, 9, 2553–2563.

45. Ducrée J., Haeberle S., Brenner T., Glatzel T., and Zengerle R., Patterning of flow and mixing in rotating radial microchannels. *Microfluid. Nanofluid.* 2006, 2, 97–105.

46. Lai S., Wang S., Luo J., Lee L.J., Yang S.T., and Madou M.J., Design of a compact disk-like microfluidic platform for enzyme-linked immunosorbent assay. *Anal. Chem.* 2004, 76, 1832–1837.

47. Du E., Ha S., Diez-Silva M., Dao M., Suresh S., Chandrakasan A.P., Electric impedance microflow cytometry for characterization of cell disease states. *Lab Chip* 2013, 13 (19), 3903–3909.

48. Burger R., Kitsara M., Gaughran J., Nwankire C., and Ducrée J., *Future Med. Chem.* 2014, 72–92.

49. Roy E., Stewart G., Mounier M., Malic L., Peytavi R., Clime L., Madou M., Bossinot M., Bergeron M.G., and Veres T., *Lab Chip* 2015, 15, 406–416.

50. Czilwik G., Messinger T., Strohmeier O., Wadle S., Von Stetten F., Paust N., Roth G., Zengerle R., and Saarinen P., Rapid and fully automated bacterial pathogen detection on a centrifugal-microfluidic LabDisk using highly sensitive nested PCR with integrated sample preparation, *Lab Chip* 2015, 15, 3749–3759.

51. Michael I.J., Kim T.H., Sunkara V., and Cho Y.K., Challenges and opportunities of centrifugal microfluidics for extreme point-of-care testing. *Micromachines* 2016, 7 (32), 1–14.

52. Ducrée J., Haeberle S., Lutz S., Pausch S., Von Stetten F., and Zengerle R., The centrifugal microfluidic platform. *J. Micromech. Microeng.* 2007, 17, S103–S115.

53. De Souza Castilho M. and Laube T., Magneto immunoassays for *Plasmodium falciparum* histidine-rich protein 2 related to malaria based on magnetic nanoparticles. *Anal. Chem.* 2011, 83 (14), 5570–5577.

54. Sharma M.K., Rao V.K., Merwyn S., Agarwal G.S., Upadhyay S., and Vijayaraghavan R., A novel piezoelectric immunosensor for the detection of malarial *Plasmodium falciparum* histidine rich protein-2 antigen. *Talanta* September 2011, 85 (4), 1812–1817.

8

Microfluidics for Tuberculosis Diagnosis: Advances, Scalability, and Challenges

Bhavna G. Gordhan and Bavesh D. Kana

CONTENTS

8.1 Background

8.1.1 Current Tuberculosis Pandemic

Tuberculosis (TB) is an infectious disease transmitted by the airborne bacterium *Mycobacterium tuberculosis* that commonly attacks the lungs but can cause disease in almost any part of the body. A healthy immune system provides adequate defense against TB disease, as 60% of infected adults are able to completely eradicate the infecting bacteria. TB disease dynamics are complex and can range from containment of the organisms in lung lesions with the absence of symptoms, referred to as latent TB infection (LTBI), to an active life-threatening contagious disease state. In the case of the latter, patients display symptoms such as coughing, fever, weight loss, fatigue, and night sweats (Dheda et al. 2016a). Clinically, LTBI is a nontransmissible state while active pulmonary TB is highly transmissible via aerosolized droplets generated during coughing and sneezing by an infected individual (Dheda et al. 2016a). In healthcare settings, the risk of the caregiver acquiring TB is managed by using protective N95 respirators/masks, ventilation systems, keeping potentially infectious patients separate from others, and the regular screening of healthcare workers for TB. A key feature that has hampered ultimate eradication of TB from human society is the lack of effective, rapid point of care (POC) diagnostics. This is evidenced by the fact that smear microscopy, a method developed a century ago, still forms the basis of most TB national priority control programs. Miniaturization of TB detection systems using microfluidic platforms holds great promise to change the landscape of modern TB, but these efforts have been hampered by the complex clinical presentation of TB and difficulty in identifying low numbers of infecting organisms. In this chapter, we provide a brief background and current status of the TB epidemic, drug treatment, vaccination, and disease manifestation in vulnerable populations, which together outline the diagnostic challenges with TB. While no microfluidic diagnostic platform has been rolled out for TB in endemic countries, significant strides have been made in the development and implementation of molecular diagnostics, which now set the scene for POC microfluidic platforms. We detail these molecular diagnostic platforms and follow this with a discussion on the state of the art for TB microfluidic diagnostics that are in development. We also outline the challenges in scaling up these interventions and integrating them into healthcare systems.

8.1.2 Epidemiology and Spread of TB Disease

In 2015, 10.4 million people fell ill with TB (5.9 million men, 3.5 million women, and 1 million children), with 1.8 million people succumbing to the disease, of which 0.4 million were HIV-coinfected (WHO 2016). In 2014, 80% of TB cases were concentrated in 22 high-burden countries with 58% of the 9.6 million new TB cases concentrated in South-East Asia and Western Pacific regions. Five countries, India, Indonesia, China, Nigeria, and Pakistan, accounted for 54% of all new cases. The African region accounted for 28% of the world's TB cases in 2014 but had the most severe burden relative to population with 281 cases for every 100,000 people, more than double the global average of 133 (WHO 2015b). Moreover, the HIV epidemic has severely fueled TB disease and accounted for 1.2 million (12%) TB infections with 0.4 million (25%) deaths in 2014 (WHO 2015a).

Increasing multi-drug resistant TB (MDR-TB) and extensively drug resistant TB (XDR-TB) cases are a constant threat to the eradication of TB and in 2015, 480,000 people developed MDR-TB although only a quarter of these cases received formal diagnosis (WHO 2016). Hundred and five countries reported XDR-TB by 2015, which comprised 9.7% of TB misdiagnosed as MDR-TB. These resistant forms of TB are equally transmissible when compared to their drug-susceptible counterparts but have lower cure rates and higher fatalities as the treatment is less effective, more toxic, expensive, and the required medicines may not be available (Raviglione 2006). Globally in 2014, only 50% of MDR-TB patients were successfully treated; however, the 2015 treatment success target of $\geq 75\%$ for MDR-TB patients was reached by 43 out of the 127 countries. XDR-TB patients failing therapy continue to transmit the infection to other patients and healthcare workers, propagating the spread of resistant strains (Gandhi et al. 2006, Harries et al. 2003, Millen et al. 2008).

Women represent a notable vulnerable population as TB is one of the top five killer diseases of women aged 20–50 years with 480,000 deaths in 2014, 140,000 of whom were co-infected with HIV. Women of reproductive age are more likely to develop TB but are less likely to seek help for TB symptoms due to various socio-cultural and socio-economic issues (Connolly and Nunn 1996). While TB treatment is safe during pregnancy, increased side effects have been reported. Maternal TB infection has also been linked to complications such as premature birth, low birth weight, and is a leading cause of death due to an infectious disease during pregnancy and delivery, especially among women living with HIV (Bekker et al. 2016).

In the face of these alarming TB death estimates, major effort has been made over the last decade to reduce and halt TB incidence. TB mortality has fallen 47% since 1990 with nearly all the improvements taking place since 2000, when the Millennium Development Goals were set. An estimated 43 million lives have been saved between 2000 and 2014 due to effective diagnosis and treatment of TB. Globally TB incidence has fallen steadily by an average of

1.5% per year since 2000, and currently it is 18% lower than that reported in 2000. Despite these advances in reducing TB mortality rates, a number of countries are still not on track to meet the UN-set goals to reduce TB infections. While 9 out of the 22 high-burden countries have met the WHO targets for reduction in TB infections and deaths ahead of the 2015 deadline, 11 countries including Russia, South Africa, and Pakistan are not on track to reduce the TB incidence, prevalence, and mortality. In 2014, 6 million new TB cases were reported to the WHO, which is less than two-thirds (63%) of the 9.6 million people estimated to have fallen sick with the disease, which suggests that globally more than a third (37%) of new cases were undiagnosed or unreported. These missed cases are a cause for concern as these individuals continue to transmit the disease. Clearly, stronger policy and health systems interventions are needed to close this gap in TB case detection.

8.1.3 Drug Treatment and Resistance

TB is curable with antibiotics and rapid diagnosis enhances cure rates and prevents transmission as an individual with untreated disease can transmit to 10–15 other people each year (WHO 2016). Standard treatment for TB involves a 6-month regimen of four first line antimicrobials that include rifampicin (RIF), isoniazid (INH), ethambutol, and pyrazinamide. Drug-resistant TB can develop owing to incorrect or incomplete treatment due to patient non-compliance, intermittent drug shortages, and poor monitoring of TB patients on chemotherapy. The protracted treatment with the four-drug combination often results in severe side effects, which deter people from completing treatment, especially if symptoms subside. Drug-resistant forms of TB have equal propensity for transmission as drug-susceptible TB but cannot be cured with the standard 6-month treatment prescribed for drug-susceptible TB (Dheda et al. 2016b, Seddon et al. 2012, Tam et al. 2009).

The TB pandemic has been defined by the occurrence of complex forms of drug resistance, which require treatment with drugs that are less effective, toxic, and costly. Moreover, treatment takes up to 2 years with low cure rates and high fatalities (Jeon et al. 2011). MDR-TB is defined as a disease causing *M. tuberculosis* strains that are resistant to INH and RIF. XDR-TB disease, often associated with a high mortality where 70% of patients die within a month of diagnosis, is not only resistant to RIF and INH but also to one fluoroquinolone and one of the three injectable second line aminoglycosides (Gandhi et al. 2006, Muller et al. 2013). For these reasons, the WHO's global plan to stop TB (2011–2015) recommended monitoring adherence of patients with drug-susceptible TB to the standardized treatment regimen through directly observed treatment (DOT), thus reducing their risk of developing MDR-TB. Limiting the spread of drug-resistant TB through strong infection control measures such as isolating infectious patients and using respirators are expected to have notable impact. Furthermore, reliable and affordable supply of high-quality drugs, particularly in high-burden countries, together with appropriate laboratory facilities to diagnose MDR-TB and XDR-TB is important for good treatment outcomes (Parsons et al. 2011).

8.1.4 Impact of HIV on TB Disease and Diagnosis

The maturation of the HIV pandemic has added to the global burden of TB and the two diseases are a lethal combination, each speeding the other's progress with deadly outcomes (Osman et al. 2015). In HIV-infected individuals, the lack of CD4+ T-cells leads to poor containment of *M. tuberculosis* to lung lesions, and as a result bacteria readily traffic out of the lungs to other compartments in the body thus giving rise to extra-pulmonary TB (Barthwal et al. 2005, Spalgais et al. 2013). Hence, sputa from HIV-infected individuals usually contain low numbers of bacteria, making diagnosis using standard culture methods challenging (Padmapriyadarsini et al. 2011). Early diagnosis of both diseases is central to reducing deaths from co-infection and requires careful management and monitoring of TB medication and antiretroviral therapy (ART) to avoid adverse drug interactions and side effects in patients (Manosuthi et al. 2016). Treatment of TB is generally more protracted in people living with HIV due to the extra-pulmonary nature of the disease. Even after treatment, these patients are more vulnerable to getting re-infected with TB. In addition, those patients who have been treated for pulmonary TB can remain infectious after treatment initiation. The tools currently available to prevent, diagnose, and treat TB are not adequate, as they do not meet the challenges posed by issues such as poverty, weak political will, substance misuse, and stigma. Hence, a coordinated approach is required to successfully tackle HIV and TB. For people living with HIV, the WHO recommends intensified case-findings and treatment of TB, TB prevention through INH preventative therapy, and early ART for control of TB infection in healthcare facilities and other settings. In people diagnosed with or suspected to have a TB infection, HIV testing and counseling to identify people with HIV co-infection is recommended (WHO 2015a). For optimal patient monitoring, it is crucial that the health services for both these diseases are integrated and based at the same, decentralized location.

People affected with TB are often victims of discrimination due to the stigma and myths that surround the illness. TB is associated with HIV, poverty, drug abuse, alcohol misuse, homelessness, and linked to prisons and refugee camps, all of which are associated with stigma. Discrimination is responsible for social isolation or shunning of individuals and/or entire families, particularly in small, impoverished communities. The impact of stigma is far reaching as the fear of discrimination results in a situation where people with TB symptoms are reluctant to seek help, until they become seriously ill. Stigma around TB can also make people unwilling to stick with the lengthy course of treatment for fear of being "discovered"; hence, they take their treatment at irregular intervals, with poor cure outcomes and an increased risk of developing drug resistance.

8.1.5 TB in Children

TB in children is often neglected as it is difficult to diagnose, so the scale of the problem in this vulnerable group is underestimated. TB affects young and weak children including those living with HIV or afflicted with other common childhood infections and the severely malnourished. Children are most likely to get infected with TB due to close contact with their infected parents and other relatives living in overcrowded conditions. The impact of TB on children is far reaching and contributes to the devastating cycle of poverty. Children also serve as sentinels for community health as sick children reflect the presence of sick adults. In 2015, the WHO estimated 1 million children were infected with TB and 210,000 succumbed to the disease (WHO 2016). A further 10 million children have been orphaned by TB, making them more likely to live in poverty and die prematurely (WHO 2015a). Moreover, children with ailing parents often are unable to attend school as they need to take on caregiving responsibilities or earn money for survival.

Unlike TB-diseased adults, children do not pose an infection risk, since they are unable to generate sufficient sputum for a productive cough; hence in resource-limited settings childhood TB is not a priority. Sadly, children are more severely disabled with TB disease as they are more vulnerable to complex clinical manifestations such as TB meningitis, causing inflammation of the membranes that surround the brain and the spinal cord (Nabukeera-Barungi et al. 2014). Moreover, until 2015 there was no child-friendly TB treatment formulation and children were compelled to take a concoction of crushed adult pills. This naturally led to drug refusal, resulting in inappropriate dosing with subsequent development of drug resistance (Murray et al. 2015, Taneja et al. 2015).

8.1.6 TB Vaccination

In addition to chemotherapy, a live attenuated vaccine in the form of Bacillus Calmette-Guerin (BCG) has been widely used around the world since 1921 (Mangtani et al. 2014, Roy et al. 2014). In children, the vaccine has been shown to protect against *M. tuberculosis* and prevents life-threatening TB meningitis in infants and young children <5 years of age but has been ineffective in controlling the global TB epidemic due to its variable efficacy (0%–80%) in adolescents and adults (Zhang et al. 2016). The reasons for this variable efficacy are currently unknown. However, a meta-analysis has indicated that the efficacy of the BCG vaccine wanes with time and the protective duration is around 10 years (Abubakar et al. 2013). As a result, most cases of transmissible pulmonary TB disease occur in adolescence and in adults (Barreto et al. 2011). As BCG is administered once at birth with no booster, it is unlikely to provide protection beyond adolescence (Zwerling et al. 2011). BCG has also proven to be less effective in children living with HIV and in equatorial regions due to the high levels of naturally occurring environmental mycobacteria (Mangtani et al. 2014). As with the chemotherapeutic drugs, the BCG vaccine was developed in an age before the emergence of the HIV pandemic; hence development of new-generation vaccines that are effective for all age groups, for all forms of TB, and are safe for people living with HIV is crucial for the elimination of TB. Recent modelling data has shown that a vaccine with just 60% efficacy delivered to 20% of adolescents and adults could prevent 30 million cases of active TB cases in the first 20 years and could prevent 35 million cases if administered to 90% of newborns (AERAS 2014, Knight et al. 2014). Thus, a vaccine targeted at adolescents and adults could have a much greater effect than vaccines targeted at infants only. The development of TB vaccine faces numerous challenges, the key one being the lack of a validated, predictive animal model to measure correlates of protection. Hence, efficacy trials that are time consuming and costly can only be carried out late in the process. Due to this, prioritization of promising candidates during early development must be carefully considered. Despite these limitations, 13 vaccine candidates are currently undergoing clinical assessment (Pai et al. 2016).

8.2 TB Diagnosis and Challenges for Microfluidics

TB diagnosis continues to pose serious problems, mainly because of the complexity of the disease. Rapid diagnosis and appropriate effective treatment of TB are important for preventing transmission. Furthermore, the early identification and treatment of individuals with LTBI, who when immunocompromised are at high risk of developing active infection, is crucial for disease control. However, current tests are poor at differentiating between patients with LTBI and those with healed lesions, BCG vaccinated individuals and unvaccinated Mantoux positive individuals (Pai et al. 2014, Pai and Sotgiu 2016). There are several methods available to diagnose TB depending on the type of TB suspected and the resources available for testing (Figure 8.1). These are described in the following text to provide some background to the challenges for miniaturization of TB diagnostics into microfluidics devices for POC applications.

8.2.1 Smear Microscopy

Conventional smear microscopy using Auramine/Ziehl–Neelsen staining is the most widely used diagnostic test for TB in resource-constrained countries as it is cheap and does not require specialized biosafety facilities or skills. The approach of identifying acid-fast bacteria microscopically was originally described by Robert Koch in the late 1800s and variations of this method forms the basis of modern-day TB diagnosis. While microscopy is effective

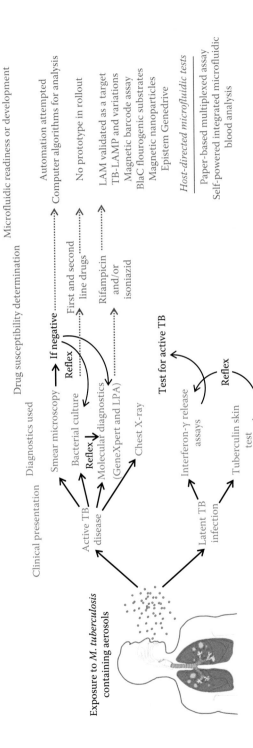

FIGURE 8.1
Diagnostic tests for TB and associated technology level readiness for microfluidic platform development. Exposure to *M. tuberculosis* can result in active disease or latent infection. The former is diagnosed with a variety of methods including smear microscopy, bacterial culture, molecular diagnostics, or chest X-ray. LTBI is detected using the tuberculin skin test (TST) or interferon-γ release assays (IGRA); a positive TST usually requires reflex to an IGRA and positive IGRAs necessitate an assessment for active TB. Negative smears require an appending culture or molecular diagnostic result to rule out TB disease. Bacterial culture methods currently are not specific for *M. tuberculosis* and require reflex testing on a molecular diagnostic for speciation. Current TB molecular diagnostics can identify rifampicin or isoniazid resistance while bacterial culture offers the option to test phenotypic susceptibility to a variety of first- and second-line TB drugs. The technology level readiness for translation onto a microfluidic platform is still in its infancy for smear and culture-based methods. However, several recent innovations have created the possibility of developing microfluidic TB diagnostics that are based on molecular testing. In addition, microfluidic tests that monitor the host health status can also be explored.

in identifying active, pulmonary TB in adults with a high bacillary load (5,000–10,000 colony forming units [CFU]/mL) in sputum, it cannot identify drug-resistant TB and lacks the sensitivity to identify TB in children, people living with HIV, and extrapulmonary TB as these individuals have fewer bacteria in their sputum (Hobby et al. 1973, Tostmann et al. 2008). Furthermore, microscopy is unable to distinguish between *M. tuberculosis* from other mycobacterial strains (*M. kansai*, *M. marinum*, and *M. avium* complex) and nontuberculosis mycobacteria (*Norcadia* sp.). The use of fluorescence staining has increased the sensitivity but requires expensive fluorescent microscopes, which are often not accessible in resource-limited settings. Consequently, these limitations result in delayed diagnosis with compromised patient healthcare and have implications for controlling the transmission of drug-sensitive and drug-resistant TB. Attempts have been made to automate smear microscopy for high throughput. TBDX is a recently developed roboticized smear platform that automates slide loading, image capture, bacterial detection, and final classification of smear status, with specificity and positive predictive value that is equivalent to a microscopist (Lewis et al. 2012). In addition, several computer algorithms have been devised to transform microscopy data for automated analysis (Chang et al. 2013).

8.2.2 Mycobacterial Culture

A more sensitive method for diagnosis is bacteriological culture, which can include testing for drug resistance, and presently this is considered the gold standard for detection of TB. However, this technique has several disadvantages as it takes weeks or months to confirm diagnosis and requires sophisticated and well-equipped laboratory infrastructure. Due to biosafety concerns, culture requires trained staff and an efficient transport system to ensure specimen viability is maintained from point of collection to delivery. Culture tests are highly reliable but building adequate culture capacity in countries with a high TB burden has been slow given the cost and infrastructural constraints. In reality, although the culture test is highly sensitive for TB diagnosis, most people will not have their test results in time to guide treatment management and prevent transmission.

To reduce the time to positivity of culture-based diagnostics, radiometric liquid culture platforms were first described in 1975 wherein radioactive palmitic acid in Middlebrook 7H12 media is metabolized by growing mycobacteria, releasing $^{14}CO_2$ as a metabolic by-product, which serves as an indicator of growth (Cummings et al. 1975). In 1977, Middlebrook described the first fully automated liquid culture system, the Bactec460, that became the most widely used culture-based diagnostic for detection of drug-sensitive and drug-resistant TB (Pfyffer et al. 1999, Roberts et al. 1983, Siddiqi et al. 1981, 1985). Over the past decade, next-generation non-radiometric platforms have superseded Bactec460 including Bactec MGIT960 (MGIT) (Hanna et al. 1999), MB Redox (Cambau et al. 1999); BacT/Alert3D (MB/BacT) (Rohner et al. 1997), and the VersaTrek (ESP Culture II) (Woods et al. 1997). The latter have similar performance characteristics to the MGIT 960 and can reliably determine first-line drug susceptibility (Garrigo et al. 2007, Ruiz et al. 2000). BacT/Alert3D has also been shown to reliably confirm second-line DST (Barreto et al. 2003). The MGIT detects *M. tuberculosis* growth using a non-radiometric ruthenium salt where the unquenched salt fluoresces under ultraviolet light as oxygen in the tube is consumed by bacterial growth. A limitation with this method is that it is not specific for *M. tuberculosis* as any bacterial species will consume oxygen during growth. Consequently, MGIT culture requires reflexing to a speciation test to confirm TB infection. These reflex tests can take the form of microscopy or molecular diagnostics (Figure 8.1). The automated MGIT has a faster time to positivity and is more sensitive than solid media but its performance is equivalent to other liquid culture techniques (Ardito et al. 2001, Garrigo et al. 2007, Hanna et al. 1999, Somoskovi et al. 2000), with reliable verification of first and second line indirect DST (Bemer et al. 2002, Kontos et al. 2004, Kruuner et al. 2006, Rusch-Gerdes et al. 2006, Scarparo et al. 2004, Tortoli et al. 2002). These developments have significantly enhanced rapid TB diagnostics, and data from MGIT implementation projects led the WHO to recommend wider implementation of liquid culture and DST in global TB control programs (WHO 2007). However, technical, infrastructural, and financial constraints limit the implementation of automated MGIT in reference laboratories in developing countries. Fortunately, the fluorescent signal of a MGIT tube can also be detected manually under an ultraviolet lamp, preventing the need for an expensive, fully automated platform and thus offering greater use of a faster TB diagnostic assay in resource-constrained countries. The performance of the manual MGIT is comparable to Bactec460 and MGIT960 providing reliable and sensitive DST (albeit indirect) for RIF and INH (Adjers-Koskela and Katila 2003). At this point, there is no microfluidic version of the MGIT available; such an intervention will enhance diagnostic capacity in high-burden countries, and culture still remains the gold standard for the foreseeablefuture.

8.2.3 Diagnosis of Latent TB Infection

8.2.3.1 Tuberculin Skin Test

Currently, there is no gold standard for the diagnosis of LTBI, and indication of prophylactic therapy is based on epidemiologic, clinical and laboratory criteria, and patient acceptance (MMWR 2000). The tuberculosis skin test (TST) first described by Koch in 1890 and developed by Mantoux in 1907 has been in use for the diagnosis of LTBI since 1910 (Figure 8.1). TST or intradermal Mantoux is the oldest diagnostic test, and despite limitations it is included in the WHO's latest recommendations for TB control (WHO 2015a). TST is based on a protein-purified derivate (PPD), from a culture filtrate of tubercle bacilli containing over 200 antigens common to BCG and most non-tuberculosis bacteria. Consequently, the TST specificity is low, with limited ability to distinguish LTBI from other similar immunological responses (Lalvani 2007, Richeldi 2006). Generally, five tuberculin units of PPD are injected intradermally, and in persons with cell-mediated immunity against these antigens a delayed-type hypersensitivity reaction will occur within 48–72 h. The size of the induration is measured and interpreted as a predictor for LTBI conversion to active TB. TST has several advantages, particularly in limited-resource settings as it has low reagent and equipment costs and limited skill and laboratory requirements. However, it has two major limitations. Firstly, consecutive TSTs can produce false-positive results because of the booster phenomenon, BCG vaccination, and sensitization with non-tuberculous mycobacteria (Farhat et al. 2006). Secondly, TST has poor predictive value, as most TST positive patients do not progress to active disease, and displays low sensitivity in HIV-infected patients due to compromised immune responses (Cobelens et al. 2006).

8.2.3.2 Interferon Gamma Release Assays

A hallmark feature of the host cellular immune response to *M. tuberculosis* infection is the release of interferon (IFN)-γ by CD4 cells (Kaufmann 2002). Interrogation of the whole genome sequence of *M. tuberculosis* has identified a specific genomic segment, referred to as the region of difference-1 (RD-1), wherein two proteins, ESAT-6 and the CFP-10, are primary immunogens that stimulate T-cell responses (Mahairas et al. 1996, Sorensen et al. 1995). Based on this antigen-specific T-cell reaction, two new diagnostic methods were developed for the detection of TB infection (Pai et al. 2004). These tests are more specific than the TST assay as the antigens are not shared with BCG and most non-tuberculosis mycobacterial species of clinical relevance (Andersen et al. 2000). The commercially available blood tests currently in use are the QuantiFERON-TB, based on whole blood ELISA developed in Australia in 1980, and the TSPOT.TB test developed in the United Kingdom in 1990. The major advantages of these blood tests are their speed and simplicity compared to microscopy or culture, their high sensitivity in the detection of false-negative TST, and their ability to discern false-positive TST in BCG-vaccinated individuals (Dheda et al. 2009, Pai et al. 2014, van Zyl-Smit et al. 2016). However, a positive result does not indicate whether the infection is active or latent and further tests are necessary to confirm infection (Figure 8.1).

8.2.4 Molecular Diagnostics for TB

Given the limitations of TST and IFN-γ release assays, extensive research has resulted in the development of new diagnostic procedures, such as the nucleic acid amplification tests (NAATs) that can be used directly on clinical specimens (Dinnes et al. 2007, Ling et al. 2008). These tests amplify target nucleic acid regions in viable or nonviable bacilli, thus uniquely identifying organisms in the *M. tuberculosis* complex. Two commercially available tests, the Amplicor MTB test (Roche diagnostics System) and the Amplifier Mycobacterial Tuberculosis Direct test (Gen Probe, Inc., San Diego), have been recently approved by the U.S. Food and Drug Administration (FDA). NAATs have high specificity and are useful to confirm a positive sputum smear result but have low sensitivity in patients with negative sputum smears (Chida and Shah 2016). The time needed for NAATs is less than sputum culture, and they can be promptly used to enroll patients with pulmonary TB infection into a treatment program. However, a major limitation of NAATs it that they do not differentiate between viable and dead bacteria, complicating the evaluation of disease progression or treatment effectiveness in patients receiving treatment. Therefore, NAAT results also require confirmation by sputum culture. Although NAATs have been shown to be more accurate than TST in patients with clinical suspicion of LTBI, they have low specificity and sensitivity for extra-pulmonary TB. While detection of mycobacterial DNA in clinical samples by polymerase chain reaction (PCR) is a promising approach for the rapid diagnosis of TB infection, the result must be controlled and corrected for the presence of PCR inhibitors and DNA contamination. These limitations suggest that NAATs still require further refinement if they are to replace sputum microscopy and culture in TB diagnosis and to evaluate treatment effectiveness.

Numerous attempts have been made to develop clinically useful serodiagnostic kits based on the detection of the antibody immune response to *M. tuberculosis* against proteinaceous and other cell wall components to improve TB diagnosis. Unfortunately, none of these assays proved to be clinically useful although they were rapid, simple, and inexpensive (Garg et al. 2003). Developing an ELISA test utilizing a suitable antigen has also proven to be difficult because *M. tuberculosis* shares a large number of antigens with other microorganisms that may or may not be pathogenic; thus, any such test would vary widely in performance and sensitivity (Dowdy et al. 2011, Steingart et al. 2011). A particularly novel approach was the combination of ELISA with NAAT detection (Gill et al. 2006).

8.2.4.1 Detection of Lipoarabinomannan

Presently, NAAT tests alone are insufficient for the accurate diagnosis of TB infection, and in 2011 the WHO advised against their use for TB diagnosis as they cannot replace sputum culture (WHO 2011a). Nevertheless, an antigen detection assay that detects lipoarabinomannan (LAM, a lipopolysaccharide component of the mycobacterial cell wall) in urine shows promise and has been used to develop a simple lateral flow assay known as Determine TB-LAM (Alere, Waltham, MA) (Lawn et al. 2012). Testing urine samples has many advantages over sputum samples, as urine is simpler to collect and safer to handle in resource-constrained settings. This kit is inexpensive (~US$3.5/test) and yields results in 30 min requiring minimal training and no complex instruments or electric supply. The test only requires a single clinic visit; thus it has the potential to be used as a POC assay (Lawn et al. 2012, Peter et al. 2012). A drawback of the test is that it has a low sensitivity of 28.2% in patients with culture-confirmed TB but studies have shown improved sensitivity to 66.7%, when the CD4+ T-cell count is below 50–200 cells/μL. This suggests that the LAM lateral flow test may add value in diagnosing TB in HIV-infected patients with advanced AIDS (Lawn et al. 2012). The LAM lateral flow test in combination with smear microscopy yielded a sensitivity equivalent to the GeneXpert MTB/RIF molecular diagnostic (discussed in the following text), particularly in the HIV-infected population (Lawn et al. 2012, Peter et al. 2012). Thus, the LAM lateral flow test has utility in the management of TB-HIV co-infection in countries burdened with these two epidemics. However, rigorous field evaluation is needed to assess the diagnostic efficacy of this test for the detection of active TB cases in various HIV-infected populations (e.g., women and children) in resource-constrained settings (Denkinger and Pai 2012, Lawn et al. 2012, Peter et al. 2012).

To respond to the growing TB problem, there has been resurgence in the development of a number of novel, rapid, and more sensitive tests for improved diagnosis that can either replace or complement the existing tests. These include molecular line probe assays and the Gene Xpert MTB/RIF® (Cepheid, United States) assay system, both of which are rapid DNA tests based on PCR that simultaneously confirm the presence of *M. tuberculosis* and detect resistance to either RIF (with mutations mapping to the RIF-resistance determining region of the *rpoB* gene) or INH (with mutations mapping to the *katG* and *inhA* genes, in addition to the *inhA* promoter region) or both. These assays are discussed in detail in the following text.

8.2.4.2 Genotype MTBDRplus Assay

The Genotype MTBDR*plus* test is a WHO-endorsed line-probe assay (LPA) for the rapid detection of *M. tuberculosis* complex bacteria and the previously mentioned mutations conferring resistance to RIF and INH. The LPA allows for the rapid diagnosis of MDR-TB in known smear positive TB cases or cultures wherein drug resistance is suspected. Additionally, the test can be used to detect mono-resistance to INH and to confirm RIF resistance identified from other tests such as Gene Xpert MTB/RIF (Barnard et al. 2012, Madhuri et al. 2015). Following the 2008 recommendation by the WHO on the utilization of LPAs for the rapid detection of RIF resistance, use of two alternative LPAs was further recommended by the WHO in 2015. The newer tests also had the ability to simultaneously detect TB and confirm RIF resistance. Subsequent to the GenoType® MTBDR*plus* assay, Hain Lifesciences developed an updated version, the Hain Version 2 assay, which allows for the identification of *M. tuberculosis* complex, and incorporates *rpoB* probes for RIF resistance detection as well as *katG* and *inhA* probes for the detection of INH resistance. In addition, Nipro Corporation, Japan, has developed an LPA that is similar to that of Hain Lifesciences (Nipro assay), which also allows for the identification of *M. tuberculosis* complex and some common non-tuberculous mycobacteria including *M. avium*, *M. intracellulare*, and *M. kansasii*. Nipro can also detect RIF and INH conferring mutations. To assess the diagnostic accuracy of these two newly available tests, in 2014 and 2015 the Foundation for Innovative New Diagnostics (FIND) coordinated a multi-center, blinded cross-sectional study to compare their performance against that of the Hain Version 1 assay. The study was carried out in two phases: phase 1 was designed to evaluate the performance of the newer assays on a wide range of clinical isolates and phase 2 to evaluate their performance on sputum specimens from patients with pulmonary TB. Using DST and DNA sequencing as reference standards, the newer LPA assays (Hain Version 2 and Nipro) demonstrated comparable performance to the Hain version 1 assay for the detection of *M. tuberculosis* and RIF resistance conferring mutations in smear-positive samples (Nathavitharanaa et al. 2016). Based on the outcomes of the FIND-coordinated study, the WHO recommended the use of Hain Version 1 assay over the Hain version 2 and Nipro assays, for the rapid detection of RIF-resistance conferring mutations in smear-positive samples and positive cultures. Complex LPAs are available that identify not only the various members of the MTB complex but up to 30 different non-tuberculous mycobacteria (NTM). A more advance LPA for the detection of resistance to second-line drugs (Hain Lifescience Genotype MTBDRsl) is also available. However, new evidence about its clinical utility is currently under review by the WHO and will be updated in 2016 (WHO 2013). Data from a systematic review and meta-analysis revealed that the LPA is highly accurate as compared to conventional culture and phenotypic DST (Ling et al. 2008). The GenoType MTBDR*plus* has an approximate sensitivity and specificity of $\geq 97\%$ and $\geq 98.7\%$, respectively, for RIF resistance and $\geq 90\%$ and $\geq 99\%$, respectively, for high-level INH resistance. Overall accuracy for detection of MDR was equally high at 99% and retained when RIF resistance alone was used as a marker for MDR.

For smear-negative samples, once the specimen is grown in culture, GenoType MTBDR*plus* can significantly shorten the time to resistance detection for RIF and INH compared to conventional DST. The assay has utility for both smear-positive and smear-negative pulmonary disease. The MTBDR*plus* test can detect resistance to both INH and RIF. There is no need for batching the GenoType MTBDR*plus* test since each test is individually packaged as a single strip, but batching may be advantageous in reducing turnaround times. It is important to note that LPAs cannot replace conventional culture and DST, as mycobacteriological culture is still required for low bacterial load/smear-negative specimens and conventional DST is still necessary for full drug panel susceptibility testing. According to a 2008 meta-analysis of published literature, the Hain GenoType MTBDR*plus* has a sensitivity of under 100% for both RIF and INH, respectively, suggesting it can miss TB cases with low bacterial loads; hence if the clinical representation is highly suggestive of TB, further conventional testing is warranted.

8.2.4.3 GeneXpert MTB/RIF®

A notable advance in TB molecular diagnostics has been the development of the GeneXpert MTB/RIF (Cepheid, Inc., Sunnyvale, CA), which is a fully automated, cartridge-based NAAT for TB diagnostics. The test is designed to simultaneously detect *M. tuberculosis* and mutations linked to RIF resistance, from sputum specimens in less than 2 h with minimal staff involvement and biosafety risk (Helb et al. 2010). More than 95% of RIF-resistant *M. tuberculosis* strains have mutations within the 81-base pair core region of the *rpoB* gene, which are absent in nearly all RIF-susceptible strains (Musser 1995). Moreover, approximately 90% of RIF-resistant *M. tuberculosis* is also resistant to INH, which makes the mutant *rpoB* gene a potential surrogate marker for a reliable measure of MDR-TB (Morgan et al. 2005). The GeneXpert MTB/RIF assay is essentially a molecular beacon-based RT-PCR that utilizes five overlapping probes spanning the 81 base pair core region of the *rpoB* gene (Piatek et al. 1998). As with LPAs, GeneXpert MTB/RIF is also reliant on PCR and results must therefore be corrected for the possible presence of inhibitors and DNA contamination from dead bacteria and/or other non-tuberculous mycobacteria. Even though GeneXpert MTB/RIF test results can be ready in 2 h, the turnaround times for communicating the results are delayed at many settings. The reasons for patients receiving their results days later often are due to sub-optimal laboratory operations, limited human resources, batching of specimens to save time and costs, and inefficient transport networks. These barriers need to be surmounted to recognize the full impact of this technology for improved TB management and eradication (Piatek et al. 1998). Despite these barriers, this advancement has potentially reduced the time of diagnosis and increased the prospect of timely treatment initiation. GeneXpert MTB/RIF is more sensitive than sputum smear microscopy and has equivalent accuracy as culture (Boehme et al. 2010, 2011). The most beneficial feature is its ability to detect smear negative TB, leading to the improvement of case identification in people living with HIV, where smear microscopy detects only 22%–43% of active TB cases (Getahun et al. 2007). A meta-analysis showed that GeneXpert MTB/RIF has a 36%–44% higher sensitivity to detect TB disease in children compared to sputum smear microscopy (Detjen et al. 2015). When compared with cultures of expectorated or induced sputum or gastric aspirates, GeneXpert MTB/ RIF has a sensitivity of 62%–66% and a specificity of 98% (Detjen et al. 2015). Hence, the Xpert MTB/RIF as recommended by the WHO for TB disease detection in children has contributed to identifying a greater number of children not only with susceptible TB but also with MDR-TB, which were previously missed (Lawn and Nicol 2011). Regardless of these advances, conventional microscopy and culture still remain necessary for monitoring treatment response and for accurately testing susceptibility to second line drugs. Use of GeneXpert MTB/RIF is relatively simple as it involves minimal specimen handling. However, there are several operational and programmatic requirements associated with the efficient implementation of the assay. From an operational perspective these include sustained power supply, adequate storage, and a waste disposal system for cartridges, ambient temperature not higher than 30°C, biosafety facilities equivalent to smear microscopy, trained laboratory and clinical staff, annual calibration of the GeneXpert MTB/RIF modules, and computer and software technical support.

The benefits of GeneXpert MTB/RIF outweighs that of smear microscopy but with a higher cost; individual cartridges cost US\$9.98 per test, a price reduced by 40% from US\$16.87 through a financial agreement with the manufacturer and the Bill and Melinda Gates Foundation, the U.S. President's Emergency Plan for AIDS Relief (PEPFAR), UNITAID, and the United States Agency for International Development (USAID). Equipment, consumable, and maintenance costs are a barrier to scaling up GeneXpert MTB/RIF in many middle- to low-income countries. Considering this, it is highly likely that in countries that have already implemented GeneXpert MTB/RIF, the machines will sit idle after the initial investment of implementation unless due attention is given to identifying sustained resources for consumables and recurrent maintenance costs (Piatek et al. 1998). Strong health systems are required to realize the full potential of this and other new technologies. One crucial need for TB diagnostics is to develop a POC test that is fast and accurate in the detection of TB and MDR-TB at community level, linked to strong laboratory and referral systems to ensure that patients have access to all required diagnostic and follow-up testing.

The WHO endorsed the use of GeneXpert MTB/RIF in December 2010, and the global TB community responded quickly to roll out and scale up this test in high burden countries. As a result, its use has since expanded with 4.8 million test cartridges procured in 2014 by 116 low- and middle-income countries at concessional prices (FIND 2012), up from 550,000 in 2011. By 2015, 69% of the countries recommended using Xpert MTB/RIF as the initial diagnostic test for people at risk of drug-resistant TB and 60% recommended it as the initial diagnostic test for people living with HIV. The GeneXpert MTB/RIF is a promising technology for rapid detection and has significantly shifted the TB diagnosis landscape with >17 million cartridges procured since its introduction in 2010 (Albert et al. 2016, WHO 2015b). In an exciting recent development, newer versions of the GeneXpert MTB/RIF are on the horizon including GeneXpert Omni, intended for POC testing, with a smaller and more streamlined design. In addition, the new GeneXpert Ultra cartridge is projected as a replacement for the GeneXpert MTB/RIF and will have a lower limit of detection (10–100 organisms with GeneXpert Ultra compared to 133 organisms with GeneXpert MTB/RIF).

To combat the TB problem, a single diagnostic test that is affordable and applicable for use throughout the developing world is desperately needed. The test results must be immediate so that the patient receives the diagnosis while at the clinic. Inefficient and expensive transport networks to centralized clinics loses people to TB services even before they can receive the diagnosis and treatment, often because they cannot afford the costs of return travel to the clinic. The test must be sensitive and specific to identify active or latent disease and predict the risk of reactivation or recurrent disease. In the modern era of genetics, combined with the development of proteomics and genomics, next-generation technologies such as DNA chip-based hybridization assays that instantly reveal mycobacterial infections/genotype are on the horizon. This timely diagnosis together with the correct treatment regimen is likely to make TB a disease of the past.

8.3 Microfluidics for Tuberculosis

Microfluidics is a multidisciplinary field that emerged in the 1980s with applications in the fields of engineering, physics, chemistry, biology, nanotechnology, and biotechnology, allowing for the design of systems to handle small volumes (μL, nL, pL, fL) of fluids saving time, money, and energy and reducing safety risk. Microfluidics in biology, often described as a laboratory-on-chip technology, allows miniaturization and integration of complex functions that facilitate their use for high throughput applications. In general, the microfluidic device comprises a micro-channel network that has been moulded to allow fluids to pass through different channels of different diameter, usually ranging from 5 to 500 μm (Whitesides 2006). The micro-channel network is specifically designed for the required application or analyses (cell culture, organ-on-a-chip, DNA analysis, etc.), making it a very attractive technology for duplication of complete laboratory protocols on a single chip of a few square centimeters. The development of one such microfluidic platform was motivated due to the difficulty in mixing aqueous cross-linking agents into droplets using conventional approaches. Land et al. reported a microfluidic device wherein channel structures were used, for two emulsions with different droplet sizes, one created on-chip, the other off-chip, to rapidly mix with each other, allowing for the mixing of the two emulsions (Land et al. 2014). To realize the WHO's goal of eliminating TB globally by 2050, effective POC TB diagnostics must be implemented to prevent delayed and/or misdiagnosis of TB, which presently fuels the epidemic with high annual mortality rates. Miniaturization of TB diagnosis by using on-chip microfluidic technologies or by integrating novel nanotechnologies could be the strategy for developing inexpensive and effective diagnostics for resource-constrained countries.

The lack of an instrument-free test, like a dipstick type POC test, continues to constrain TB disease management, thus demanding the development of a simple, inexpensive, sensitive, and portable assay for the detection of active disease (Wang et al. 2013). Ideally, the diagnostic and therapeutic design of the POC device should be a sensitive and robust platform that does not require bacterial isolation and/or culturing. Intense research effort has been invested to develop platforms that meet these requirements, some of which are discussed in the following text and shown in Figure 8.1. POC microfluidic devices can be split into small handheld ones including quantitative and qualitative strips and larger bench-top devices with more complex built-in fluidics, often miniature variants of ones used in conventional laboratories. Numerous lateral flow immunoassay (LFIA) test strips have been developed and established as POC testing platforms for diagnosis of infectious diseases such as the LAM test (discussed earlier) to detect *M. tuberculosis* in the urine sample of patients infected with HIV, as well as a range of disease-associated biomarkers, for example, in cardiac disease and cancer for countries where timely medical care remains a challenge (St John and Price 2014). A key barrier for progress in the development of POC TB diagnostic assays has been the lack of reliable and validated host or pathogen-derived markers (biomarkers) for the detection of active TB and identification of LTBI. Limited understanding of the complexity of TB disease pathogenesis, host–pathogen interactions, and protective immune responses during infection is responsible for this. Furthermore, different disease states in individuals such as latent infection/re-infection or with different immunization profiles results in varied immune responses that may confound the interpretation of immunoassay results.

An ideal POC microfluidic test for TB diagnosis in a resource-limited setting should detect early infection/disease through the use of multiple biomarkers for increased sensitivity and specificity. For effective linkage to care, minimum sputum processing, a single sample (without the need for a follow-up sample), and rapid turnaround times are essential for initiation of appropriate treatment. Given the extra-pulmonary nature of TB in HIV-infected individuals and the requirement to use gastric aspirates in children, any POC would need to use a variety of specimen types and detect paucibacillary disease (Sharma et al. 2015). Proactive, rapid diagnosis of patients at an early stage of disease that are smear negative would definitely be advantageous, as these patients may yield better treatment outcomes and consequently are less contagious, thus reducing overall TB morbidity and mortality (Siddiqi et al. 2003). While simple microfluidic POC diagnostics for TB might not be in the pipeline for the near future, the prospect is looking promising for a more decentralized, field-friendly, affordable molecular test that can be used at the clinical interface to reduce diagnostic delays. These include the POC manual NAATs such as the loop-mediated isothermal amplification (TB-LAMP) from Eiken/FIND and a handheld NAAT device from Epistem (Genedrive MTB/RIF) developed in the United Kingdom for implementation in India by Xcelris (Pai and Pai 2012, WHO 2011b).

8.3.1 Loop-Mediated Isothermal Amplification Platform

FIND and Eiken Chemical Company (Eiken), Tokyo, Japan, have been collaborating to develop an assay for TB diagnosis that could replace microscopy to improve the accuracy of TB detection using a loop-mediated isothermal amplification platform (LAMP). The principle of the LAMP assay is based on using primers that bind to at least six sites in a target sequence. The addition of loop primers, with two complementary regions in the template, and a template displacing polymerase results in products that are able to form hairpin structures and subsequently amplify through a similar mechanism. This leads to rapid amplification (10^9–10^{10} times) of double-stranded DNA in a short period of time (as little as 15 min). These products can then be detected by using dyes such as SYBR green, or detecting turbidity caused by precipitating magnesium pyrophosphate, or using a non-inhibitory fluorescing reagent that is quenched in the presence of divalent cations.

LAMP shows great promise to serve as the basis of a microfluidic detection system for many diseases as it is sensitive, rapid, inexpensive, and robust, together with the added benefits of high specificity and sensitivity (Ahmad and Hashsham 2012, Mori and Notomi 2009, Njiru 2012).

This is evidenced by reports that describe the integration of LAMP onto microfluidic chips for the detection of bacterial and viral pathogens at POC. Sample volumes were in the µL range, with assay times as short as 1 h and a limit of detection of 10 fg of DNA (Fang et al. 2010). These platforms can be streamlined by enhancing methods of detection such as the use of electrochemistry for real-time quantification of DNA. With this approach, as little as 19 copies of Salmonella DNA can be detected within an hour (Hsieh et al. 2012). For waterborne pathogens, real-time fluorescence LAMP (microRT$_f$-LAMP) was conducted on cyclic olefin polymer microchips. When combined with the SYTO-82 dye and detection using a charge-coupled device (CCD) camera, this test was able to detect single genomes of *Campylobacter jejuni* within 19 min (Ahmad et al. 2011). LAMP can also be applied in a multiplexed format to detect different bacterial pathogens as demonstrated by the detection of *Neisseria gonorrhoeae*, *Salmonella enterica*, and methicillin-resistant *Staphylococcus aureus* in a single reaction, completed in less than 20 min. In this, the detection limit varied between organisms ranging from 10 CFUs for *S. aureus* and *S. enterica* to 100 CFUs for *N. gonorrhoeae* (Kersting et al. 2014).

8.3.2 TB-LAMP

The TB-LAMP assay is fast, isothermal (requiring only a heat block), robust to inhibitors and reaction conditions that usually adversely affect PCR methods, and do not require sophisticated equipment. The result can be detected with the naked eye, making it attractive as a diagnostics platform for resource-poor settings. The initial format of the TB-LAMP assay did not take the form of a microfluidic platform; however new iterations of this approach have allowed for miniaturization.

During the development of the TB-LAMP assay, a number of important design changes were made to try to make the test equal or superior to sputum smear microscopy in ease-of-use, speed, sensitivity, and specificity. Briefly, the current assay involves transfer of a small volume of sputum to a heating tube already containing lysis mix, followed by removal of amplification inhibitors and transfer of DNA into a reaction tube containing lyophilized reagents. Validation of the assay involved 170 patients at two hospital settings in Japan where 320 TB-LAMP tests were performed of which 205 were positive. The sensitivity of TB-LAMP was 98.2% among smear-positive/culture-positive samples and 55.6% among smear-negative/culture-positives and the specificity for TB diagnosis was 93.9% (Mitarai et al. 2011). These data supported registration of the TB-LAMP assay in Japan. Subsequently, a series of clinical studies, coordinated by FIND, were carried out in reference centers and in high-burden TB countries to determine the performance and applicability of the assay relative to microscopy, with conventional culture as the reference standard. Multi-center evaluation studies involving 1061 patients at reference laboratories in Brazil, India, Peru, South Africa, and Vietnam showed that TB-LAMP detected almost 97% of smear-positive/culture-positive patients and 53% of smear-negative/culture-positive patients with very low indeterminate rates (<0.2%) (WHO 2013). False-positive results arose from contamination after exposure of the reaction tubes to humidity. Consequently, changes in packaging were made and evaluation studies were carried out in 11 rural or urban microscopy centers in India, Uganda, and Peru (Gray et al. 2016). In these settings, 1741 patients with a final diagnosis with microscopy, liquid, and solid culture from a reference laboratory were enrolled in the study. In this cohort of patients, the TB-LAMP performed slightly better than the earlier studies in reference laboratories, detecting 97% of smear-positive patients and 62% of smear-negative TB (Gray et al. 2016). Indeterminate rates (1.5%) were slightly higher than previous studies in reference settings. The specificity of TB-LAMP (96.3%) was lower than that of microscopy (97.3%) (Gray et al. 2016). A survey of TB-LAMP users suggested strong support for implementation of the assay in routine laboratories as it was less complex and faster than smear microscopy. However, the same users also pointed out some disadvantages of the test such as the possible risks for cross-contamination, false-positive results, the dependence of TB-LAMP results on a trained user, and the need for comprehensive training and quality assurance, which together with cost could pose to be obstacles for widespread implementation (WHO 2013).

8.3.2.1 Next-Generation LAMP Technologies for TB

To address some of the challenges arising from field testing of TB-LAMP, newer versions of LAMP-based assays in microfluidics format have been developed. In one such development, the LAMP principle was applied to detect *M. tuberculosis* in semisolid polyacrylamide gel arrays, with 670 nL test volume. The detection of amplified DNA was achieved through the use of an LCGreen Plus+ fluorescent dye, polymerized with the gel, which is detected with a CCD camera. The limit of detection was 13 mycobacterial genomes with a test time of 75 min (Manage et al. 2013). To further advance the approach, LAMP was conducted in droplets contained within capillaries, for efficient temperature control, yielding a diagnostic test with 96.8% sensitivity on clinical samples, with a specificity of 100%. The test took 50 min to complete with a limit of detection of 10 organisms (Liu et al. 2013). Using an analogous method, LAMP amplification of DNA in capillaries, for less than 15 min, yielded a turbidimetric diagnostic test with 90% sensitivity and 95% specificity on clinical specimens. The method was able to detect as little as 1 pg/mL with no contribution from non-specific DNA (Rafati and Gill 2015). Other variations of LAMP tests for TB include targeting the *hspX* gene for detection of the *M. tuberculosis* complex with a high degree of specificity with no false positives from non-tuberculosis mycobacteria (Bi et al. 2012).

8.3.3 Magnetic Barcode Assay

Liong et al. developed a platform in which all components were integrated into a single, small microfluidic cartridge for streamlined on-chip operation that detects nucleic acids using a magnetic barcoding strategy (Liong et al. 2013). The methodology is based on PCR-amplification of mycobacterial genes that are sequence-specifically captured on microspheres, labeled with a pair of complementary oligo-nucleotides, conjugated to microspheres and magnetic nanoprobes. These are then detected by nuclear magnetic resonance (NMR) systems (Haun et al. 2011, Issadore et al. 2011, Lee et al. 2009). This platform was able to detect *M. tuberculosis* with higher sensitivity than smear microscopy and identified drug-resistant strains based on single-nucleotide polymorphisms in target genes from mechanically processed sputum samples within 2.5 h. This was significantly shorter than the time required for culture. The specificity of the magnetic barcode assay for *M. tuberculosis* was confirmed by comprehensive characterization of the target gene from sputum samples using a panel of unrelated, clinically relevant bacterial strains (*Streptococcus pneumoniae*, *Pseudomonas aeruginosa*, *Staphylococcus aureus*, *Escherichia coli*, and *Haemophilus influenzae*). Signals from tuberculous sputum samples containing high concentration (10^6 CFU/mL) of these unrelated species were nearly equivalent to those from sputa only, indicating that non-specific amplification and/or binding of the primers to unrelated bacteria was negligible. The assay had the potential to detect a single bacterium and this high level of specificity is necessary for accurate detection from complex sputum specimens, which may be overpowered with several upper respiratory tract bacterial species. The sensitivity was evaluated in *M. tuberculosis* smear positive patient sputum and in "sputa" from healthy patients as controls. The magnetic barcode assay was highly specific as *M. tuberculosis* was detected in all TB-positive patient samples only and the control samples displayed a signal at baseline level. The assay was also able to detect TB in patients co-infected with HIV (Liong et al. 2013). As current standard approaches are insensitive for detection of low bacterial load in this group of individuals, the magnetic barcode assay is a significant advance for TB diagnostics in HIV-infected individuals. Furthermore, detection of higher bacterial loads with this assay correlates with studies that have shown that HIV and *M. tuberculosis* co-infection display synergistic effect at the cellular level and mutually accelerate the growth of each other (Diedrich et al. 2010, Pathak et al. 2010, Pawlowski et al. 2012). The magnetic barcode assay was further optimized for rapid detection of single-nucleotide polymorphisms in the 81 bp RIF resistance determining region of the *rpoB* gene. The focus was initially on the C → T mutation in codon 531 (S531L, *E. coli* numbering) as it is the most common amino acid substitution responsible for RIF resistance and accounts for 70% of drug-resistant strains detected in clinics (Barnard et al. 2008). These strains are also reported to have a high fitness level (Gagneux et al. 2006). Through multichanneled measurements using wild type and mutant-specific probes directed to the *rpoB* gene, the ratio between RIF-resistance and susceptible *M. tuberculosis* can be determined. This is a highly useful capability of the magnetic barcode assay as it could potentially aid in the study of bacterial mutation rate during antibiotic treatment (Ford et al. 2011). One limitation of the magnetic barcode assay is that sputum samples need to be processed off-chip for DNA extraction from *M. tuberculosis* using a simple mechanical method based on vigorous mixing with glass beads. Ideally, the magnetic barcode assay should be further optimized to incorporate this aspect of the protocol within the closed portable system (as with GeneXpert MTB/RIF) if it is to become a sensitive, high-throughput, and low-cost platform for POC TB diagnostic.

8.3.4 BlaC-Specific Fluorogenic Substrates

In another platform, a naturally occurring enzyme in *M. tuberculosis*, β-lactamase, encoded by *blaC*, belonging to the class A β-lactamase family (Flores et al. 2005, Hugonnet et al. 2009) capable of hydrolyzing all classes of β-lactam substrates, including cephalosporin's, was exploited to develop a microfluidic assay. The mechanism of cephalosporin hydrolysis by β-lactamases yields hydrolyzed β-lactam, concomitant with the loss of a 3' leaving group (Boyd and Lunn 1979, Faraci and Pratt 1985). This characteristic was used to develop several fluorogenic and bioluminogenic probes for the detection of β-lactamase activity *in vitro*, in living cells, and even in whole animals (Gao et al. 2003, Rukavishnikov et al. 2011, Xing et al. 2005, Yao et al. 2007, Zlokarnik et al. 1998). Kong et al. developed a BlaC-specific fluorogenic substrate, chemically linked to a quencher that enabled the sensitive detection of *M. tuberculosis* and BCG *in vitro* and in mice (Kong et al. 2010). However, these probes lacked specificity for BlaC in *M. tuberculosis* as the common TEM-1 β-lactamase (TEM-1 Bla) in gram-negative bacteria is also capable of generating fluorescence. This reduces the utility of the test for TB diagnosis. These earlier probes were also generally large and displayed slow hydrolytic kinetics for BlaC; hence using a rational design approach that took advantage of the unique flexibility of the BlaC substrate-specificity loop, a series of chemically modified fluorescent probes were developed. Enzymatic kinetics, structural analyses, and whole-cell assays revealed that these second-generation probes gained greater specificity and sensitivity compared to their precursors and did not detect the class A homologue TEM-1 Bla and β-lactamases produced by *Pseudomonas*, *Staphylococcus*, and the environmental mycobacterium *M. smegmatis* (Xie et al. 2012). Less than 100 BCG bacilli were detected directly in unprocessed patient sputum with a simple, inexpensive imaging system of a cellular phone. Using the improved BlaC probe, Rosenfeld et al. recently developed a method for rapid detection of TB from picoliter droplets of *M. tuberculosis* (Rosenfeld et al. 2014). The close proximity of the quencher prevents fluorescence of the substrate, with a fluorescent product generated only after cleavage of the linker due to the hydrolysis of β-lactam. The emission was increased >200-fold compared to the un-cleaved product indicating the high sensitivity for detection. Such a catalytic reporter is highly sensitive as it is not dependent on the number of tagged molecules that can be delivered to the cell but instead the fluorescent probe can be continuously produced to increase the signal as long as the substrate is available. Moreover, since BlaC is surface localized, the probe does not have to cross the bacterial cell wall in order to be cleaved, making this marker ideal for rapid diagnosis of TB (Kong et al. 2010).

8.3.5 Magnetic Nanoparticles

Chung et al. developed a more generic, accurate POC platform for the detection of several clinical pathogens (Chung et al. 2013). The assay makes use of magnetic nanoparticles (MNPs) and oligonucleotide probes to specifically detect the16S rRNA (a component of the 30S small subunit of bacterial ribosomes) as the target marker from the pathogen since a single bacterium contains many 16S rRNA strands (Yang et al. 2002). Moreover, the 16S rRNA has a high degree of sequence consensus across species allowing for general bacterial detection as well as species-specific variable regions that allow for speciation (Rajendhran and Gunasekaran 2011, Woo et al. 2008). Drug resistance phenotypes were identified by targeting specific mRNA sequences, which were sequenced with primers and probes that amplify and detect specific regions of interest within common bacterial types. The signal was interpreted using a miniaturized micro-NMR system, which requires only small volumes of sample for detection (2 mL), thus able to support rapid, high-throughput operations in POC settings (Haun et al. 2010, Lee et al. 2008, 2009). This study was developed for Gram-negative human pathogens, but as extensive sequence databases are available for several mycobacterial species, such a strategy can be adopted to develop a robust, fast, sensitive, and accurate POC diagnostic tool for TB detection.

8.3.6 Epistem Genedrive

The Epistem Genedrive test uses a simple paper-based DNA extraction method coupled with PCR amplification and detection on an Epistem's Genedrive instrument, a lightweight, portable, bench-top PCR platform with real-time PCR and melting temperature analysis capabilities. The assay targets two different regions of the *M. tuberculosis* complex genome, a short repetitive region, rep13E12, and a segment of the *rpoB* gene, containing the RIF resistance determining region (Castan et al. 2014, Gordon et al. 1999, Lee et al. 1997). This test is available in European Economic Area (EEA) member states and was launched for distribution in India. However, the test was not approved by the Indian Council of Medical Research and the Revised National TB Control Program (*DDNews* August 2011, Epistem 2012, Labmate 2015). Furthermore, the clinical and analytical performance of the test was not been extensively evaluated apart from a single study published by the manufacturer and collaborators (Castan et al. 2014). To address this, Shenai et al. assessed the analytical performance, biosafety, and diagnostic accuracy of the Genedrive assay for detection of *M. tuberculosis* in a multicenter prospective diagnostic accuracy clinical study (Shenai et al. 2016). The analytical limit of detection of the Genedrive PCR amplification was tested with genomic DNA and the specificity was tested using common respiratory pathogens and non-tuberculosis mycobacteria. A clinical evaluation involved enrolment of 504 adults with suspected pulmonary TB and the accuracy of Genedrive was compared to that of GeneXpert MTB/RIF using *M. tuberculosis* cultures as a reference standard. The Genedrive assay had a limit of detection of 1 pg/µL (100 genomic DNA copies/reaction) and 2.5×10^5 CFU/mL. False-positive *rpoB* probe signals were observed in 3/32 (9.4%) negative controls as well as for 3 non-tuberculosis mycobacterial strains (*M. abscessus*, *M. gordonae*, and *M. thermoresistibile*). In the analysis population, the 336 participants analyzed showed overall sensitivities for TB case detection of 45.4%, 91.8%, and 77.3% using Genedrive, GeneXpert MTB/RIF, or smear microscopy, respectively (Shenai et al. 2016). The sensitivity of Genedrive and GeneXpert MTB/RIF for detection of smear negative TB cases was 0% and 68.2%, respectively. The sample processing volumes were insufficiently miniaturized to declare the diagnostic test bio-safe, thus necessitating BSLIII infrastructure or at least a BSLII facility with a Biosafety-2 cabinet to process samples. Further treatment of all sample processing cassettes with 20% bleach or other acceptable decontaminants for 20–30 min was necessary before discarding. Considering this, the Genedrive assay does not meet WHO-recommended performance standards as a test to replace smear microscopy. Hence, the Genedrive assay needs further optimization and development to address these challenges with adequate validation trials before implementation in India. Premature implementation of the Genedrive test could have drastic consequences for TB patients, as low sensitivity of the test will result in missed diagnoses.

8.3.7 Other Developments

Alternative microfluidic platforms for detection of mycobacteria in the environment are also being developed. As an example, Jing et al. coupled an on-chip airborne bacteria capture system and a rapid bacteriological immunoassay into an automated microfluidic system that was able to detect the pathogen in 50 min, eliminating the need of a culturing step (Jing et al. 2014). Prior to this, another group developed an airborne capture device that was able to harvest *E. coli* and *Mycobacterium smegmatis* with an efficiency of 100% in 9 min.

Despite these advances in the last couple of decades, to date these microfluidic devices have still not met the criteria for implementation in the developing world and most of them remain in a proof-of-concept state mainly as they lack the clinical trials needed for approval of the tests. However, further development and modifications of these interventions are likely to close the gaps in the pipeline of POC TB diagnostics.

8.3.8 Host-Directed Microfluidic Tests for TB

8.3.8.1 Paper-Based Multiplexed Microfluidic Assay

In developed nations, monitoring for drug-induced hepatotoxicity by serial measurements of serum transaminases (aspartate aminotransferase [AST] and alanine aminotransferase [ALT]) in individuals at risk is the standard of care. However, monitoring for drug-related hepatotoxicity in resource-limited settings is often inadequate or completely absent due to cost and logistical issues. The Diagnostics for All (DFA) founded in 2007 by George Whitesides and his group at Harvard University demonstrated the potential of a 3D device made from layering patterned paper for monitoring drug-induced liver injury in individuals being treated for TB and/or HIV (Pollock et al. 2012). The paper-based, multiplexed microfluidic assay designed for a finger stick specimen consisted of layers of patterned paper using a wax-based printer and a heat source to print the microfluidic, hydrophilic paths within the paper. This allows the flow to be directed to specific detection zones enabling rapid, semi-quantitative measurement of AST and ALT within 15 min (Pollock et al. 2012). The test also contains three control zones to ensure performance reliability, and each test zone has a unique environment (pH, buffer, reagents, etc.) that ensures specificity. The AST assay chemistry is based on the sulfonation of methyl green, which results in a visual transformation from blue to pink as the dye becomes colorless, thus revealing the pink background color (Rhodamine B). The ALT assay chemistry is based on the conversion of L-alanine to pyruvate, the subsequent oxidation of pyruvate by pyruvate oxidase, and the utilization of the liberated hydrogen peroxide by horseradish peroxidase to generate a red dye (Pollock et al. 2012). These reactions generate visual colorimetric signals that can be interpreted and semi-quantified using a visual "read guide" that was generated using device images obtained from a desktop scanner and image analysis software (Pollock et al. 2012). A validation study conducted on 223 clinical specimens obtained by venipuncture together with 10 finger stick specimens from healthy volunteers showed that the assay has the capability to visually measure AST and ALT in whole blood or serum with >90% accuracy. These data suggest that the ultimate POC finger stick device will have high impact on TB/HIV patient care in low-resource settings.

8.3.8.2 Self-Powered Integrated Microfluidic Blood Analysis System

Another host-directed platform is the self-powered integrated microfluidic blood analysis system (SIMBAS), wherein filter trenches separate plasma from whole blood, eliminating the need for any external connections, tethers, or tubing to deliver and analyze a raw whole-blood sample. Red and white blood cells are removed by trapping them in an integral trench structure. Furthermore, the device design has five parallel channels allowing for the simultaneous performance of five complete biotin-streptavidin sample-to-answer assays, within 10 min with a limit of detection of 1.5 pM (Dimov et al. 2011). SIMBAS is a model design example toward the development of POC molecular diagnostics with integration of the minimal number of components without sacrificing effectiveness in performing rapid, complete bioassays.

8.3.8.3 Cellular Telephone Technology

Given the widespread use of cell phones across the developing world, a colorimetric detection system integrated with a mobile cell phone application will eliminate the need for specialized expensive detection equipment to obtain results. On-chip ELISAs coupled with a cell phone detection system have been developed for detection of an ovarian cancer biomarker from clinical urine samples (Wang et al. 2011). Similarly, portable microchip-based approaches can be potentially developed to detect biomarkers specific for *M. tuberculosis*.

8.4 Scalability and Challenges

A number of microfluidic platforms for rapid detection of infectious diseases have been developed and offer great promise as diagnostic tools to improve human health in low-resource settings. However, not many have been scaled as POC tests. There are still numerous hurdles for the application of microfluidics in routine diagnostic devices as many prototypes still use complex detection methods requiring expensive equipment, which limits the use of these devices as POC detection in low-resource settings (Milat et al. 2013). For example, the GeneXpert MTB/RIF assay has transformed TB diagnostics and can be used outside a laboratory setting. However, while it is "close to patient," it is still unsuitable for POC implementation, particularly in low-income countries mainly due to the high costs involved (Pai 2011). In South Africa, the GeneXpert MTB/RIF scale up initiative carried out by the National Health Laboratory Service (NHLS) has highlighted several other barriers for POC testing. The NHLS is unable to monitor any external testing and is also grappling with issues such as training, quality assurance, maintenance, management, and ownership of the POC program (Schnippel et al. 2012). Furthermore, from their experience the NHLS has also established that implementation of the GeneXpert MTB/RIF test at the POC is more costly than placing within the NHLS laboratories (Meyer-Rath et al. 2012, Schnippel et al. 2012). Hence, these factors need careful consideration for sustained implementation of microfluidics as POC. Nevertheless, the rollout of GeneXpert MTB/RIF has provided useful insights for future implementation of molecular and microfluidics-based TB diagnostics.

Apart from the requirement of financial resources for implementation of new health interventions, non-financial resources, such as skilled human resource, are crucial for the process to be successful. Gaps created by lack of skilled personnel cannot be easily closed with money, thus restricting scaling up. Human capacity can be built either by simplifying and standardizing procedures such that the service can be delivered by less skilled staff or aggressively training unskilled staff to carry out more complex tasks. Prior to implementation, it is important to assess the feasibility of the implementation process based on the technical complexity of the intervention and the institutional capacity. Another key factor for consideration is the political feasibility and committed health policy decision-making (Yamey 2012). Reducing the technical complexity of interventions will not only promote wider implementation of the microfluidics at POC but will also meet the TB Millennium Development Goals. However, prioritizing and planning the implementation of health interventions in resource-poor countries is challenging as accurate evidence for scale up is not available, analytical tools to assess the feasibility according to its complexity are limited, mechanisms for identifying priorities are lacking, and governmental support for decision-making and implementation of policies are often absent (Gericke et al. 2005). A good balance between technical complexity and capacity will support implementation, but if complexity exceeds capacity, this creates a capacity gap that will affect feasibility with a consequent negative impact on scaling up (Milat et al. 2015). Feasibility assessments of the intervention must also take into account the POC setting, and for successful implementation of new innovations, primary healthcare facilities or centralized hospitals may need strengthening. Successful implementation is also dependent on strong collaborative associations between various governmental and health sectors, between government and the public, as well as between government and external funding agencies, increasing the scale and adoption of population health interventions: experiences and perspectives of policy makers, practitioners, and researchers (Milat et al. 2014). Countries with weak governmental support are often reliant on nongovernmental organizations (NGOs). However, for long-term sustainability, developed countries will have to continue investing in TB research and provide new financial mechanisms to support TB control efforts in low-income countries who paradoxically also carry the highest burden of TB (Pai et al. 2016).

8.5 Advocacy for TB Research and Development

Comparative analysis of the progress in HIV and TB diagnostics clearly indicates that the diagnostic and prophylactic prowess of the latter epidemic has lagged behind HIV. TB disease has plagued humanity for the last century, yet the research and development (R&D) has not met the needs for TB control (Harrington 2010). Success in the HIV field is owed to patients, providers, and activists who have played a major role in pushing for innovations in HIV diagnosis and treatment, and moreover they actively lobbied for price reductions and generic products thus making drugs, diagnostics, and vaccines affordable in low-resource countries. As the HIV epidemic also affected the developed world, much of the R&D products were transferred to benefit the developing world. R&D in the HIV field has also been heavily supported by the pharmaceutical industry as HIV is a chronic disease that requires lifelong management, ensuring a sustainable market for HIV diagnostics and antiretroviral drugs. On the contrary, R&D, and more importantly advocacy for TB, has been weak with very little interest from the private industry and funders (Harrington 2010). Investors do not see huge profitability in the discovery of novel TB diagnostics or chemotherapeutics as these products will ultimately need to be cheap to serve poorly resourced countries.

The Global Plan to Stop TB 2011–2015 estimated a sum of US$9.8 billion for TB R&D to reach the targets of 50% reduction in TB prevalence and mortality by 2015 (WHO 2010). However, the analyses undertaken by the Treatment Action Group (TAG) and Stop TB Partnership (STP) revealed that globally TB research remained grossly underfunded with a total funding gap of US$6.4 billion (64%) over the 5 years (2011–2015). The 2011, TAG and STP funding report also highlighted that TB funding for basic science research was on the decline over this period (Treatment Action Group 2011, WHO 2015a). Without a fresh injection of new sustained funding, progress in the area of microfluidics and basic research for the development of POC tests will be severely hampered. As an alternative strategy, to circumvent the lack of funding and industry interest in TB R&D, attention is now shifting to Brazil, Russia, India, China, and South Africa (BRICS) for leadership to provide definitive direction and development of affordable healthcare technologies for the management of TB (Engel et al. 2012). Several of the BRICS countries have been identified to have the technical resources and intellectual capacity to develop solutions to support the much-need next-generation innovations (Small and Pai 2010). Furthermore, countries such as China and India have a strong growing biotechnology industry and therefore are in good stead to bring new TB drugs, vaccines, and diagnostics to the fore (Frew et al. 2008).

The 2030 targets set out in the WHO End TB strategy proposes a 80% reduction in TB incidence and a 90% reduction in the number of deaths compared to levels in 2015 (WHO 2014). These statistics can only be reached with greater engagement and involvement of industry, funders, governments, and researchers. More importantly, the lessons learned from the successes with the HIV epidemic must be considered to intensify advocacy for R&D for improved tools for TB care and control. If we are to win the battle against TB, clearly more needs to be done on all fronts to eradicate this dreaded disease. The scene is set for microfluidics to revolutionize TB diagnostics.

Acknowledgments

This work was supported by funding from an International Early Career Scientist Award from the Howard Hughes Medical Institute (to BDK), the South African National Research Foundation (to BDK and BGG), the South African Medical Research Council (to BDK), and the National Health Laboratory Services Research Trust (to BDK and BGG).

References

Abubakar, I., L. Pimpin, C. Ariti, R. Beynon, P. Mangtani, J. A. Sterne, P. E. Fine et al. 2013. Systematic review and meta-analysis of the current evidence on the duration of protection by Bacillus Calmette-Guerin vaccination against tuberculosis. *Health Technol Assess* 17 (37):1–372.

Adjers-Koskela, K. and M. L. Katila. 2003. Susceptibility testing with the manual mycobacteria growth indicator tube (MGIT) and the MGIT 960 system provides rapid and reliable verification of multidrug-resistant tuberculosis. *J Clin Microbiol* 41 (3):1235–1239.

AERAS. 2014. TB vaccine research and development: A business case for investment. Available at http://www.aeras.org/pdf/TB RD Business Case Draft 3.pdf. Accessed November 2016.

Ahmad, F. and S. A. Hashsham. 2012. Miniaturized nucleic acid amplification systems for rapid and point-of-care diagnostics: A review. *Anal Chim Acta* 733:1–15.

Ahmad, F., G. Seyrig, D. M. Tourlousse, R. D. Stedtfeld, J. M. Tiedje, and S. A. Hashsham. 2011. A CCD-based fluorescence imaging system for real-time loop-mediated isothermal amplification-based rapid and sensitive detection of waterborne pathogens on microchips. *Biomed Microdevices* 13 (5):929–937.

Albert, H., R. R. Nathavitharana, C. Isaacs, M. Pai, C. M. Denkinger, and C. C. Boehme. 2016. Development, roll-out and impact of Xpert MTB/RIF for tuberculosis: What lessons have we learnt and how can we do better? *Eur Respir J* 48 (2):516–525.

Andersen, P., M. E. Munk, J. M. Pollock, and T. M. Doherty. 2000. Specific immune-based diagnosis of tuberculosis. *Lancet* 356 (9235):1099–1104.

Ardito, F., B. Posteraro, M. Sanguinetti, S. Zanetti, and G. Fadda. 2001. Evaluation of BACTEC Mycobacteria Growth Indicator Tube (MGIT 960) automated system for drug susceptibility testing of *Mycobacterium tuberculosis*. *J Clin Microbiol* 39 (12):4440–4444.

Barnard, M., H. Albert, G. Coetzee, R. O'Brien, and M. E. Bosman. 2008. Rapid molecular screening for multidrug-resistant tuberculosis in a high-volume public health laboratory in South Africa. *Am J Respir Crit Care Med* 177 (7):787–792.

Barnard, M., N. C. Gey van Pittius, P. D. van Helden, M. Bosman, G. Coetzee, and R. M. Warren. 2012. The diagnostic performance of the GenoType MTBDRplus version 2 line probe assay is equivalent to that of the Xpert MTB/RIF assay. *J Clin Microbiol* 50 (11):3712–3716.

Barreto, A. M., J. B. Araujo, R. F. de Melo Medeiros, and P. C. de Souza Caldas. 2003. Evaluation of indirect susceptibility testing of *Mycobacterium tuberculosis* to the first- and second-line, and alternative drugs by the newer MB/BacT system. *Mem Inst Oswaldo Cruz* 98 (6):827–830.

Barreto, M. L., S. M. Pereira, D. Pilger, A. A. Cruz, S. S. Cunha, C. Sant'Anna, M. Y. Ichihara, B. Genser, and L. C. Rodrigues. 2011. Evidence of an effect of BCG revaccination on incidence of tuberculosis in school-aged children in Brazil: Second report of the BCG-REVAC cluster-randomised trial. *Vaccine* 29 (31):4875–4877.

Barthwal, M. S., K. E. Rajan, R. B. Deoskar, and S. K. Sharma. 2005. Extrapulmonary tuberculosis in human immunodificiency virus infection. *Med J Armed Forces India* 61 (4):340–341.

Bekker, A., H. S. Schaaf, H. R. Draper, M. Kriel, and A. C. Hesseling. 2016. Tuberculosis disease during pregnancy and treatment outcomes in HIV-infected and uninfected women at a referral hospital in Cape Town. *PLoS One* 11 (11):e0164249.

Bemer, P., F. Palicova, S. Rusch-Gerdes, H. B. Drugeon, and G. E. Pfyffer. 2002. Multicenter evaluation of fully automated BACTEC Mycobacteria Growth Indicator Tube 960 system for susceptibility testing of *Mycobacterium tuberculosis*. *J Clin Microbiol* 40 (1):150–154.

Bi, A., C. Nakajima, Y. Fukushima, A. Tamaru, I. Sugawara, A. Kimura, R. Kawahara, Z. Hu, and Y. Suzuki. 2012. A rapid loop-mediated isothermal amplification assay targeting hspX for the detection of *Mycobacterium tuberculosis* complex. *Jpn J Infect Dis* 65 (3):247–251.

Boehme, C. C., P. Nabeta, D. Hillemann, M. P. Nicol, S. Shenai, F. Krapp, J. Allen et al. 2010. Rapid molecular detection of tuberculosis and rifampin resistance. *N Engl J Med* 363 (11):1005–1015.

Boehme, C. C., M. P. Nicol, P. Nabeta, J. S. Michael, E. Gotuzzo, R. Tahirli, M. T. Gler et al. 2011. Feasibility, diagnostic accuracy, and effectiveness of decentralised use of the Xpert MTB/RIF test for diagnosis of tuberculosis and multidrug resistance: A multicentre implementation study. *Lancet* 377 (9776):1495–1505.

Boyd, D. B. and W. H. Lunn. 1979. Electronic structures of cephalosporins and penicillins. 9. Departure of a leaving group in cephalosporins. *J Med Chem* 22 (7):778–784.

Cambau, E., C. Wichlacz, C. Truffot-Pernot, and V. Jarlier. 1999. Evaluation of the new MB redox system for detection of growth of mycobacteria. *J Clin Microbiol* 37 (6):2013–2015.

Castan, P., A. de Pablo, N. Fernandez-Romero, J. M. Rubio, B. D. Cobb, J. Mingorance, and C. Toro. 2014. Point-of-care system for detection of *Mycobacterium tuberculosis* and rifampin resistance in sputum samples. *J Clin Microbiol* 52 (2):502–507.

Chang, J., P. Arbelaez, N. Switz, C. Reber, A. Tapley, J. L. Davis, A. Cattamanchi, D. Fletcher, and J. Malik. 2013. Automated tuberculosis diagnosis using fluorescence images from a mobile microscope. *Med Image Comput Comput Assist Interv* 15 (Pt 3):345–352.

Chida, N. and M. Shah. 2016. Infectious diseases (ID) learning unit: How rapidly to evaluate for active tuberculosis disease in low-prevalence settings. *Open Forum Infect Dis* 3 (2):ofw058.

Chung, H. J., C. M. Castro, H. Im, H. Lee, and R. Weissleder. 2013. A magneto-DNA nanoparticle system for rapid detection and phenotyping of bacteria. *Nat Nanotechnol* 8 (5):369–375.

Cobelens, F. G., S. M. Egwaga, T. van Ginkel, H. Muwinge, M. I. Matee, and M. W. Borgdorff. 2006. Tuberculin skin testing in patients with HIV infection: Limited benefit of reduced cutoff values. *Clin Infect Dis* 43 (5):634–639.

Connolly, M. and P. Nunn. 1996. Women and tuberculosis. *World Health Stat Q* 49 (2):115–119.

Cummings, D. M., D. Ristroph, E. E. Camargo, S. M. Larson, and H. N. Wagner, Jr. 1975. Radiometric detection of the metabolic activity of *Mycobacterium tuberculosis*. *J Nucl Med* 16 (12):1189–1191.

DDNews. August 2011. Epistem and Xcelris lab partner on TB diagnostics. Available at http://www.ddn-news.com/index.php/newsarticle=5251. Accessed November 2016.

Denkinger, C. M. and M. Pai. 2012. Point-of-care tuberculosis diagnosis: Are we there yet? *Lancet Infect Dis* 12 (3):169–170.

Detjen, A. K., A. R. DiNardo, J. Leyden, K. R. Steingart, D. Menzies, I. Schiller, N. Dendukuri, and A. M. Mandalakas. 2015. Xpert MTB/RIF assay for the diagnosis of pulmonary tuberculosis in children: A systematic review and meta-analysis. *Lancet Respir Med* 3 (6):451–461.

Dheda, K., C. E. Barry, 3rd, and G. Maartens. 2016a. Tuberculosis. *Lancet* 387 (10024):1211–1226.

Dheda, K., K. C. Chang, L. Guglielmetti, J. Furin, H. S. Schaaf, D. Chesov, A. Esmail, and C. Lange. 2016b. Clinical management of adults and children with MDR and XDR-TB. *Clin Microbiol Infect* 23(3):131–140.

Dheda, K., R. van Zyl Smit, M. Badri, and M. Pai. 2009. T-cell interferon-gamma release assays for the rapid immunodiagnosis of tuberculosis: Clinical utility in high-burden vs. low-burden settings. *Curr Opin Pulm Med* 15 (3):188–200.

Diedrich, C. R., J. T. Mattila, E. Klein, C. Janssen, J. Phuah, T. J. Sturgeon, R. C. Montelaro, P. L. Lin, and J. L. Flynn. 2010. Reactivation of latent tuberculosis in cynomolgus macaques infected with SIV is associated with early peripheral T cell depletion and not virus load. *PLoS One* 5 (3):e9611.

Dimov, I. K., L. Basabe-Desmonts, J. L. Garcia-Cordero, B. M. Ross, Y. Park, A. J. Ricco, and L. P. Lee. 2011. Stand-alone self-powered integrated microfluidic blood analysis system (SIMBAS). *Lab Chip* 11 (5):845–850.

Dinnes, J., J. Deeks, H. Kunst, A. Gibson, E. Cummins, N. Waugh, F. Drobniewski, and A. Lalvani. 2007. A systematic review of rapid diagnostic tests for the detection of tuberculosis infection. *Health Technol Assess* 11 (3):1–196.

Dowdy, D. W., K. R. Steingart, and M. Pai. 2011. Serological testing versus other strategies for diagnosis of active tuberculosis in India: A cost-effectiveness analysis. *PLoS Med* 8 (8):e1001074.

Engel, N., J. Kenneth, and M. Pai. 2012. TB diagnostics in India: Creating an ecosystem for innovation. *Expert Rev Mol Diagn* 12 (1):21–24.

Epistem. 2012. *Epistem Signs Tuberculosis Channel Partner Agreement*. Epistem Plc., Manchester, U.K. Available at http://www.epistem.co.uk/press-release/EpistemPressReleaseTBCollaborationAgreement05Mar12.pdf.   Accessed November 2016.

Fang, X., Y. Liu, J. Kong, and X. Jiang. 2010. Loop-mediated isothermal amplification integrated on microfluidic chips for point-of-care quantitative detection of pathogens. *Anal Chem* 82 (7):3002–3006.

Faraci, W. S. and R. F. Pratt. 1985. Mechanism of inhibition of the PC1 beta-lactamase of *Staphylococcus aureus* by cephalosporins: Importance of the 3′-leaving group. *Biochemistry* 24 (4):903–910.

Farhat, M., C. Greenaway, M. Pai, and D. Menzies. 2006. False-positive tuberculin skin tests: What is the absolute effect of BCG and non-tuberculous mycobacteria? *Int J Tuberc Lung Dis* 10 (11):1192–1204.

FIND. 2012. Negotiated prices for XpertH MTB/RIF. Available from http://www.finddiagnostics.org/about/what_we_do/successes/find-negotiated-prices/xpert_mtb_rif.html. Accessed November 2016.

Flores, A. R., L. M. Parsons, and M. S. Pavelka, Jr. 2005. Genetic analysis of the beta-lactamases of *Mycobacterium tuberculosis* and *Mycobacterium smegmatis* and susceptibility to beta-lactam antibiotics. *Microbiology* 151 (Pt 2):521–532.

Ford, C. B., P. L. Lin, M. R. Chase, R. R. Shah, O. Iartchouk, J. Galagan, N. Mohaideen et al. 2011. Use of whole genome sequencing to estimate the mutation rate of *Mycobacterium tuberculosis* during latent infection. *Nat Genet* 43 (5):482–486.

Frew, S. E., H. E. Kettler, and P. A. Singer. 2008. The Indian and Chinese health biotechnology industries: Potential champions of global health? *Health Aff (Millwood)* 27 (4):1029–1041.

Gagneux, S., C. D. Long, P. M. Small, T. Van, G. K. Schoolnik, and B. J. Bohannan. 2006. The competitive cost of antibiotic resistance in *Mycobacterium tuberculosis*. *Science* 312 (5782):1944–1946.

Gandhi, N. R., A. Moll, A. W. Sturm, R. Pawinski, T. Govender, U. Lalloo, K. Zeller, J. Andrews, and G. Friedland. 2006. Extensively drug-resistant tuberculosis as a cause of death in patients co-infected with tuberculosis and HIV in a rural area of South Africa. *Lancet* 368 (9547):1575–1580.

Gao, W., B. Xing, R. Y. Tsien, and J. Rao. 2003. Novel fluorogenic substrates for imaging beta-lactamase gene expression. *J Am Chem Soc* 125 (37):11146–11147.

Garg, S. K., R. P. Tiwari, D. Tiwari, R. Singh, D. Malhotra, V. K. Ramnani, G. B. Prasad et al. 2003. Diagnosis of tuberculosis: Available technologies, limitations, and possibilities. *J Clin Lab Anal* 17 (5):155–163.

Garrigo, M., L. M. Aragon, F. Alcaide, S. Borrell, E. Cardenosa, J. J. Galan, J. Gonzalez-Martin et al. 2007. Multicenter laboratory evaluation of the MB/BacT Mycobacterium detection system and the BACTEC MGIT 960 system in comparison with the BACTEC 460TB system for susceptibility testing of *Mycobacterium tuberculosis*. *J Clin Microbiol* 45 (6):1766–1770.

Gericke, C. A., C. Kurowski, M. K. Ranson, and A. Mills. 2005. Intervention complexity—A conceptual framework to inform priority-setting in health. *Bull World Health Organ* 83 (4):285–293.

Getahun, H., M. Harrington, R. O'Brien, and P. Nunn. 2007. Diagnosis of smear-negative pulmonary tuberculosis in people with HIV infection or AIDS in resource-constrained settings: Informing urgent policy changes. *Lancet* 369 (9578):2042–2049.

Gill, P., R. Ramezani, M. V. Amiri, A. Ghaemi, T. Hashempour, N. Eshraghi, M. Ghalami, and H. A. Tehrani. 2006. Enzyme-linked immunosorbent assay of nucleic acid sequence-based amplification for molecular detection of M. tuberculosis. *Biochem Biophys Res Commun* 347 (4):1151–1157.

Gordon, S. V., B. Heym, J. Parkhill, B. Barrell, and S. T. Cole. 1999. New insertion sequences and a novel repeated sequence in the genome of *Mycobacterium tuberculosis* H37Rv. *Microbiology* 145 (Pt 4):881–892.

Gray, C. M., A. Katamba, P. Narang, J. Giraldo, C. Zamudio, M. Joloba, R. Narang et al. 2016. Feasibility and operational performance of tuberculosis detection by loop-mediated isothermal amplification platform in decentralized settings: Results from a multicenter study. *J Clin Microbiol* 54 (8):1984–1991.

Hanna, B. A., A. Ebrahimzadeh, L. B. Elliott, M. A. Morgan, S. M. Novak, S. Rusch-Gerdes, M. Acio et al. 1999. Multicenter evaluation of the BACTEC MGIT 960 system for recovery of mycobacteria. *J Clin Microbiol* 37 (3):748–752.

Harries, A. D., T. E. Nyirenda, P. Godfrey-Faussett, and F. M. Salaniponi. 2003. Defining and assessing the maximum number of visits patients should make to a health facility to obtain a diagnosis of pulmonary tuberculosis. *Int J Tuberc Lung Dis* 7 (10):953–958.

Harrington, M. 2010. From HIV to tuberculosis anhd back again: A tale of activism in 2 pandemics. *Clin Infect Dis* 50 (Suppl 3):S260–S266.

Haun, J. B., C. M. Castro, R. Wang, V. M. Peterson, B. S. Marinelli, H. Lee, and R. Weissleder. 2011. Micro-NMR for rapid molecular analysis of human tumor samples. *Sci Transl Med* 3 (71):71ra16.

Haun, J. B., N. K. Devaraj, S. A. Hilderbrand, H. Lee, and R. Weissleder. 2010. Bioorthogonal chemistry amplifies nanoparticle binding and enhances the sensitivity of cell detection. *Nat Nanotechnol* 5 (9):660–665.

Helb, D., M. Jones, E. Story, C. Boehme, E. Wallace, K. Ho, J. Kop et al. 2010. Rapid detection of *Mycobacterium tuberculosis* and rifampin resistance by use of on-demand, near-patient technology. *J Clin Microbiol* 48 (1):229–237.

Hobby, G. L., A. P. Holman, M. D. Iseman, and J. M. Jones. 1973. Enumeration of tubercle bacilli in sputum of patients with pulmonary tuberculosis. *Antimicrob Agents Chemother* 4 (2):94–104.

Hsieh, K., A. S. Patterson, B. S. Ferguson, K. W. Plaxco, and H. T. Soh. 2012. Rapid, sensitive, and quantitative detection of pathogenic DNA at the point of care through microfluidic electrochemical quantitative loop-mediated isothermal amplification. *Angew Chem Int Ed Engl* 51 (20):4896–4900.

Hugonnet, J. E., L. W. Tremblay, H. I. Boshoff, C. E. Barry, 3rd, and J. S. Blanchard. 2009. Meropenem-clavulanate is effective against extensively drug-resistant *Mycobacterium tuberculosis*. *Science* 323 (5918):1215–1218.

Issadore, D., C. Min, M. Liong, J. Chung, R. Weissleder, and H. Lee. 2011. Miniature magnetic resonance system for point-of-care diagnostics. *Lab Chip* 11 (13):2282–2287.

Jeon, D. S., D. O. Shin, S. K. Park, J. E. Seo, H. S. Seo, Y. S. Cho, J. Y. Lee et al. 2011. Treatment outcome and mortality among patients with multidrug-resistant tuberculosis in tuberculosis hospitals of the public sector. *J Korean Med Sci* 26 (1):33–41.

Jing, W., X. Jiang, W. Zhao, S. Liu, X. Cheng, and G. Sui. 2014. Microfluidic platform for direct capture and analysis of airborne *Mycobacterium tuberculosis*. *Anal Chem* 86 (12):5815–5821.

Kaufmann, S. H. 2002. Protection against tuberculosis: Cytokines, T cells, and macrophages. *Ann Rheum Dis* 61 Suppl 2:ii54–ii58.

Kersting, S., V. Rausch, F. F. Bier, and M. von Nickisch-Rosenegk. 2014. Multiplex isothermal solid-phase recombinase polymerase amplification for the specific and fast DNA-based detection of three bacterial pathogens. *Mikrochim Acta* 181 (13–14):1715–1723.

Knight, G. M., U. K. Griffiths, T. Sumner, Y. V. Laurence, A. Gheorghe, A. Vassall, P. Glaziou, and R. G. White. 2014. Impact and cost-effectiveness of new tuberculosis vaccines in low- and middle-income countries. *Proc Natl Acad Sci USA* 111 (43):15520–15525.

Kong, Y., H. Yao, H. Ren, S. Subbian, S. L. Cirillo, J. C. Sacchettini, J. Rao, and J. D. Cirillo. 2010. Imaging tuberculosis with endogenous beta-lactamase reporter enzyme fluorescence in live mice. *Proc Natl Acad Sci USA* 107 (27):12239–12244.

Kontos, F., M. Maniati, C. Costopoulos, Z. Gitti, S. Nicolaou, E. Petinaki, S. Anagnostou, I. Tselentis, and A. N. Maniatis. 2004. Evaluation of the fully automated Bactec MGIT 960 system for the susceptibility testing of *Mycobacterium tuberculosis* to first-line drugs: A multicenter study. *J Microbiol Methods* 56 (2):291–294.

Kruuner, A., M. D. Yates, and F. A. Drobniewski. 2006. Evaluation of MGIT 960-based antimicrobial testing and determination of critical concentrations of first- and second-line antimicrobial drugs with drug-resistant clinical strains of *Mycobacterium tuberculosis*. *J Clin Microbiol* 44 (3):811–818.

Labmate. 2015. India approves licence for TB diagnosis. Available at http://www. labmate-online.com/news/news-and-views/5/epistem_ltd/india_approves_ lincence_for_tb_diagnosis/34643. Accessed November 2016.

Lalvani, A. 2007. Diagnosing tuberculosis infection in the 21st century: New tools to tackle an old enemy. *Chest* 131 (6):1898–1906.

Land, K. J., M. Mbanjwa, and J. G. Korvink. 2014. Microfluidic channel structures speed up mixing of multiple emulsions by a factor of ten. *Biomicrofluidics* 8 (5):054101.

Lawn, S. D., A. D. Kerkhoff, M. Vogt, and R. Wood. 2012. Diagnostic accuracy of a low-cost, urine antigen, point-of-care screening assay for HIV-associated pulmonary tuberculosis before antiretroviral therapy: A descriptive study. *Lancet Infect Dis* 12 (3):201–209.

Lawn, S. D. and M. P. Nicol. 2011. Xpert(R) MTB/RIF assay: Development, evaluation and implementation of a new rapid molecular diagnostic for tuberculosis and rifampicin resistance. *Future Microbiol* 6 (9):1067–1082.

Lee, H., E. Sun, D. Ham, and R. Weissleder. 2008. Chip-NMR biosensor for detection and molecular analysis of cells. *Nat Med* 14 (8):869–874.

Lee, H., T. J. Yoon, J. L. Figueiredo, F. K. Swirski, and R. Weissleder. 2009. Rapid detection and profiling of cancer cells in fine-needle aspirates. *Proc Natl Acad Sci USA* 106 (30):12459–12464.

Lee, T. Y., T. J. Lee, J. T. Belisle, P. J. Brennan, and S. K. Kim. 1997. A novel repeat sequence specific to *Mycobacterium tuberculosis* complex and its implications. *Tuber Lung Dis* 78 (1):13–19.

Lewis, J. J., V. N. Chihota, M. van der Meulen, P. B. Fourie, K. L. Fielding, A. D. Grant, S. E. Dorman, and G. J. Churchyard. 2012. "Proof-of-concept" evaluation of an automated sputum smear microscopy system for tuberculosis diagnosis. *PLoS One* 7 (11):e50173.

Ling, D. I., A. A. Zwerling, and M. Pai. 2008. GenoType MTBDR assays for the diagnosis of multidrug-resistant tuberculosis: A meta-analysis. *Eur Respir J* 32 (5):1165–1174.

Liong, M., A. N. Hoang, J. Chung, N. Gural, C. B. Ford, C. Min, R. R. Shah et al. 2013. Magnetic barcode assay for genetic detection of pathogens. *Nat Commun* 4:1–9.

Liu, D., G. Liang, Q. Zhang, and B. Chen. 2013. Detection of *Mycobacterium tuberculosis* using a capillary-array microsystem with integrated DNA extraction, loop-mediated isothermal amplification, and fluorescence detection. *Anal Chem* 85 (9):4698–4704.

Madhuri, K., S. Deshpande, S. Dharmashale, and R. Bharadwaj. 2015. Utility of line probe assay for the early detection of multidrug-resistant pulmonary tuberculosis. *J Glob Infect Dis* 7 (2):60–65.

Mahairas, G. G., P. J. Sabo, M. J. Hickey, D. C. Singh, and C. K. Stover. 1996. Molecular analysis of genetic differences between *Mycobacterium bovis* BCG and virulent *M. bovis*. *J Bacteriol* 178 (5):1274–1282.

Manage, D. P., L. Chui, and L. M. Pilarski. 2013. Sub-microliter scale in-gel loop-mediated isothermal amplification (LAMP) for detection of *Mycobacterium tuberculosis*. *Microfluid Nanofluidics* 14 (3):731–741.

Mangtani, P., I. Abubakar, C. Ariti, R. Beynon, L. Pimpin, P. E. Fine, L. C. Rodrigues et al. 2014. Protection by BCG vaccine against tuberculosis: A systematic review of randomized controlled trials. *Clin Infect Dis* 58 (4):470–480.

Manosuthi, W., S. Wiboonchutikul, and S. Sungkanuparph. 2016. Integrated therapy for HIV and tuberculosis. *AIDS Res Ther* 13:22.

Meyer-Rath, G., K. Schnippel, L. Long, W. MacLeod, I. Sanne, W. Stevens, S. Pillay, Y. Pillay, and S. Rosen. 2012. The impact and cost of scaling up GeneXpert MTB/RIF in South Africa. *PLoS One* 7 (5):e36966.

Milat, A. J., A. Bauman, and S. Redman. 2015. Narrative review of models and success factors for scaling up public health interventions. *Implement Sci* 10:113.

Milat, A. J., L. King, A. E. Bauman, and S. Redman. 2013. The concept of scalability: Increasing the scale and potential adoption of health promotion interventions into policy and practice. *Health Promot Int* 28 (3):285–298.

Milat, A. J., L. King, R. Newson, L. Wolfenden, C. Rissel, A. Bauman, and S. Redman. 2014. Increasing the scale and adoption of population health interventions: Experiences and perspectives of policy makers, practitioners, and researchers. *Health Res Policy Syst* 12:18.

Millen, S. J., P. W. Uys, J. Hargrove, P. D. van Helden, and B. G. Williams. 2008. The effect of diagnostic delays on the drop-out rate and the total delay to diagnosis of tuberculosis. *PLoS One* 3 (4):e1933.

Mitarai, S., M. Okumura, E. Toyota, T. Yoshiyama, A. Aono, A. Sejimo, Y. Azuma et al. 2011. Evaluation of a simple loop-mediated isothermal amplification test kit for the diagnosis of tuberculosis. *Int J Tuberc Lung Dis* 15 (9):1211–1217, i.

MMWR. 2000. Targeted tuberculin testing and treatment of latent tuberculosis infection. In American Thoracic Society. MMWR Recommendation and Reports. www.cdc.gov/mmwr/preview/mmwrhtml/rr4906a1.htm. Accessed June 09, 2000, 49 (RR06):1–54

Morgan, M., S. Kalantri, L. Flores, and M. Pai. 2005. A commercial line probe assay for the rapid detection of rifampicin resistance in *Mycobacterium tuberculosis*: A systematic review and meta-analysis. *BMC Infect Dis* 5:62.

Mori, Y. and T. Notomi. 2009. Loop-mediated isothermal amplification (LAMP): A rapid, accurate, and cost-effective diagnostic method for infectious diseases. *J Infect Chemother* 15 (2):62–69.

Muller, B., V. N. Chihota, M. Pillay, M. Klopper, E. M. Streicher, G. Coetzee, A. Trollip et al. 2013. Programmatically selected multidrug-resistant strains drive the emergence of extensively drug-resistant tuberculosis in South Africa. *PLoS One* 8 (8):e70919.

Murray, S., L. McKenna, E. Pelfrene, and R. Botgros. 2015. Accelerating clinical drug development for children with tuberculosis. *Int J Tuberc Lung Dis* 19 (Suppl 1):69–74.

Musser, J. M. 1995. Antimicrobial agent resistance in mycobacteria: Molecular genetic insights. *Clin Microbiol Rev* 8 (4):496–514.

Nabukeera-Barungi, N., J. Wilmshurst, M. Rudzani, and J. Nuttall. 2014. Presentation and outcome of tuberculous meningitis among children: Experiences from a tertiary children's hospital. *Afr Health Sci* 14 (1):143–149.

Nathavitharanaa, R. R., D. Hillemann, S. G. Schumacher, B. Schlueter, N. Ismail, S. V. Omar, W. Sikhondze et al. 2016. Multicenter noninferiority evaluation of Hain GenoType MTBDRplus Version 2 and Nipro NTM+MDRTB Line Probe Assays for detection of rifampin and isoniazid resistance *J Clin Microbiol* 54 (6):1624–1630.

Njiru, Z. K. 2012. Loop-mediated isothermal amplification technology: Towards point of care diagnostics. *PLoS Negl Trop Dis* 6 (6):e1572.

Osman, M., J. A. Seddon, R. Dunbar, H. R. Draper, C. Lombard, and N. Beyers. 2015. The complex relationship between human immunodeficiency virus infection and death in adults being treated for tuberculosis in Cape Town, South Africa. *BMC Public Health* 15:556.

Padmapriyadarsini, C., G. Narendran, and S. Swaminathan. 2011. Diagnosis & treatment of tuberculosis in HIV co-infected patients. *Indian J Med Res* 134 (6):850–865.

Pai, M. 2011. Improving TB diagnosis: Difference between knowing the path and walking the path. *Expert Rev Mol Diagn* 11 (3):241–244.

Pai, M., M. A. Behr, D. Dowdy, K. Dheda, M. Divangahi, C. C. Boehme, A. Ginsberg et al. 2016. Tuberculosis. *Nat Rev Dis Primers* 2:1–23.

Pai, M., C. M. Denkinger, S. V. Kik, M. X. Rangaka, A. Zwerling, O. Oxlade, J. Z. Metcalfe et al. 2014. Gamma interferon release assays for detection of *Mycobacterium tuberculosis* infection. *Clin Microbiol Rev* 27 (1):3–20.

Pai, M., L. W. Riley, and J. M. Colford, Jr. 2004. Interferon-gamma assays in the immunodiagnosis of tuberculosis: A systematic review. *Lancet Infect Dis* 4 (12):761–776.

Pai, M. and G. Sotgiu. 2016. Diagnostics for latent TB infection: Incremental, not transformative progress. *Eur Respir J* 47 (3):704–706.

Pai, N. P. and M. Pai. 2012. Point-of-care diagnostics for HIV and tuberculosis: Landscape, pipeline, and unmet needs. *Discov Med* 13 (68):35–45.

Parsons, L. M., A. Somoskovi, C. Gutierrez, E. Lee, C. N. Paramasivan, A. Abimiku, S. Spector, G. Roscigno, and J. Nkengasong. 2011. Laboratory diagnosis of tuberculosis in resource-poor countries: Challenges and opportunities. *Clin Microbiol Rev* 24 (2):314–350.

Pathak, S., T. Wentzel-Larsen, and B. Asjo. 2010. Effects of *in vitro* HIV-1 infection on mycobacterial growth in peripheral blood monocyte-derived macrophages. *Infect Immun* 78 (9):4022–4032.

Pawlowski, A., M. Jansson, M. Skold, M. E. Rottenberg, and G. Kallenius. 2012. Tuberculosis and HIV co-infection. *PLoS Pathog* 8 (2):e1002464.

Peter, J. G., G. Theron, R. van Zyl-Smit, A. Haripersad, L. Mottay, S. Kraus, A. Binder, R. Meldau, A. Hardy, and K. Dheda. 2012. Diagnostic accuracy of a urine lipoarabinomannan strip-test for TB detection in HIV-infected hospitalised patients. *Eur Respir J* 40 (5):1211–1220.

Pfyffer, G. E., D. A. Bonato, A. Ebrahimzadeh, W. Gross, J. Hotaling, J. Kornblum, A. Laszlo et al. 1999. Multicenter laboratory validation of susceptibility testing of *Mycobacterium tuberculosis* against classical second-line and newer antimicrobial drugs by using the radiometric BACTEC 460 technique and the proportion method with solid media. *J Clin Microbiol* 37 (10):3179–3186.

Piatek, A. S., S. Tyagi, A. C. Pol, A. Telenti, L. P. Miller, F. R. Kramer, and D. Alland. 1998. Molecular beacon sequence analysis for detecting drug resistance in *Mycobacterium tuberculosis*. *Nat Biotechnol* 16 (4):359–363.

Pollock, N. R., J. P. Rolland, S. Kumar, P. D. Beattie, S. Jain, F. Noubary, V. L. Wong, R. A. Pohlmann, U. S. Ryan, and G. M. Whitesides. 2012. A paper-based multiplexed transaminase test for low-cost, point-of-care liver function testing. *Sci Transl Med* 4 (152):152ra129.

Rafati, A. and P. Gill. 2015. Microfluidic method for rapid turbidimetric detection of the DNA of *Mycobacterium tuberculosis* using loop-mediated isothermal amplification in capillary tubes. *Microchimica Acta* 182 (3):523–530.

Rajendhran, J. and P. Gunasekaran. 2011. Microbial phylogeny and diversity: Small subunit ribosomal RNA sequence analysis and beyond. *Microbiol Res* 166 (2):99–110.

Raviglione, M. 2006. XDR-TB: Entering the post-antibiotic era? *Int J Tuberc Lung Dis* 10 (11):1185–1187.

Richeldi, L. 2006. An update on the diagnosis of tuberculosis infection. *Am J Respir Crit Care Med* 174 (7):736–742.

Roberts, G. D., N. L. Goodman, L. Heifets, H. W. Larsh, T. H. Lindner, J. K. McClatchy, M. R. McGinnis, S. H. Siddiqi, and P. Wright. 1983. Evaluation of the BACTEC radiometric method for recovery of mycobacteria and drug susceptibility testing of *Mycobacterium tuberculosis* from acid-fast smear-positive specimens. *J Clin Microbiol* 18 (3):689–696.

Rohner, P., B. Ninet, C. Metral, S. Emler, and R. Auckenthaler. 1997. Evaluation of the MB/BacT system and comparison to the BACTEC 460 system and solid media for isolation of mycobacteria from clinical specimens. *J Clin Microbiol* 35 (12):3127–3131.

Rosenfeld, L., F. Lyu, Y. Cheng, J. Rao, and S. K. Y. Tang. 2014. Rapid detection of tuberculosis using droplet based microfluidics. *18th International Conference on Miniaturized Systems for Chemistry and Life Sciences*, San Antonio, TX, October 26–30, 2014.

Roy, A., M. Eisenhut, R. J. Harris, L. C. Rodrigues, S. Sridhar, S. Habermann, L. Snell et al. 2014. Effect of BCG vaccination against *Mycobacterium tuberculosis* infection in children: Systematic review and meta-analysis. *BMJ* 349:g4643.

Ruiz, P., F. J. Zerolo, and M. J. Casal. 2000. Comparison of susceptibility testing of *Mycobacterium tuberculosis* using the ESP culture system II with that using the BACTEC method. *J Clin Microbiol* 38 (12):4663–4664.

Rukavishnikov, A., K. R. Gee, I. Johnson, and S. Corry. 2011. Fluorogenic cephalosporin substrates for beta-lactamase TEM-1. *Anal Biochem* 419 (1):9–16.

Rusch-Gerdes, S., G. E. Pfyffer, M. Casal, M. Chadwick, and S. Siddiqi. 2006. Multicenter laboratory validation of the BACTEC MGIT 960 technique for testing susceptibilities of *Mycobacterium tuberculosis* to classical second-line drugs and newer antimicrobials. *J Clin Microbiol* 44 (3):688–692.

Scarparo, C., P. Ricordi, G. Ruggiero, and P. Piccoli. 2004. Evaluation of the fully automated BACTEC MGIT 960 system for testing susceptibility of *Mycobacterium tuberculosis* to pyrazinamide, streptomycin, isoniazid, rifampin, and ethambutol and comparison with the radiometric BACTEC 460TB method. *J Clin Microbiol* 42 (3):1109–1114.

Schnippel, K., G. Meyer-Rath, L. Long, W. MacLeod, I. Sanne, W. S. Stevens, and S. Rosen. 2012. Scaling up Xpert MTB/RIF technology: The costs of laboratory- vs. clinic-based roll-out in South Africa. *Trop Med Int Health* 17 (9): 1142–1151.

Seddon, J. A., R. M. Warren, D. A. Enarson, N. Beyers, and H. S. Schaaf. 2012. Drug-resistant tuberculosis transmission and resistance amplification within families. *Emerg Infect Dis* 18 (8):1342–1345.

Sharma, S., J. Zapatero-Rodriguez, P. Estrela, and R. O'Kennedy. 2015. Point-of-Care diagnostics in low resource settings: Present status and future role of microfluidics. *Biosensors (Basel)* 5 (3):577–601.

Shenai, S., D. T. Armstrong, E. Valli, D. L. Dolinger, L. Nakiyingi, R. Dietze, M. P. Dalcolmo et al. 2016. Analytical and clinical evaluation of the Epistem Genedrive assay for detection of *Mycobacterium tuberculosis*. *J Clin Microbiol* 54 (4):1051–1057.

Siddiqi, K., M. L. Lambert, and J. Walley. 2003. Clinical diagnosis of smear-negative pulmonary tuberculosis in low-income countries: The current evidence. *Lancet Infect Dis* 3 (5):288–296.

Siddiqi, S. H., J. E. Hawkins, and A. Laszlo. 1985. Interlaboratory drug susceptibility testing of *Mycobacterium tuberculosis* by a radiometric procedure and two conventional methods. *J Clin Microbiol* 22 (6):919–923.

Siddiqi, S. H., J. P. Libonati, and G. Middlebrook. 1981. Evaluation of rapid radiometric method for drug susceptibility testing of *Mycobacterium tuberculosis*. *J Clin Microbiol* 13 (5):908–912.

Small, P. M. and M. Pai. 2010. Tuberculosis diagnosis—Time for a game change. *N Engl J Med* 363 (11):1070–1071.

Somoskovi, A., C. Kodmon, A. Lantos, Z. Bartfai, L. Tamasi, J. Fuzy, and P. Magyar. 2000. Comparison of recoveries of *Mycobacterium tuberculosis* using the automated BACTEC MGIT 960 system, the BACTEC 460 TB system, and Lowenstein-Jensen medium. *J Clin Microbiol* 38 (6):2395–2397.

Sorensen, A. L., S. Nagai, G. Houen, P. Andersen, and A. B. Andersen. 1995. Purification and characterization of a low-molecular-mass T-cell antigen secreted by *Mycobacterium tuberculosis*. *Infect Immun* 63 (5):1710–1717.

Spalgais, S., A. Jaiswal, M. Puri, R. Sarin, and U. Agarwal. 2013. Clinical profile and diagnosis of extrapulmonary tb in HIV infected patients: Routine abdominal ultrasonography increases detection of abdominal tuberculosis. *Indian J Tuberc* 60 (3):147–153.

St John, A. and C. P. Price. 2014. Existing and emerging technologies for point-of-care testing. *Clin Biochem Rev* 35 (3):155–167.

Steingart, K. R., L. L. Flores, N. Dendukuri, I. Schiller, S. Laal, A. Ramsay, P. C. Hopewell, and M. Pai. 2011. Commercial serological tests for the diagnosis of active pulmonary and extrapulmonary tuberculosis: An updated systematic review and meta-analysis. *PLoS Med* 8 (8):e1001062.

Tam, C. M., W. W. Yew, and K. Y. Yuen. 2009. Treatment of multidrug-resistant and extensively drug-resistant tuberculosis: Current status and future prospects. *Expert Rev Clin Pharmacol* 2 (4):405–421.

Taneja, R., A. J. Garcia-Prats, J. Furin, and H. K. Maheshwari. 2015. Paediatric formulations of second-line anti-tuberculosis medications: Challenges and considerations. *Int J Tuberc Lung Dis* 19 (Suppl 1):61–68.

Tortoli, E., M. Benedetti, A. Fontanelli, and M. T. Simonetti. 2002. Evaluation of automated BACTEC MGIT 960 system for testing susceptibility of *Mycobacterium tuberculosis* to four major antituberculous drugs: Comparison with the radiometric BACTEC 460TB method and the agar plate method of proportion. *J Clin Microbiol* 40 (2):607–610.

Tostmann, A., S. V. Kik, N. A. Kalisvaart, M. M. Sebek, S. Verver, M. J. Boeree, and D. van Soolingen. 2008. Tuberculosis transmission by patients with smear-negative pulmonary tuberculosis in a large cohort in the Netherlands. *Clin Infect Dis* 47 (9):1135–1142.

Treatment Action Group, Stop TB Partnership. 2011. Tuberculosis research and development: 2011 Report on tuberculosis research funding trends, 2005–2010. Available at http://www.stoptb.org/news/stories/2012/ns12_067.asp.

van Zyl-Smit, R. N., R. J. Lehloenya, R. Meldau, and K. Dheda. 2016. Impact of correcting the lymphocyte count to improve the sensitivity of TB antigen-specific peripheral blood-based quantitative T cell assays (T-SPOT.((R))TB and QFT-GIT). *J Thorac Dis* 8 (3):482–489.

Wang, S., F. Inci, G. De Libero, A. Singhal, and U. Demirci. 2013. Point-of-care assays for tuberculosis: Role of nanotechnology/microfluidics. *Biotechnol Adv* 31 (4):438–449.

Wang, S., X. Zhao, I. Khimji, R. Akbas, W. Qiu, D. Edwards, D. W. Cramer, B. Ye, and U. Demirci. 2011. Integration of cell phone imaging with microchip ELISA to detect ovarian cancer HE4 biomarker in urine at the point-of-care. *Lab Chip* 11 (20):3411–3418.

Whitesides, G. M. 2006. Overview. The origins and the future of microfluidics. *Nature* 442:368–373.

WHO. 2007. Strategic TB Advisory Group (STAG-TB). Report on conclusions and recommendations. Available at http://www.who.int/tb/events/stag_report_2007.pdf. World Health Organization, Geneva, Switzerland.

WHO. 2010. Global plan to stop tuberculosis 2011–2015. Available at http://www.who.int/nmh/events/ncd_action_plan/en/. World Health Organization, Geneva, Switzerland.

WHO. 2011a. Commercial sero-diagnostic tests for diagnosis of tuberculosis. Available at http://whqlibdoc.who.int/publications/2011/9789241502054_eng.pdf. Accessed November 2016.

WHO. 2011b. Global tuberculosis control 2011. Available at http://www.who.int/tb/publications/global_report/en/. Accessed November 2016.

WHO. 2013. The use of a commercial loop-mediated isothermal amplification assay (TB-LAMP) for the detection of tuberculosis. Available at http://www.stoptb.org/wg/gli/documents.asp. Accessed October 2016.

WHO. 2014. The end TB strategy. Available at http://www.who.int/tb/strategy/end_tb/en/. Accessed November 2016.

WHO. 2015a. Global tuberculosis report. Available at https://www.health-e.org.za/wp-content/uploads/2015/10/Global-TB-Report-2015-FINAL-2.pdf. World Health Organization, Geneva, Switzerland.

WHO. 2015b. WHO monitoring of of Xpert MTB/RIF roll out. Available at http://www.who.int/tb/areas-of-work/laboratory/mtb-rif-rollout/en/. Accessed November 2016.

WHO. 2016. Global tuberculosis report. Available at http://www.who.int/tb/publications/global_report/en/. World Health Organization, Geneva, Switzerland.

Woo, P. C., S. K. Lau, J. L. Teng, H. Tse, and K. Y. Yuen. 2008. Then and now: Use of 16S rDNA gene sequencing for bacterial identification and discovery of novel bacteria in clinical microbiology laboratories. *Clin Microbiol Infect* 14 (10):908–934.

Woods, G. L., G. Fish, M. Plaunt, and T. Murphy. 1997. Clinical evaluation of difco ESP culture system II for growth and detection of mycobacteria. *J Clin Microbiol* 35 (1):121–124.

Xie, H., J. Mire, Y. Kong, M. Chang, H. A. Hassounah, C. N. Thornton, J. C. Sacchettini, J. D. Cirillo, and J. Rao. 2012. Rapid point-of-care detection of the tuberculosis pathogen using a BlaC-specific fluorogenic probe. *Nat Chem* 4 (10):802–809.

Xing, B., A. Khanamiryan, and J. Rao. 2005. Cell-permeable near-infrared fluorogenic substrates for imaging beta-lactamase activity. *J Am Chem Soc* 127 (12):4158–4159.

Yamey, G. 2012. What are the barriers to scaling up health interventions in low and middle income countries? A qualitative study of academic leaders in implementation science. *Global Health* 8:11.

Yang, S., S. Lin, G. D. Kelen, T. C. Quinn, J. D. Dick, C. A. Gaydos, and R. E. Rothman. 2002. Quantitative multiprobe PCR assay for simultaneous detection and identification to species level of bacterial pathogens. *J Clin Microbiol* 40 (9):3449–3454.

Yao, H., M. K. So, and J. Rao. 2007. A bioluminogenic substrate for in vivo imaging of beta-lactamase activity. *Angew Chem Int Ed Engl* 46 (37):7031–7034.

Zhang, L., H. W. Ru, F. Z. Chen, C. Y. Jin, R. F. Sun, X. Y. Fan, M. Guo et al. 2016. Variable virulence and efficacy of BCG vaccine strains in mice and correlation with genome polymorphisms. *Mol Ther* 24 (2):398–405.

Zlokarnik, G., P. A. Negulescu, T. E. Knapp, L. Mere, N. Burres, L. Feng, M. Whitney, K. Roemer, and R. Y. Tsien. 1998. Quantitation of transcription and clonal selection of single living cells with beta-lactamase as reporter. *Science* 279 (5347):84–88.

Zwerling, A., M. A. Behr, A. Verma, T. F. Brewer, D. Menzies, and M. Pai. 2011. The BCG World Atlas: A database of global BCG vaccination policies and practices. *PLoS Med* 8 (3):e1001012.

Section III

Practical Aspects of Developing a Commercial Diagnostic Device

9

Starting with the End in Mind by Developing Diagnostics around User Needs

Mark David Lim

CONTENTS

"A couple drops of blood is all that is needed to diagnose a patient's health or disease" is a frequently used headline describing the aspirations for many new diagnostic tools in which both simple collection of small specimen volumes and rapid turn-around-time of test results aim to increase patient compliance and accuracy of treatment. The physician office is often the target market in higher-income countries and private healthcare systems, with recent interest in moving these capabilities closer to the patient in retail settings such as the corner pharmacy. The global health community is another target for these technologies; a healthcare setting is often depicted with images of a minimally trained community health worker who travels extreme distances, solely equipped with a backpack full of drugs and tests administered "under a tree."

Developing diagnostic tools that meet the needs of these settings—a physician office, a pharmacy, and a backpack—seems simple enough. Yet, the fast pace of diagnostics-focused innovations in microfluidics, signal transduction, and multiplexing is faced with an asymmetric adoption rate in any of these settings. Beyond the simplest format, the lateral flow rapid diagnostic test (RDT), and complex cartridges that operate on laboratory-based instruments such as Cepheid's GeneXpert system, there is a paucity of other microfluidic formats that have been implemented at significant scale.

As discussed in this chapter, the commercialization and adoption bottle-necks for these moderately complex diagnostics cannot be overcome by technological innovation alone, particularly in the highly regulated and payer-limited healthcare and public health markets. Diagnostics, unlike other clinical products, is not an intervention but a decision-aid that guides the use (or nonuse) of an intervention. It is important that the value proposi-tion for any technology-centric innovation in diagnostics include a strong link to a gained efficiency in making a specific decision. Any assay devel-oped without context to the system, users, decision points, and downstream interventions resembles one that is more targeted to the research community, rather than clinical care or public health.

This chapter highlights considerations for designing a diagnostic for use on individual patients or populations by assessing and incorporating the answers to two fundamental questions—who is asking for the test and how do test results guide a decision—questions that cannot be addressed in isolation of the user community. The methodology described is a best-practice for assessing and ensuring that user needs are central to the design, development, and eval-uation of a new diagnostic tool. The assessment starts with a clear intended-use statement that is centered around an actionable decision and justifies the time and cost to obtain a diagnosis. This definition is used to frame use-cases and user scenarios that identify users and describe how the test will be imple-mented, as well as criteria for generating an actionable test result. All three of these assessments are then used to create a list of product attributes that are required to meet the needs of an end user. The diagnostic developer plays a convening or observer role in the market assessment up until this point but has an active role in defining the technical performance specifications for a prod-uct that can satisfy the criteria described in these requirements. This process may be laborious, but centering design principles and functionality around user-needs avoids the creation of a proverbial hammer looking for that nail.

9.1 Defining How the Test Guides a Clinical or Public Health Decision: Intended-Use

Oftentimes, the value proposition for a new test is described through improve-ments in physical operability, speed, and ease of use, with little details on how test results improve a clinical or public health decision. Designing a new diagnostic should always start and remain accountable to a clearly defined "intended-use" that is grounded by the utility of the test's results, framed by an agreed-upon decision algorithm that links a patient encounter with a deci-sion to prescribe or not prescribe a specific intervention (see Box 9.1).

Clinical utility includes circumstance, decision, and action: definitions that justify the use of a test, presentation of test results to a user (e.g., qualitative,

---

BOX 9.1 DIAGNOSTIC ALGORITHMS

The absence of a decision tree or algorithm is a good indicator that the tool is more appropriate for research use instead of the clinical market. It is important to remember that diagnostic tools are used to guide a decision for individual clinical care or population-based public health. For instance, a diagnostic intended for measuring disease prognosis often results in a decision to monitor individuals more or less frequently with another test, depending on the interpretation test results in context of predetermined risk criteria. Similarly, results from a diagnostic used to measure the presence of an infection guide decisions on the course of intervention—using these types of diagnostics without access to treatment options could be considered unethical. Public health diagnostics could be used to monitor the resurgence of a previously quenched disease within a given population; positive results might be weighed with other considerations, such as population mobility, to guide a decision to test each individual with a more specific (and oftentimes more expensive) secondary diagnostic.

These decision trees are often published by a group of disease specialists convened by an overarching organization. Most global health communities, reference guidelines, recommendations, and policies are provided by global or regional departments of the World Health Organization (WHO) and/or by the ministries of health at the country or subnational levels. The algorithms integrate all healthcare tools—diagnostics and treatment—relying on evidence that assures safety and effectiveness for each recommended decision. Health economics also plays a large part in the rationale for these algorithms in which cost-effectiveness includes the resources required to perform the test, test performance, and availability of tools for intervention, considerations that are important for the resource-constrained global health market.

---

semiquantitative, and quantitative), and types of measurements needed to produce interpretable test results. Defining the patient's situation provides criteria that justifies a decision-maker to administer the test such as presentation of symptoms, ongoing treatment (such as a companion diagnostic), or other risk-associated factors such as geography, environment, or disposition. The action could be prescription or modification of a therapy, additional testing (such as subtyping or confirmatory testing), increased frequency of testing, or a public health action such as quarantine, vector control measure, or mass drug administration.

These attributes—clinical utility, presentation of test results, and interpretation to inform a specific decision—form the two to three sentences that comprise an intended-use statement. This statement should match an existing clinical or public health practice, not a hypothetical or aspirational workflow, as these also describe the targeted commercial market and regulatory pathway. It is an uphill battle if a developer envisions that a new technology will change guidelines and workflows because of placement of a new technology in a clinical care or public health program.

In addition to identifying the market, the intended-use statement is central to the design, development, and evaluation of a diagnostic by separating "nice-to-have" technical attributes from "must haves." The latter are the bare minimum requirements to successfully meet the needs of an end user in which every claim in the intended-use statement needs to be validated with clinical evidence. One should be critical of these intended-use claims, remembering that analytical validation studies are much simpler to perform and demonstrate compared to clinical validation studies. For example, if quantitative test results are essential for guiding a decision, studies can demonstrate analytical feasibility using spiked or contrived specimens. However, clinical feasibility must be demonstrated using nonaltered specimen from patient populations representative of the actual intended use, with statistically structured studies that evaluate the ability of the test to reproducibly provide quantitative results relevant to the decision. Challenges could include access to specimens annotated with this level of quantitative data as well as lack of a quantitative gold standard comparator, and it is important to assess the availability of these resources during the planning process of the project. Alternatively, the bar for validating a test's ability to reliably provide a qualitative "yes/no" result may be easier to cross, particularly if this type of test result is all that is needed to guide a specific decision; in this example, quantitation may be a "nice-to-have" that does not impact the final decision.

9.2 Defining How a Test Will Be Used: Use-Cases

The intended-use statement is a generalizable description that is enriched with use-cases and user-scenarios to add context to the decision algorithm. The goal of this exercise is to systematically identify how a test will be implemented and used, details that define requirements for getting a test used successfully. By weaving together details that identify users, workflows, and the settings in which the test is performed, the use-case and scenarios detail the "needs" that a test should address from the perspective of the user(s) within a defined healthcare system or public health program.

It is important to note that each use-case does not equate to a single independent test; one diagnostic tool can solve the needs of many use-cases. However, a test developer should demonstrate feasibility against one use-case and then consider expanding to other use-cases. It would be detrimental to develop a diagnostic that is not accountable to an intended use and associated use-case, or resource-intensive to simultaneously address multiple use-cases.

As mentioned earlier, a use-case is not developed by a test developer as these descriptions are inherently technology agnostic and should be developed by a community of end users to reflect current clinical or public health practice. At a high level, use-cases include details specific to the targeted patient population, decision-maker (user), healthcare or public health system, and linkage between the specific decision and interpretation of test results.

Use-cases always start with identifying the patient population targeted by the diagnostic and expand on the short description used in the intended-use statement. These include patient characteristics that trigger the use of a test by a decision-maker, such as symptoms, ongoing treatment, associated risk factors, etc. Additional details include potential coinfections or other factors that define eligibility or ineligibility for a test such as behavior, lifestyle, geography, environmental exposure, etc.

It is also important to understand the patient situation. For example, some patients and their families might have made substantial effort to seek healthcare and thus may resist the concept that a test will determine if they receive treatment, particularly if the testing adds out-of-pocket cost or time. It is also important to understand the role of culture for a specific patient population—a positive test result may result in stigma or isolation, rather than seeking care. If properly identified, many of these risks can be mitigated in the design or implementation of a test. For instance, there may be different ease-of-use considerations if a tribal healer is more effective at obtaining patient compliance for testing compared to a healthcare worker. It may also be important that testing staff include resources for proper counseling if a patient will be informed about their test results.

Another component of the use-case is the identity of the user, the individual responsible for making the clinical or public health decision with authority and resources to act on the test results, in accordance to a decision algorithm. By identifying the user, one can also deduce their workload. For instance, a clinician with a significant patient load might prefer prescribing treatment rather than waiting for test results. The user should not be confused with the test operator who performs the test, a role that is defined in the user scenarios.

These details include circumstances for "why" the user seeks the test results, "what" decisions are made by the user, and "how" test results guide their decision. In many public health programs, the user may be a program manager who is only interested in aggregated diagnostic results of a population, whereas a clinician or healthcare worker may be interested in the test results of an individual patient. Details may also include incentives or challenges for administering the test, such as cost or program achievements. Designing a test that addresses the pressures, incentives, and circumstance of the user are important not only for adoption by a healthcare or public health system, but also routine use. Table 9.1 lists some assumptions about the user that should be defined in a use-case.

Use-cases also include how the test will be interpreted, framing the criteria for making the results meaningful to the decision faced by the user. These details provide context to the decision algorithm by describing the type of analysis (e.g., organisms/molecules) and measurement parameters necessary for making a decision (e.g., level of quantitation). Natural history of disease can also be included if aspects such as stage or progression of disease are essential considerations for making a decision. This component of the use-case should also include integration with other data sources if the decision requires consideration of nondiagnostic data.

Severity of risk to a patient's health from an inaccurate result or diagnosis should also be elucidated, as related to the unintended misuse of an intervention. Defining the implications of an inaccurate result to a patient's health sets the threshold for allowable false positive or negative results, which are statistically inevitable but can be mitigated through the use of controls, processes, and other design criteria.

Details about the healthcare system or public health program frame the resources available for administering the test and the prioritization of a specific test in competition with other strategic priorities. It also describes institutional buy-in for using a test, availability and adherence to guidelines or recommendations (see Box 9.1), infrastructure for both administration and sustainable operation of the test, identity of a payer for the test results, and

TABLE 9.1

Assumptions That Need to Be Evaluated

Patient	• Stigma of diagnosis by social circles (family, friends, community) • Methods for seeking care (traditional healers, spiritual, clinical) • Cultural/spiritual beliefs with collecting specimens • Privacy considerations for non-blood-based specimens (urine, stool, genital swabs)
Community healthcare worker	• Confidence in operating new technology • Vulnerability to robbery/theft with more valuable technology • Off-label use of technology • Incentives • Proficiency testing • Turnover and training
Decision maker	• Patient load • Incorporation of test into clinical standard-of-care workflow • Demographics of patients • Incentives • Off-label use of technology • Proficiency testing

the regulatory pathway required for implementation. For instance, a public health program focused on a specific global health disease may dedicate resources (infrastructure, labor, funding, supply chain) into a specific testing program and also require that the test is evaluated through the World Health Organization's (WHO) prequalification program[1] to ensure that the test is manufactured using quality assurance processes and appropriate for use in the global health setting. Conversely, a primary healthcare system may have to balance their services among several disease priorities and may not be able to adequately resource or incentivize the use of a test. These components of the use-case can help forecast and mitigate several potential implementation challenges. Using these examples, a multipathogen platform may be the advantageous route for implementing a diagnostic in the primary healthcare setting but not practical for a disease-focused public health program. Common assumptions that many test developers take are listed in Table 9.2.

TABLE 9.2

Assumptions about the Healthcare System That Need to Be Evaluated

Lack of testing is due to lack of access/availability of an easily performed test.	• Identify who recommends the testing of a patient population. Design the performance and usability of a test around a treatment or decision algorithm, which often describes settings for the testing and are described in policy or guidelines authored by a country's Ministry of Health, or at a higher level by the World Health Organization. • Identify who pays for the test, these usually fall under the auspices of a country's Ministry of Finance or nongovernment procurers such as The Global Fund to fight AIDS, tuberculosis, and malaria.
Lack of testing is due to high costs of existing test.	• Cost of goods should reflect costs and ability to manufacture a design-locked device at scale, not costs reflecting construction of alpha-prototype. • Costs should not be limited to the test/device by itself, but should include all costs to perform the test. In many instances, costs for training, proficiency testing, and infrastructure to implement a new test may outweigh its technological benefits. • Components with low cost of goods may not be able to be manufactured at scale or under quality assurance requirements for in vitro diagnostics.
Regulatory approval is simpler for global health diagnostics because of the unmet need.	• Diagnostics that guide the clinical course for an individual patient often require the evaluation by a stringent regulatory body and/or prequalification by the World Health Organization. • Diagnostics that guide public health programs often follow recommendations, guidelines, or policies at the country level, or by the appropriate department of the World Health Organization.

The details described in this chapter only scratch the surface for developing use-cases, and additional considerations relevant to the implementation of a specific test should be documented as part of the market assessment. As decision-aids, diagnostic tools are an essential part of a healthcare or public health system, and it is important to do these assessments and unpack a list of requirements for integrating a new test into these systems as part of the planning process.

9.3 Defining Where a Test Will Be Used: User-Scenarios

A use-case should be further enriched with the depiction of a user-scenario, a series of storyboards that describe "how" a test will be implemented and performed. These storyboards describe the resources needed to perform the test successfully by generalizing the testing workflow. Often a use-case is accompanied by several scenarios, a selection of which represent current practice and others that may require slight changes to the current workflow as necessary compromises for implementing a "better" test. It may be possible to adjust the workflow in small pilot studies, but use of the test broadly and at significant scale requires that the test developer engage the related guideline and payer communities early in the planning process.

This exercise may also reveal that scenarios are dependent on the healthcare systems within a specific geography. By defining as many scenarios as possible, a test developer is given the choice to determine those that align with their business strategy and customize the design of the test around the circumstances of the physical operating environment. As with the use-cases, a test that can be used in all scenarios is likely one that is not perfect for any of them.

At a high level, user scenarios include:

- Patient flow: Mechanism of patient encounter, number of patients seen over a set period of time (hours/days), and workload (patients arrive at one time or over a period of time). These considerations are used to define throughput for the test, batching requirements, and turnaround time for test results. For example, a patient seeking care in a dedicated facility complicates predictions on total throughput, making random access more amenable to this scenario. Conversely, if the patient encounter is through a door-to-door public health campaign, total batch size and turnaround times are dependent on coverage and defined logistics, making these requirements more predictable.

- Testing environment: Examples include testing at the point of contact, transporting a medium-throughput mobile laboratory in proximity to a patient population (e.g., via a van), or collecting the specimens with shipment to a semi/centralized laboratory. These considerations are used to define the operational conditions and environments to frame the physical format, availability of resources (running water, electricity, etc.), turnaround time, and accessories necessary for performing the test.

- Staffing: Linked to the patient flow and workflow, this accounts for all individuals who interact with the patient—from preparation of the patient, collection and processing of the specimen, and operating the test. If applicable, it should also identify who provides counsel to the patient on their test results. The education and proficiency for performing these duties should be described as all of these considerations guide ease-of-use and training requirements. These details also inform throughput, batching requirements, turnaround time, and presentation of test results.

- Location of decision-maker (user): Describes whether the decision is made at the same location of the test or if interpretation is made remotely. These considerations are used to define turnaround time and presentation of test results, and data-transmission requirements. For example, a rapid result may not be necessary if, for logistical or cost reasons, the interpretation and intervention options are located in a different location than the test.

- Specimen custody: Details whether the specimen is acquired in a patient's home, in the same location as the test, or is collected remotely and transported to a central laboratory. These details inform the need for additional consumables, such as specimen collection and preservation accessories, and define logistics requirements for batching, shipping, and receiving specimens for testing.

- Test deployment: Resources that a program or healthcare system dedicates to train and prepare test operators and users, assurances for steady supply chain of reagents and equipment maintenance, and infrastructure for transporting test equipment not used in a central location. These details could include procurers, storage, customs regulations, and transportation requirements.

9.4 Translating Intended-Use, Use-Cases, and Scenarios into Product Requirements

The last phase of the user assessment is the development of product requirements. This is one of the hardest exercises as it involves compromise between "must have" requirements with "nice to have" attributes. The "must have" product requirements are the minimal criteria to meet end-user needs. They also set the bar for the performance of the test, as the final developed prototype must meet all minimum requirements. As with the intended-use, use-cases, and user-scenarios, the product requirements should be defined in collaboration with the end user and technology agnostic.

Compromises are inevitable in the creation of product requirements as they take into context end-user constraints or technical feasibility. For instance, in the global health setting, WHO has defined that the ideal test follows ASSURED criteria (affordable, sensitive, specific, user-friendly, robust and rapid, equipment-free, and deliverable to those who need them).[2] Each of those criteria have dependencies on each other. For instance, a highly sensitive and specific test may not be affordable or equipment-free, and it is up to the user-community to prioritize these attributes and define them as part of the product requirements.

Product requirements are meant to evolve over time, and it is important to assess any impact of changes to the user scenarios, use-cases, and intended use. It is important to document any change to the original product requirements by their causes and downstream implications to user acceptance.

9.5 Translating Product Requirements into Technical Performance Specifications

The product requirements set the goal for any new test, and it is now the responsibility of the developer to create the performance specifications that are achievable using their own technical approaches. This is the step where multiplexing, signal transduction, fluid manipulation, etc., can be incorporated as long as these components improve the ability to meet the product requirements. As mentioned earlier, it may be possible that the original product requirements are difficult to meet with a technical solution, and it is up to the developers to engage the end users to identify implications for compromising these requirements.

9.6 Concluding Thoughts

Starting with the end in mind, where end user needs are central to design and development of novel products are the best practices for most sectors outside of biomedicine. As described throughout this chapter, user needs for diagnostics is multifactorial because of the dependencies on both the specific decision and intervention, infrastructure required for implementing the test, and constraints from the regulatory and payer pathways. However, it is important to define criteria for a successful test before designing a new diagnostic from the onset because the opposite approach of forcing a technology into the complexities of a healthcare or public health system without this context will likely fail to have meaningful impact.

References

1. World Health Organization. Prequalification of in vitro diagnostics, http://www.who.int/diagnostics_laboratory/evaluations/en/, accessed on October 2016.
2. Peeling R.W., Holmes K.K., Mabey A. *Sex Transm Infect*, 82, 2006, 1–6.

10

Incorporating the Needs of Users into the Development of Diagnostics for Global Health: A Framework and Two Case Studies

Jacqueline C. Linnes, Elizabeth Johansen, and Ashok A. Kumar

CONTENTS

10.1 Introduction

Technologies created with users in mind are more innovative, require fewer resources to develop, and have better chance of making an impact (Griffin and Hauser 1993; Maidique and Zirger 2013). A canonical example of the importance of design is the Apple iPod; few consumer companies are as synonymous with the word "design" as Apple. The size, click wheel control, and LCD screen all enabled a user experience that ensured the iPod became the dominant player in the market despite not having a "first mover" advantage in the space of portable MP3 players. Moreover, competitors' designs took cues from the iPod, leading to a convergence in design (Peng and Sanderson 2014). Similarly in diagnostic technology, adoption and implementation improve with thoughtful design; it impacts both initial uptake as well as continued use (Langhan et al. 2015). No matter how sensitive or specific a diagnostic is, if users are frustrated by the device (e.g., the results of a colorimetric test are too subtle to interpret) or the device is difficult to fit into the clinical workflow (e.g., the time for the test is significantly longer than the average provider visit), it will have trouble achieving widespread use and competing devices with poorer technical performance but better user-design may be adopted instead.

Increasingly, designing with end-user needs in mind is not only important for adoption but also for patient safety and for regulatory approval. The U.S. Food and Drug Agency (FDA) provides examples of medical emergencies caused by devices developed for the wrong patient populations (e.g., critically ill hospital patients receiving the wrong insulin doses because blood glucose monitors were designed and tested for patients in-home, not in-hospital intensive care units) (FDA 2014). Accordingly, the FDA now provides specific guidance for human-factors studies for medical devices (FDA 2016). Similarly, the European CE Mark requires compliance with ISO/EN 62366, which includes usability testing. The FDA provides additional recommendations and instructions for diagnostic tests designed for point-of-care use according to the 1988 Clinical Laboratory Improvement Amendments (CLIA) to ensure that the tests are suitable for the lay user (FDA 2008; Kingsley and Backinger 1993). Although regulatory approval requirements vary from country to country, U.S. FDA approval or CE Marking can often assist with speedy approval in other countries.

Engineers and scientists are perfectly placed to address both the technical requirements and the needs of device users to develop new global health technologies. In fact, the Accreditation Board for Engineering and Technology (ABET), the body responsible for accrediting engineering training programs around the world, recognizes the integral role that design plays in technology development (ABET 2015). In their criteria for student outcomes in all areas (engineering programs, computing programs, engineering technology programs, and applied science programs), ABET student outcomes include "an ability to design a system, component, or process to meet desired needs within realistic constraints such as economic, environmental, social, political, ethical, health and safety, manufacturability, and sustainability."

This chapter focuses on understanding and designing for the needs of the patients and caregivers who will actually use diagnostic technologies.

Using the framework of human-centered design (HCD), we lay out techniques for applying this framework to diagnostic design and follow these methods with two case studies in which these methods are used in the field. Finally, we address some of the most common myths and misconceptions preventing test developers from using HCD.

10.1.1 General Embodiments and Framework of HCD

The scene in the comic in the figure below is all too familiar. As scientists and engineers, we are comfortable solving a technical problem and spend a long time perfecting a potential solution before sharing it with the world. However, the solution suffers because it has not benefited from the feedback of real end-users and stakeholders in the problem.

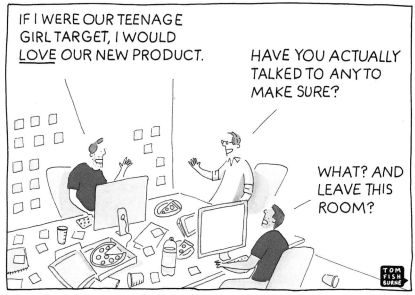

Failing to incorporate end users into a design. (From Fishburne, T., in: Constable, G., *Talking to Humans*, Edited by Rimalovski, F., 2014.)

HCD is a framework for developing in-depth understanding and addressing the needs of all stakeholders taking part in a product, service, or experience. In terms of diagnostic development, device users, their use environment, and their motivations and expectations are taken into account during development. HCD includes a mix of empathic design, user-centered design, and participatory design techniques (Seshadri et al., 2014). The HCD process encourages a team to develop empathy by understanding the big picture of a user's life including hopes, dreams, and emotions. This empathy fuels inspiring ideas that lead to a well-received, holistic product experience. HCD incorporates user-centered design by emphasizing iterative user feedback with prototypes. Finally, HCD contains participatory design elements that invite users themselves to design and prototype aspects of the product, service, or experience. In HCD many team members, not just a specialized designer, should understand and represent the user's point of view (Peace Corps 2007; Sanders 2002; UX Mastery Community 2016).

In diagnostic development, user needs are one of the most difficult aspects to integrate during the long, often laboratory-based, creation process. We seek to lay out benefits and example methods for closely integrating user needs into the technical diagnostics development process yielding better health outcomes for fewer dollars spent. This integration is especially valuable in global health, where funding can be scarce and health impact is paramount. Several excellent examples of point-of-care diagnostic development integrating user needs in different countries have been described in other articles (Derda et al. 2015; Kumar et al. 2015; Laksanasopin et al. 2015; Oden et al. 2010). Here, we provide an introduction to the HCD framework, step-by-step techniques, and case studies to further illustrate how these techniques improve diagnostic devices.

10.1.2 HCD Can Be Incorporated throughout the R&D Process

A typical diagnostic development process takes 2–5 years depending on technical novelty. This process is described in the 2004 United States FDA/Industry In Vitro Diagnostic (IVD) Roundtable as consisting of seven phases: (1) viability/feasibility, (2) planning, (3) development, integration, and verification, (4) internal validation, (5) external study validation, (6) launch readiness and release, and (7) sustaining engineering (Phillips et al. 2006).

By engaging with users through activities during the feasibility, planning, and development phases, test developers can increase certainty around their assumptions that

- The correct target users have been identified.
- The target users will be able to use the diagnostic correctly and effectively.
- The diagnostic will be well adopted by the target users.

As seen in the following figure, there are numerous opportunities to increase certainty about the user needs surrounding a diagnostic, or other medical technology, throughout a device's development. Those in the middle of the ladder of certainty (field partner feedback, in-context user feedback, and working prototype field demonstrations) are often overlooked ways to learn about the target usage despite being economical alternatives to waiting until a resource-intensive human factor trials for validation, when the cost of failure is much higher.

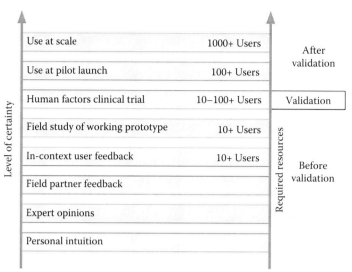

Ladder of certainty. Activities to increase knowledge of a medical technology's fit for the user.

10.2 Techniques

This section describes techniques to include HCD in the development of diagnostics. The techniques listed here are by no means exhaustive. For additional ideas, consider referencing materials from design consultancies IDEO and IDEO.org, Design that Matters, and the Stanford D. School (IDEO.org 2015; Plattner 2011; Prestero 2010; Stout 2003).

The following figure shows a process loop for learning about the target user. It is used throughout the chapter and can be adapted to any stage of product development. Activities are centered around developing and iterating on a product hypothesis—a description of the relationship between the user, context, and diagnostic need. A cycle of three activities continually improves the product hypothesis. First, *prepare* to engage with stakeholders by defining with whom to meet, planning the type of information you wish to gather and how it will be acquired, as well as obtaining required approvals. Then *engage* with your users to develop empathy for their experiences and understand the context in which your potential solutions will be applied. Finally, *synthesize* what was learned to refine ideas for potential solutions, embody these ideas in a way that users can respond to, and then put the simulated devices and kits in front of users to empathize once again. An R&D team might iterate through this HCD loop dozens of times during the normal multiyear diagnostic development process.

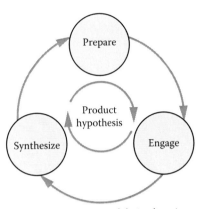

Cycle of human-centered design learning.

10.2.1 Initial Product Hypothesis

A product hypothesis is the embodiment of the most important assumptions surrounding the users, the context of use, and need that a product will solve. To develop an initial product hypothesis, create a list of assumptions surrounding the product. This list should detail all of the users who will come in direct contact with a diagnostic device, the important qualities of the contexts where the device will be operated, and the needs being satisfied. The list may also include specific needs, users, and contexts that will not be satisfied by this product. After the list of assumptions is created, summarize this in a single statement of the most important assumptions including the users, context, and need

A particular group(s) of users

—NEED—

A solution to their specific problem within the context of important identified constraints

Below is an example of a product hypothesis from Design that Matters' Firefly Phototherapy project to treat newborn jaundice. The resulting medical device is now treating newborns with jaundice in 22 developing countries.

Low-resource hospitals providing overnight care that wish to improve treatment outcomes and reduce newborn referrals

—NEED—

A cost-effective, durable tool that is intuitive for nurses and that can be placed in the mother's room to provide individual infant phototherapy to otherwise healthy newborns with mild to severe jaundice while allowing infant warming.

Here, the need is to improve treatment outcomes for newborns with jaundice and reduce newborn referrals to higher level hospitals. Satisfying this need will reduce newborn mortality through successful treatment of more newborns and reduce the burden on higher-level hospitals so they can focus on more complex newborn conditions. The users include the specific patients (otherwise healthy newborns with jaundice) and the operators (nurses and potentially mothers). The context is low-resource hospitals providing overnight care.

Additional examples can be found in the case studies within this chapter, as well as from author E. Johansen's workshop at the 2016 Unite for Sight Conference (Johansen 2016).

10.2.2 Prepare

Address the who, what, where, when, why, and how of engaging users before you begin in order to get the best results. Many teams working in global health will find themselves interacting with end users who do not speak the same language and are from different cultures. In addition, users may have different professional experience from the team. Planning to visit users early and often can ensure proper time is taken to overcome these potential barriers. The following table provides tips to help teams prepare to engage users in a global health setting.

Method	Description
Who to visit	• *Extreme users and extreme contexts*: Visit a small number of users and contexts that represent a wide variety of needs and uses (the extremes). If the diagnostic technology satisfies these extreme needs, then it will probably work well for those in the middle of the bell curve. • *Number of users*: Depending on the technique used, 3–20 extreme users will give enough information to inspire the design direction.
What to ask	Before engaging any users, write down a list of potential questions and activities. This kind of document is often called a protocol in HCD, but it will only be a starting point, not a rigid script the way that a protocol is designed for in-lab verification test or a clinical trial. Questions should include basic background information, information about daily life and personal goals, and feedback about existing devices or representations of the new technology.
How to protect participants	Organizational approvals may be required before engaging users to protect study participants from risks to privacy or mental, physical, or emotional health. It is important when the information will be disseminated, published, or used for regulatory approval processes. Consider Institutional Review Board (IRB), Institutional Animal Care and Use Committee (IACUC), or FDA approvals based on the policies of your organization, as well as funders, and field partners (Varricchione 2016).

(Continued)

Method	Description
How to choose team roles	Having at least two core team members enables more thorough documentation, brings multiple viewpoints to bear, and increases safety in any context in the team's home country or abroad. However, bringing more than 3 or 4 people can be overwhelming when speaking with an individual. Assign the roles of moderator, note-taker, photographer, prototype handler, and observer to each team member.
How to document	• *Notes*: Include user quotes written verbatim, layout sketches of important rooms/locations, narratives of user actions during a usability evaluation, and/or potential error modes. • *Photos*: Take as many photos as possible during user interactions. Include portrait shots of all users, existing devices and prototypes in use, and indoor and outdoor surroundings. Do not worry about a camera being conspicuous; user evaluations are already a spectacle.
Obtaining user permission	In all cases, it is important to obtain permission to gather feedback from and take photos of users. Funders, organizations, and field partner hosts may already have guidelines to follow. Here are some guidelines to consider: • Ask for permission to take photos and notes. Do not take photos or ask questions until permission is granted. Take photos that depict people with dignity. • If the team takes photos with a variety of different permission levels (for publication, for internal use only, etc.), a photo management system, such as a set of folders that helps keep track of different levels of permission, should be used. • More examples of photo permission policies as well as methods for informed consent can be found in Corti et al. (2000) and Gardner (2015).
Access users via a field partner	• *Field partner*: To provide feedback before, during, and after travel, hosts in-country travel, and potential future partner for clinical studies and implementation. • *Qualities of a great field partner*: Ability to grant access to users in context and obtain any government or institutional permissions. See Kumar et al. (2015) for more suggestions on forging field partnerships.
Qualities of a great translator	Experience translating in a conversational setting and knowledge of relevant medical terms.
Preparing the translator for HCD	• *Big picture and specifics*: The team is looking to learn about users' lives broadly, as well as get specific feedback about ideas. • *Don't filter*: Give the literal translation of what a user says when possible. Paraphrasing or interpreting while taking notes can lose the original information and miss critical insights that are not apparent until later. • *Save advice and training to the end*: The translator may be a professional whose job is to educate users. It is, however, important for the team to understand the user's perspective, especially if this information is incomplete or incorrect.

10.2.3 Engage

Once preparation is complete, the team is ready to engage users. There are many ways to efficiently learn from users. Four basic techniques are highlighted in this text: in-context interviews, usability evaluations, observations, and techniques to supplement in-field visits. Within each technique is a list of methods that have been used specifically to gain insights for diagnostic technology development. In some cases, not all techniques may be appropriate for use depending on the cultural context or other barriers. Maintaining flexibility to adjust for new information about context or culture is important in all the techniques described in the following text.

10.2.3.1 In-Context Interview

During an in-context interview, the team spends 1–2 h interacting with users in the context where they will eventually operate the diagnostic device. Environments could be as diverse as a clinic exam room, a pop-up tent, an intensive care unit, an emergency room, a mobile or stationary lab, or a home. The goal is to move beyond what a user simply says, to understand what they think, feel, and actually do. The below table provides helpful methods to use during in-context interviews.

Method	Description
Open-ended questions	Questions that require more than just a "yes" or "no" answer. They encourage storytelling to reveal the motivations, desires, and feelings of users.
The five whys	Following an open-ended question with up to five follow-up questions to clarify motivations.
Tour	A great way to start an interview, whether in a home or clinic setting. Follow a patient journey from registration to departure, or a diagnostic from storage to disposal. Meet potential interview subjects and collect existing technology for product comparison activities.
Show and tell	This method is helpful for learning how the user interacts with current technology. Example activities include operating the user's diagnostic equipment, packing a bag with diagnostic technology or samples for transport, or storing equipment or samples. Ask the user to narrate what they are doing and ask questions during the process.
Usability evaluation	A usability evaluation can take place in the latter half of an interview and is described further in the next section.
Product qualities ranking and comparison	With existing commercialized technology, prototypes, simulated devices, and sketches as prompts, ask the user to list the most important qualities of the diagnostic. Example qualities include accurate, rapid, easy to use, few parts, shelf stable, and professional looking. Have the user sort the qualities from most important to least important and then sort each technology from best to worst fit for each quality.

(Continued)

Method	Description
Design the ideal diagnostic	Ask the user which features of existing technologies or simulated devices they would combine to make their ideal diagnostic experience.
User-made prototype	Ask the user to make a sketch or prototype showing how one or more aspects of the diagnostic experience could be improved. This could mean modifying an existing prototype, or making something new in order to gain further insight into user pain points and possible experience improvements. Consider sample collection, consumables, fluid handling, electronics, instructions, and packaging.

10.2.3.2 User Observation

One of the best ways to understand how the diagnostic technology will fit into the context is to see the target users performing daily routines using existing diagnostic technology as well as other tools of the trade. Observations can be punctuated with questions to understand why a target user is completing the current actions. The following table describes three methods for user observations that can be used.

Method	Description
Fly on the wall	Spend from 30 min to several hours observing the activities taking place and technology being used in a single room in a context such as a clinic or diagnostic test lab.
Shadow	Follow a target user such as a healthcare worker as they go about their daily routine.
Benchmark observation	Spend a day at a hospital, clinic, or diagnostic lab close to where the team works, even if the context is very different. Observe any challenges in how state-of-the-art diagnostic technologies are being used in well-resourced contexts. Many of the features that are hard to use in this environment will be even more difficult to use in a lower-resource environment.

10.2.3.3 Usability Evaluation

Usability evaluations help to pinpoint specific aspects of the diagnostic that can lead to user error or are undesirable to users. During a usability test, a user operates one or more diagnostic tools while the team observes and documents the interaction. The tools could be a combination of simulation devices, working prototypes, off-the-shelf components, or devices currently on the market. If the test cannot be performed in the actual use environment, the team simulates aspects of the actual use environment as closely as possible, including but not limited to the location, environmental conditions, sense of urgency, lighting, and training. The user is asked to narrate aloud what they are doing while they do it. The team might ask questions while the user performs the task only as long as they pertain to the step currently being completed and do not detract from or contribute to the correct use of the test.

It is valuable to mock up the diagnostic experience even in the earliest stages of development before the assay is completed. A combination of off-the-shelf and custom components can be used to simulate all or part of a diagnostic use experience in the earliest stages. The below table includes ideas for prototyping diagnostic experiences.

Component	Method for Simulation
Sample collection	
Sample matrix	The viscosity and color are the most important features of a sample matrix in a usability simulation. For example, blood can be simulated by mixing water, red food coloring, and cornstarch.
Fingerstick	Various lancing devices can be compared by using them on a piece of fruit. A drop of simulated blood can be placed on a finger protected by a glove, and then touched directly to a sample pad or a capillary device.
Device	
Lateral flow and dipstick	Existing off-the-shelf test strips such as a $1 pregnancy test can stand-in for a future test by still performing the functions of absorbing the fluid and developing while the user waits. Alternately, build a device with multiple control lines to simulate the presence of one or more lines as a result.
Colorimetric and novel paper devices	A simulation device that performs basic functions of absorbing the fluid and having similar graphics and colors as the potential final design. Urinalysis dipstick pads or water quality pads can be used to simulate results.
Instrument-based or digital reader	Simulate the experience by creating a set of models mocking up each user interaction with the consumables and the instrument or reader. The outer form of the instrument might be 3D printed or cardboard. Buttons and display can be mocked up with a cell phone embedded in the housing. Existing programs like InVision App, Origami, or Pixate can take a set of images and turn them into clickable screens that take a user through the device states ultimately displaying results. A commercialized digital reader or existing instrument can be used to run simulated tests, even if the end results display reads an error. Explain why the reading returned an error and tell the user the typical range of results.

(Continued)

Component	Method for Simulation
Liquid reagents and handling	
Reagents and wash	Simulate viscosity and color using water, food coloring, and corn starch or surfactant as needed.
Handling	Off-the-shelf containers and dispensers such as dropper bottles, microcentrifuge tubes, and disposable transfer pipettes are a great start. Some custom items can be prototyped using 3D printing, or by modifying off-the-shelf parts.
Packaging	
Primary packaging	Determining the most user-appropriate primary packaging early helps stability testing in the long term. Off-the-shelf vials with desiccant lids and heat-sealable foil pouches are readily available, affordable, and invaluable in user tests. Foil pouches can be used to package test strips, consumables, and even vials of reagent.
Secondary packaging	Secondary packaging such as boxes and bags holds kit supplies together and custom labels add to the user experience.
Instructions and read guide	
Print	If the final design is likely to be laminated to increase durability, consider printing on a glossy business flier paper or using a laminator.
Digital	For digital instructions, software packages can enable teams to create app or web prototypes from a series of images.

Below is an example introduction to a usability evaluation with a simulated whole blood diagnostic device that authors A. Kumar and E. Johansen have used in the company Jana Care. This method of introduction was also used by Diagnostics For All in the case study described in Section 10.3.

> We have a simulation of the test we are developing. We would love for you to try it and give us some feedback. Can you please lead us to the location where you would most likely use this test if you had purchased it? (walk to area) We don't have a final product yet, so we made these simulation devices you can use with water instead of blood to see what it might be like to use this test. We are not going to show you how to use it, rather we want to see if the instructions and materials we have provided would be enough to tell you how to do it. This is a test for us—not for you—a test of how well we have designed this diagnostic to ensure you can use it easily. Now is the time when we can still make changes, so we look forward to your feedback.

The following table outlines some of the available methods for performing a usability evaluation. Additional material can be found in introductory anthropology textbooks and qualitative research design resources, such as *Introduction to Qualitative Research Methods: A Guidebook and Resource* by Taylor, Bogdan, and Devalt (Taylor et al. 2015).

Method	Description
In-context evaluations	Ask target users to operate one or more simulation diagnostic devices that provide the experience of using a finished device. Ask them to perform the evaluation in the context where they would anticipate using the test. Between users, change which option is tried first to decrease the effect of order on the feedback. The goal is to give the user very little instructions on how to use the test to highlight any difficulties in following the instructions.
Hallway evaluations	Chances to interact directly with actual users are infrequent, yet it is important to iterate rapidly toward a user-friendly solution. Hallway evaluations are an affordable way to test usability in between field visits.
	Recruit a small number of users who are unfamiliar with the diagnostic by walking down a hallway in the lab or office. Find some users with characteristics similar to your target user such as nontechnical background, eyesight, medical training, literacy level, and even culture and language. Perform usability evaluations with these users.
	Hallway evaluations highlight aspects of the diagnostic experience that are clearly *not* easy to use. However, if the diagnostic is easy to use for hallway test subjects, it still may not be easy enough to use for the target user. The ultimate proof will be testing with the target users in their context of use.
Follow-up questions	At the end of each test run, ask the user • What are your favorite and least favorite features? • Which step is easiest and which is most difficult? • What would you never do or use?
Product qualities ranking and comparison	Follow the product qualities ranking and comparison described in the in-context interview section to compare multiple simulated devices to each other and to other existing technology.

If there is no time to create simulated devices and the diagnostic is still in its earliest stages, having other tangible items will help the conversation. Possibilities include samples or photos of competitor devices, or diagnostics from different domains that may deliver a very similar user experience. The user may also have devices in their context that can be used to react and give feedback. Devices already owned by the user, such as old glucose monitors at a diabetic's home, can be brought together for conversation and comparison.

10.2.3.4 Techniques to Supplement In-Field Visits

Especially for global health projects, it can be difficult to travel to the actual sites of expected device use. The team can gain an initial understanding of the context and target use environment by interviewing global health experts who have experience serving the target users. However, these experts can supplement but not replace an in-context experience. A phone or video conference can also be a good way to check in with key users before and between field visits to the target context of use. Video has the advantage of being able to assess the user's reactions. Techniques for phone interviews include asking open-ended questions, the five whys, showing digital images of competitor products and new technology concepts, and product quality ranking.

10.2.4 Synthesize

The purpose of synthesis is to turn learnings into action. The team must summarize in a way that gives other team members and partners a feel for who was visited and what was learned. It is important to also give the extended team access to raw information such as photos and user quotes so they may bring their own insights to bear. Providing summary information in combination with raw data also enables the team to more easily ramp on new team members, partners, or contractors in future phases of the project.

Summarizing information during synthesis can involve a wide variety of techniques (see the below table). More details about the techniques listed here appear in the case studies.

Method	Description
Techniques to use after every engagement	
Critical assumptions	A list of critical assumptions about the user, context, and need being addressed.
Product hypothesis	A one-sentence summary of the product's user, context, and the need being addressed.
Product requirements	A living document listing all requirements for the diagnostic kit to be successful (Mallette 2016). These include • Features and functions supporting user needs and intended use • Performance requirements and characteristics • Physical characteristics and exterior design • Product configurations and external interfaces • Packaging and shipping • Service and installation • Labeling and product documentation
Photo bank	Create a folder in the team's project workspace to collect all photos. At the end of each day, transfer all photos taken into a new sub-folder with date and title. As a bonus, copy the best photos of the day into a best-of sub-folder for easier future reference.
Quotes and notes	Create a folder in the team's project workspace to collect direct quotes and notes. Create one file for each in-context interview, phone interview, observation, or usability evaluation. Scan in hand-written notes. As a bonus, pull together quotes and organize them by theme.
Optional additional techniques for synthesis	
Use cases	Describes each use case for the diagnostic technology including target user, value proposition, and other stakeholders involved.
User journey maps	A step-by-step map for each important use case. Consider steps like awareness, selection, purchase, use, disposal, and repeat purchase.
Pugh chart	A chart that enables a team to weigh the importance of different features to resolve conflicting requirements (e.g., of models and quality of inputs)

10.3 Case Studies

In this section, we share two case studies to illustrate different ways to incorporate some of the techniques described in the previous section in the context of developing two specific diagnostic tests: (1) a progesterone test for cows—work that author E. Johansen was involved in while working at Diagnostics For All, and (2) a diagnostic test for sickle cell disease—work that author A. A. Kumar led while at Harvard University.

10.3.1 Case Study 1: User Feedback on a Bovine Progesterone Diagnostic Test in Kenya

The context: In Kenya, the majority of dairy cattle are owned by smallholder farmers on farms of less than 2 ha, with an average herd size of 2–4 cows (Thorpe et al. 2000). Selling milk is often the only source of income for these families. Optimal milk production requires a cow to be pregnant once every 15 months. Currently, a farmer observes behavioral changes in the cow that indicate ovulation and then calls for artificial insemination (AI) services. Depending on behavioral observations alone, cows in Kenya are dry (not producing milk) approximately 40% of the time (Odima et al. 1994; Waithaka et al. 2002). By better predicting heat in cows, U.S. dairy farms are able to minimize dry time to 15% on average.

With support from the Bill & Melinda Gates Foundation, Diagnostics For All (DFA) has been developing a bovine progesterone rapid diagnostic test to help identifying cows in heat. DFA is a 501c3 nonprofit developing point of care diagnostics to benefit low-resource communities in the developing world. The test is a whole blood progesterone lateral flow dipstick test. High or low progesterone is indicated by the presence of one or two lines. When low progesterone is accompanied by behavioral signs of heat, the cow is likely to be ready for insemination. A progesterone test has the potential to help farmers avoid costly unsuccessful insemination attempts, reducing unprofitable dry time, and increasing farmer income by as much as $50/year/cow.

This case study illustrates some of the HCD techniques used during and insights derived from a 7-day field evaluation in Kenya. This field evaluation took place mid-way through the feasibility phase for the progesterone diagnostic. The project team during this visit included Director of Product Design Elizabeth Johansen, Senior Scientist Dr. William Matthew Dickerson, and Research Associate Kendall Milkey.

Using HCD techniques to engage users directly, the team discovered the primary target users would be artificial insemination technicians instead of farmers, the sample collection method would be venous draw instead of ear stick, the strips should be packaged in foil pouches instead of vials, and the total cost for the kit could potentially be $3 instead of $0.50 leaving more room for innovation. The product hypothesis and assumptions from before and after the visit to Kenya are summarized in the following table.

Before the Visit	After the Visit
Product hypothesis	
Dairy farmers in Kenya and East Africa with fewer than 5 cows.	Dairy farmers in Kenya and East Africa with fewer than 5 cows.
—NEED—	—NEED—
A <$0.50 progesterone test kit that is easy for farmers to use on the farm to identify cows ready for artificial insemination, <u>decreasing</u> dry time, and ultimately increasing farmer income.	*A <$3 progesterone test kit that is easy for AI techs to* use on the farm to *help* identify cows ready for artificial insemination, decreasing dry time, and ultimately increasing farmer income.
Critical assumptions	
The need	
With current methods of heat detection, dairy cows are not operating at optimal milk production.	No change.
More efficient heat detection in cows could lead to greater milk productivity and more income.	No change.
The test must be sold for less than US$0.50 per kit to be affordable and lead to significant increased income.	The test must be sold for less than *US$3* per kit to be affordable and lead to significant increased income.
The user	
The test will be performed by a farmer drawing blood from the cow by lancing the ear.	The test will *primarily* be performed by *AI techs who are trained to perform venous blood draw.*
A farmer will be able to correctly interpret the results of a lateral flow test on the farm and have the confidence to decide whether to call for an AI tech.	*AI techs will have sufficient vision to correctly interpret the test results on the farm and confidence to decide whether to administer AI.*
The context	
The test will be performed on a farm in East Africa, with a particular focus on Kenya.	No change.
There will be a safe place on the farm to put the test while waiting for the results to develop.	*The kit will include component(s) to keep the strip safe* while waiting for results to develop.
Test kits will be sold at local agricultural and veterinarian supply and service shops (Agro-Vets).	No change.
Strips will be packaged in vials of 10–20 to reduce costs.	*Each strip will be sealed in a foil pouch with desiccant to increase affordability and right-sizing for portability.*

Prepare: To prepare for the Kenya field visit, the DFA team began by generating a list of critical assumptions using the methods (literature, expert phone interviews, etc.) described in Section 10.2. These assumptions were summarized in a product hypothesis shown in the above table. The team also developed a recruiting plan, which included a request to visit at least five smallholder dairy farmers, at least three AI technicians, as well as veterinarians and others who handle cows. The team also specified extremes including location and size of farm, level of experience, and level of success in farming.

In order to test these assumptions, the DFA team engaged Sidai Africa Ltd., a field partner from prior project visits. Sidai is a social enterprise revolutionizing livestock and veterinary services through a network of franchised and branded Livestock Service Centres in Kenya. The team set up a series of calls with Sidai executives and coordinated closely with Sidai's Technical Director, Dr. Odede Ochieng, to discuss the recruiting plan and field visit plan. Dr. Odede Ochieng also became the team's host and translator during the visit. As a veterinarian, his role included forming relationships with farmers and Agro-Vet shops across Kenya.

Engage: During this visit to Kenya, the team performed in-context interviews of potential users, usability evaluations embedded in the interviews, and observations. Highlights of the visit that led to important insights are detailed in the following text.

The team wanted to test the assumption that farmers would be comfortable drawing blood from their own cows. The use of open-ended questions followed by the five whys helped generate an important learning during an interview with one smallholder farmer.

Moderator: Have you ever drawn blood from your cows for any reason? (yes/no question)

Farmer: Yes we have.

Moderator: Could you tell a story of a time you took blood? (open-ended question)

Farmer: One time the vet came and took blood from the jugular vein of one cow, then she made a smear and took it to the lab to diagnose tick-born infection. I asked how to take blood myself in the future in case the vet was unavailable in the future.

Moderator: Why did you ask to do the blood draw yourself? (first why)

Farmer: Well, I have never personally taken blood, but I had one of my farm hands learn how. I wanted him to know how to take blood in case the vet was unavailable in the future.

Moderator: Why didn't you do the blood draw yourself? Why did you ask a farm hand? (second why)

Farmer: I am not comfortable treating my animals on my own because of the sympathy and pain I have for them. That's why I get other people to care for them.

Without asking why several times, the team would not have realized the farmer had never drawn blood from his own cows and did not wish to. The team might have left this interview feeling validated in their approach to have farmers run the diagnostic test on their own cows. Receiving similar answers from other farm visits, as well as expert opinions from veterinarians and Agro-Vet shop owners led the team to consider artificial insemination service providers as the primary users for this test.

Asking users to try a simulation diagnostic test kit helped test assumptions about whether users can correctly interpret the results, how test strips should be packaged, and the cost of the test kit. The progesterone test was still in the feasibility phase at the time of this visit, so the team had to come up with a way to mimic the potential use experience. Dr. William Matthew Dickerson and Kendall Milkey conceived of and created simulation lateral flow strips that would show one or two control lines with application of water.

During the second half of each in-context interview, the team gave farmers, AI techs, and other stakeholders an opportunity to try two different simulation test kits reflecting a variety of packaging, procedure, and results. Each user was given a basic introduction to the purpose of the test without any verbal instructions on how to conduct the test. They were asked to perform the test in the most likely context they would use it on the farm (see figure below).

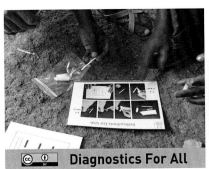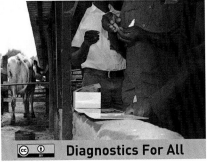

Users from two different farms try the simulated progesterone test kit in the context where they would eventually use it. (Courtesy of Diagnostics For All, Salem, MA.)

Through observations of use of the simulated kits, the team quickly learned that a single strip in a foil pouch is preferred over strips packaged in vials. While using a simulated diagnostic kit, a manager at a large farm opened a vial of 10 test strips; three fell onto the dirt floor. He indicated he much preferred the individually pouched strips he saw in the second simulation kit as he was less likely to waste extra test strips. In addition, after trying the simulation kits, a smallholder farmer noted he may never have enough money to buy 10 tests all at once. He preferred individually pouched strips for affordability because he could purchase one at a time.

Asking users to interpret the simulation tests highlighted the difficulty of reading the strip in a shady farm building. In addition, the team discovered that many farmers will not be able to correctly read the strips due to uncorrected vision impairments. On a visit to one smallholder farm, three herdsboys tried the simulated diagnostic kits. When it came time to read the results in the shade of the barn, one herdsboy said, "I can see two lines on the strong results strip, and one line on the negative results. The middle strip looks plain to me." In fact the middle strip had two lines, including a control line and a light test line (see figure below). He was still unable to see a line even in the sun. This same issue of readability occurred on other farms as well. Reading was not as difficult for AI techs who already had to see small markings and labels to perform artificial insemination.

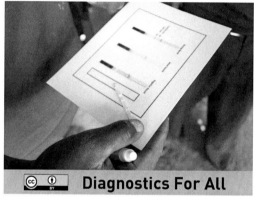

Laminated read guide showing images of what a strip looks like with a positive, negative, or invalid result. (Courtesy of Diagnostics For All, Salem, MA.)

Enabling the farmers to experience a simulation kit also opened a doorway to discuss pricing. After observing his son try two simulation kits, one smallholder farmer said, "How accurate is the kit? It must be very certain to be worth it. I would pay $5 USD if the kit was certain." This feedback along with similar feedback from other farmers and AI techs gave the team preliminary evidence that a $5 diagnostic service including $3 test kit may be affordable for farmers and still yield reasonable service fees for AI techs. Note that pricing feedback from a handful of people is difficult to depend on; the team could increase certainty by following up with a market study of price sensitivity performed with partner Sidai Africa Ltd.

The team had the opportunity to shadow two different artificial insemination providers to several service calls from farmers. The team asked for the AI techs to try fitting a range of potential diagnostic packaging into their equipment backpacks and comment on which would be the preference. Packing options included strips in a vial, strips in individual foil pouches, kits in plastic Ziploc bags, and kits in paperboard boxes. One AI provider summed it up the best: "I like the tests in individual packs instead of getting many tests in a box. The box won't fit in my backpack that carries the liquid nitrogen canister. The foil pouch saves us space. I would carry it in the front pocket of my bag. Carrying up to ten would be manageable, but it would also allow me to carry fewer if that's all I need."

One user-created prototype highlighted the need to find a good, safe place on the farm for the test to stay while waiting for results. After trying a simulation kit, the team asked one AI tech to use nearby materials to make something to keep the test strip safe on the farm. The AI tech found a piece of wood on the ground and said, "When you're on the farm, animals are moving around. I think a heavy stand like this wood block would be better and would allow an AI provider to help the farmer while waiting for the results." See figure below.

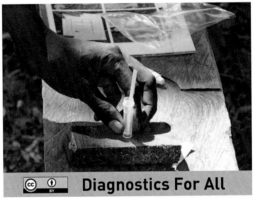

User supplying their own prototype to support the device in the field. (Courtesy of Diagnostics For All, Salem, MA.)

Synthesize: The first step upon returning from Kenya was to generate a revised product hypothesis and set of critical assumptions seen in the previous table. Findings from the trip also provided guidance on how to modify the diagnostic kit components going forward. Updated product requirements are shown in the following table.

Component	Requirement
Test strip	Sample collection method will be venous blood draw into a vacationer instead of ear prick. Development will not require any ear stick samples.
	Preferred strip packaging is individually sealed foil pouches. Stability trials should be performed in this packaging.
	Waiting for results is a challenge; time to result should be limited.
Supplies	The test needs one or more component(s) to protect it while it runs and keep in a conspicuous place so users remember to come back and read the result at the right time.
	The cost of the kit must include sample collection supplies to avoid accidental introduction of an interfering substance such as an anticoagulant in a locally sourced supply.

(Continued)

Component	Requirement
Instructions and read guide	Include a warning to read the test in good lighting.
Packaging	Test strips will be individually packaged in foil pouches with desiccant.
	All supplies and instructions required to run one test will be contained in a plastic bag to minimize kit size and enable sales of individual kits.

The team also mapped out a step-by-step user journey map to help gauge the potential effect of changes to the kit (see the following figure). This journey map also helped partners envision how the strip would be used in the market.

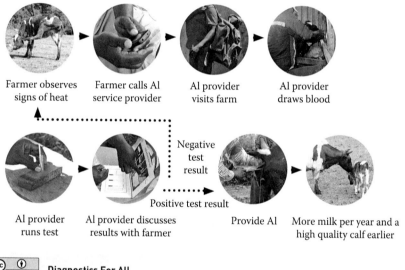

Diagnostics For All

Bovine progesterone test user journey map: confirming signs of heat. (Courtesy of Diagnostics For All, Salem, MA.)

Armed with the new learnings about the target user, sample collection method, user-preferred packaging, keeping the strip safe during wait time, and affordable kit cost, the team returned to complete the feasibility phase of development.

10.3.2 Case Study 2: End-User Feedback on a Diagnostic Test for Sickle Cell Disease in Rural Zambia

The context: Sickle cell disease is a genetic blood disorder affecting roughly 300,000 children born each year (Piel et al. 2013; Serjeant 2010). The vast majority of children born with sickle cell disease are in sub-Saharan Africa and India. Untreated, sickle cell disease leads to increased risk for bacterial infection, body pain, and potentially stroke. Although many of these risks can be mitigated by simple interventions—prophylactic penicillin or pneumococcal vaccine, hydration, and parental education—a lack of early diagnosis is an important contributor to the estimated 50%–90% mortality rate for children under 5 born with sickle cell disease in sub-Saharan Africa (Emond et al. 1985; Hankins and Ware 2009).

A team of scientists under the direction of Prof. George M. Whitesides at Harvard University developed a low-cost diagnostic to screen for sickle cell disease in point-of-care settings using the density of red blood cells to distinguish between normal, healthy blood, and blood with sickle cell disease that is characteristically accompanied with high density red blood cells (Bartolucci et al. 2012; Fabry et al. 1984). The technology uses a small capillary with liquid polymers and a simple centrifuge to perform the density-based separation. The team previously described the technology (Kumar et al. 2014b), clinical trials (Kumar et al. 2014a), and the process of developing the technology (Kumar et al. 2015) in detail. For the purposes of this discussion on HCD, we will focus on the user evaluation done by the team in rural Zambia. Before beginning field work, the team had developed a first iteration of a product hypothesis drawing on the previous experience of A. A. Kumar who had served as a Peace Corps Volunteer in rural South Africa, had attended a winter school in India on technology in rural areas, and had visited health facilities in Kenya to assess diagnostic needs. The team also relied on the knowledge of Dr. Thomas P. Stossel, a hematologist who had spent over a decade doing work with a nonprofit in rural Zambia and initiated programs to treat sickle cell disease in Zambia. These personal experiences complemented the literature to create a set of assumptions about the need for a diagnostic test for sickle cell disease (which would later be modified after the field study) (see the following table).

Before the Visit	After the Visit
Product hypothesis	
Rural health centers in Zambia —NEED—	Rural health centers in Zambia —NEED—
A <$1 diagnostic test for sickle cell disease to screen newborns, identify common genotypes, and takes less than 20 min to perform.	A <$1 diagnostic test for sickle cell disease to screen *young children at the time of routine vaccinations (6–12 months), which is simple to interpret* and takes less than 20 min to perform.
Critical assumptions	
The need	
There is a high prevalence of undiagnosed sickle cell disease in rural Zambia.	There is a high prevalence of undiagnosed sickle cell disease in rural *and urban* Zambia.
Simple interventions to treat sickle cell disease are available at rural health centers.	No change.

(Continued)

Before the Visit	After the Visit
The test must be sold for less than US$1 per test.	No change.
The user	
The test will be performed by a nurse or a community health worker or paramedical staff.	The test will *primarily* be performed by a community health worker or paramedical staff.
Health staff are comfortable performing fingersticks.	No change.
The context	
The test will be performed in rural health centers in Zambia and reference labs are available in urban centers.	The test will be performed in rural *and urban areas* in Zambia, and *reference labs are generally unavailable (only identified two in the whole country at the time of the study)*.
Power is generally unavailable in rural Zambia.	*Limited power is generally available in rural Zambia through car batteries charged with solar panels.*
Diagnostic tests must provide results in under 20 min to fit into the workflow of rural clinics and to ensure follow up.	Diagnostic tests must provide results *in 20–30 min to* fit into the workflow of rural clinics and to ensure follow up.

Prepare: Through Dr. Stossel's previous work in Zambia, the Harvard team connected with a team of clinicians, led by Dr. Catherine Chunda-Liyoka, at the University Teaching Hospital (UTH) in Lusaka, Zambia. Working together, the expanded team crafted a grant proposal to develop the rapid test for sickle cell disease that was funded by the Harvard Office of Technology Development. This grant included support for fieldwork to test the performance of a density-based assay to detect sickle cell in patients in Zambia. One of the justifications for a field trial fairly early in the research process was that there was a much higher frequency of sickle cell patients in Zambia. In addition to the plans to test the performance of the device, the team also made plans to test the usability of the device in rural health centers in Zambia. An additional grant from the Harvard Global Health Institute enabled the team to spend time and resources on human factors work that leveraged the networks built in Zambia for the clinical study.

To take advantage of this funding, the team carried out three steps in preparation of doing a rural survey: (1) worked with experts and local stake-holders to identify appropriate participants, (2) defined the types of information to be collected, and (3) practiced demonstrations before going to the field. Specifically, the team identified the Northern Province of Zambia as a geography with a potentially high concentration of sickle cell disease by talking with local experts at the University Teaching Hospital in Zambia, including Dr. Chifumbe Chintu and Dr. Chunda-Liyoka. The team then connected with the local Peace Corps office in Zambia to identify rural health centers with volunteers who would be amenable to hosting researchers.

Working with the Peace Corps, we prepared sites in advance of our visit in order to have a large attendance of community health workers. Peace Corps Volunteers and their counterparts at each site assisted in translating and getting stakeholder buy-in during the evaluations.

Ahead of the trip to the rural site, the team worked with our Zambian counterparts at the University Teaching Hospital (UTH) in Lusaka to create surveys to assess knowledge about sickle cell disease, familiarity with rapid diagnostic tests, and feedback on our prototype of a rapid test for sickle cell disease. Along with the team member from Harvard, a nurse from UTH planned to travel to the rural sites. The team also took all the equipment thought necessary to run the test in rural areas, including a small hematocrit centrifuge and a car battery for power.

Engage: The materials developed were used at two separate rural health centers to perform in-context interviews that consisted of a general education session about sickle cell disease, a presentation and demonstration of our prototype diagnostic (see a and b in the figure below), a tour of health facilities, and a survey of health workers that later evolved into interviews with individual health workers (see c in the figure below). During the tour of each facility, we took pictures of anything that could be of relevance: hand washing stations, solar refrigerators for vaccines, storage rooms, and patient waiting areas. During demonstrations, we had volunteers come and try the test procedure to see how easy or difficult it was and we observed and noted the results (see a and b in the figure below).

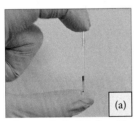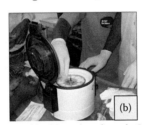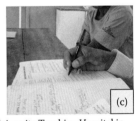

A team of scientists from Harvard and health workers from the University Teaching Hospital in Zambia did usability testing of a density-based rapid test for sickle cell disease (a). Community health workers and nurses tried using the diagnostic procedures (b). In-context, individual interviews captured insights into clinical workflow and design constraints for repid tests (c).

We also practiced observations and shadowing by embedding the nurse from our team into the clinical work at each rural health center for a day. This allowed our team to better understand the workflow at the rural sites and the challenges they faced. It also enhanced stakeholder acceptance as the clinic staff saw that we were not just taking information from them but also providing assistance while we were there. Observations of patients coming to the clinic helped us to understand that the main doctor or nurse generally only gets to spend 20–30 min to see patients and that patients often sit in a line outside the clinic for 20–30 min. Afterwards, patients would generally return home (sometimes traveling many kilometers on foot).

At the first health center, written questionnaires were given to health workers to fill out (see c in the figure on the previous page). We soon realized that they saw it more as an assessment of their understanding rather than a feedback tool; many of them showed stress trying to provide the "right" answer and we had to assure them that we wanted whatever answer they gave and there was no right or wrong answer. To remedy this situation at the second health center, we used the surveys to perform individual interviews. This format allowed the investigator to clarify answers and push for more thorough responses by adding open-ended questions and asking "why" certain responses were given.

Synthesize: After the study at the two sites, we were able to tally responses from surveys and interviews, review photographs and notes, and discuss observations. This time spent digesting the information yielded several insights.

Time requirement: During observations and in-context interviews, we created an informal map of the typical flow of patients (i.e., creating a journey map): (1) check in and wait (and get rapid tests done), (2) see a nurse or a clinical officer for consultation, and (3) go to the dispensary to collect any medications or receive shots. In order to maximize the workflow at the clinics, the staff members ran rapid tests for malaria on most febrile patients that were waiting to be seen. The time waiting before seeing a nurse or doctor is a useful time to perform rapid tests as the information from the tests can be used to inform clinical decisions, such as what medications to give the patient. To fit into the workflow at the clinics we visited, the longest time a test can take is roughly 20–30 min.

Power requirements: In the United States, there is much speculation that a manual centrifuge is better than a battery-powered centrifuge in low-resource settings (Brown et al. 2011; Saad Bhamla et al. 2016; Wong et al. 2008). The reasoning put forward is that electrical power is unreliable and batteries are not easily available, so power-free options are required. Some of these assumptions require significant caveats. Manually pedaling a bicycle, spinning a salad spinner, or cranking an eggbeater may be effective methods to achieve centrifugation, but one would be hard pressed to find the volunteer or health care provider in a rural clinic who can afford to spend 10 min in manual labor for every sample to be processed. In interviews, health worker after health worker described their ideal test as one you set, maybe press a button, and leave until it is time to read it. A battery-powered centrifuge meets this requirement but a manual centrifuge does not. If one considers batteries, the type of battery is important. In rural Zambia, AA and AAA batteries required a trip to the main town. The Hemocue Hemoglobin Analyzer at one clinic we visited was not being used, partly because the batteries were dead. In both villages, however, there were cars and, thus, car batteries. Moreover, car batteries connected to solar panels were often found in enterprising households to charge cell phones (sometimes for a small fee). When we ran our centrifuge from a car battery, it was not out of the ordinary.

Level of differentiation required: Two versions of the sickle cell test were developed. One test was simple and only differentiated between sickle cell disease (of any genotype) and non-sickle cell disease (normal hemoglobin or sickle cell trait). The other test additionally provided differentiation between the two main genotypes of sickle cell disease, but the reagent was slightly more complex. Based on observations and interviews at the rural health centers, we concluded that basic care and simple, yet important, interventions (i.e., folate, hydration, parental education, pneumococcal vaccine for children, prophylactic penicillin) could be given for patients with sickle cell disease. Differentiated care for subtypes of sickle cell disease would be difficult to implement and is not even common practice in well-resourced settings. Strategically, we decided to focus further development on the simpler test that did not differentiate subtypes.

Perception of the problem: Sometimes, the information we received was contradictory. When asked about whether health workers believed sickle cell disease was a major issue in their area, some were certain that it was while others were adamant that no sickle cell disease was present in their community. With our counterpart Zambian nurse spending a day in clinic, meeting patients and speaking with locals, we identified a potentially significant burden of sickle cell disease based on symptomatic patients. We concluded that the conflicting information we received from health workers was potentially a perception and education issue. Any new diagnostic in these areas would, thus, need to be accompanied by education programs to help improve understanding of the disease and its treatment.

Following the field study in Zambia, the lessons learned from the field study were combined with the scientific knowledge gained from clinical trials to develop a next generation diagnostic test for sickle cell disease.

10.4 Top 5 Misconceptions about HCD in Diagnostic Development

Bringing Human-Centered Design (HCD) into the practice of diagnostic development is extremely rewarding, but it also has its challenges. The following list includes some of the common misconceptions surrounding creating a diagnostic device that will be easy to use and adopted by users.

1. *If my device passes a human factors usability trial at the end of my development process, it will be well adopted by users.*

   If the team has not explored diagnostic use in the market with end users before the validation phase, it is possible for the diagnostic to fail the human factors trial. Even worse, it is possible to set up such a trial that does not test the diagnostic in a way it will actually be used in the market. In fact, even the U.S. FDA recognized that most study evaluations occur in idealized conditions (FDA 2014). The diagnostic might pass with flying colors only to enter the market and fail through user error or lack of demand.

2. *Doing a user evaluation with a small number of users won't yield actionable information; the sample size is just too small.*

Engaging small numbers of users iteratively with HCD before a product hits the market dramatically increases the chance of user acceptance and correct use. However, the information gained through HCD techniques will be qualitative, not quantitative. Users may give conflicting information. No diagnostic device will satisfy everyone and no device will ever be perfect. The benefit of HCD is to dramatically increase the chance of user acceptance and correct use before it hits the market. Ultimately, the team must make the call about how to interpret the learnings. Some information will lead to new solutions, and other information is okay to ignore. Learning and applying HCD takes time, patience, and bravery.

3. *The technology is too constrained, we are already in the middle of R&D: there isn't any leeway for user-driven changes.*

It is never too early and never too late to get value from HCD. Some teams will not engage users for fear they will learn something to which the diagnostic cannot respond. Please trust that the team is more creative and resourceful than imagined! There is a solution to most user challenges, but the team must be brave enough to look the challenges in the eye in order to generate a solution. Remember, responding to a user challenge does not always require changing the core technology; there are many challenges that can be mitigated by better user instructions, packaging, training, or selecting a better off-the-shelf fluid dispenser.

4. *I can't show a simulated device to users or field partners because it would be misconstruing that we have a working device.*

Depends on the audience and the simulated device. It is possible to explain, even across languages and cultures, that the diagnostic is just at the idea phase. Thank the user or partner for being part of the earliest development stages and help them understand the feedback they give will help bring shape to the product, which will in turn bring positive impact to many people. In this way, the team builds a cohort of cheerleaders who want the product to come to market and are happy to give ongoing feedback and even partner for activities such as clinical trials, distribution, or manufacturing.

5. *HCD is about using personal intuition to create a better product.*

A key tenet of HCD is that the team's intuition, free from interaction with users, is insufficient. In global health diagnostic development, team members may be very different from the target user along dimensions of culture, lifestyle, socioeconomics, education, profession, and more. The methods and techniques listed here have been honed as efficient ways of yielding relevant user information with a small investment of time and resources. In particular, the HCD techniques and methods listed here have shown preliminary usefulness in diagnostics development. For further learning, the Acumen Fund and IDEO.org provide a free online course called Design Kit, which teaches HCD methods (http://plusacumen.org/).

10.5 Conclusions

HCD is a process and set of methods for getting a nuanced, in-depth understanding of the needs of users and other relevant stakeholders. The HCD framework and accompanying case studies provide detailed examples of critical insights into diagnostic users and other relevant stakeholders that cannot be gained through any amount of test development in the lab. These insights are crucial to designing a diagnostic test that meets the needs of users in order to prevent test failures, misdiagnoses, or lack of test adoption.

Acknowledgments

The authors thank and acknowledge the many people behind the technologies and field visits described in the case studies. In particular, we thank the Diagnostics For All colleagues who worked tirelessly on the bovine progesterone test project over the years, featured in Case Study 1, including (alphabetical): Patrick Beattie, Dr. William Matthew Dickerson, Marcus Lovell Smith, Sahil Khullar, Kendall Milkey, Dr. Jason Rolland, Dr. Una Ryan, Dr. Jeremy Schonhorn, Paul Shaw, Dr. Matthew Stewart, Dr. Christina Swanson, and Michelle D. Wong. In addition, the partners who made this work possible include Dr. Odede Ochieng of Sidai Africa Ltd.; Professor Victor Tsuma and Dr. Wilkister Kelly Nakami of University of Nairobi; and Dr. Odipo Osano of University of Eldoret. Case Study 1 is based on research funded in part by Global Development Grant # OPP102219, an initiative of the Bill & Melinda Gates Foundation. The findings and conclusions contained within are those of the authors and do not necessarily reflect positions or policies of the Bill & Melinda Gates Foundation. The authors also thank those involved in the development of the rapid test for sickle cell disease including Dr. Carlo Brugnara, Dr. Catherine Chunda-Liyoka, Gaetana D'Alesio-Spina, Jonathan

Hennek, Dr. Julie Kanter, Si Yi Ryan Li, Dr. Hamakwa Mantina, Matthew R. Patton, Dr. Thomas P. Stossel, Prof. George M. Whitesides, the rest of the staff at the University Teaching Hospital and the rural health centers visited in Zambia, and the Peace Corps in Zambia. The sickle cell fieldwork was funded by a Biomedical Accelerator Grant from the Harvard University Office of Technology Development and by a Research Fellowship by the Harvard Global Health Institute.

E. Johansen would also like to thank colleagues at IDEO for teaching the techniques of HCD and Design that Matters for evolving its application to technology for global health.

References

ABET. 2015. 2016–2017 Criteria for accrediting engineering programs. Baltimore, MD: Engineering Accreditation Commission. ABET. http://www.abet.org/wp-content/uploads/2015/10/E001-16-17-EAC-Criteria-10-20-15.pdf.

Bartolucci, P., C. Brugnara, A. Teixeira-Pinto, S. Pissard, K. Moradkhani, H. Jouault, and F. Galacteros. 2012. Erythrocyte density in sickle cell syndromes is associated with specific clinical manifestations and hemolysis. *Blood* 120 (15): 3136–3141.

Brown, J., L. Theis, L. Kerr, N. Zakhidova, K. O'Connor, M. Uthman, Z.M. Oden, and R. Richards-Kortum. 2011. A hand-powered, portable, low-cost centrifuge for diagnosing anemia in low-resource settings. *The American Journal of Tropical Medicine and Hygiene* 85 (2): 327–332.

Constable, G. 2014. *Talking to Humans*. Edited by F. Rimalovski. Giff Constable.

Corti, L., A. Day, and G. Backhouse. 2000. Confidentiality and informed consent: Issues for consideration in the preservation of and provision of access to qualitative data archives. *Forum, Qualitative Social Research/Forum, Qualitative Sozialforschung* 1 (3), Article ID 7. http://www.qualitative-research.net/index.php/fqs/article/viewArticle/1024.

Derda, R., J. Gitaka, C.M. Klapperich, C.R. Mace, A.A. Kumar, M. Lieberman, J.C. Linnes et al. 2015. Enabling the development and deployment of next generation point-of-care diagnostics. *PLoS Neglected Tropical Diseases* 9 (5): e0003676.

Emond, A.M., R. Collis, D. Darvill, D.R. Higgs, G.H. Maude, and G.R. Serjeant. 1985. Acute splenic sequestration in homozygous sickle cell disease: Natural history and management. *The Journal of Pediatrics* 107 (2): 201–206.

Fabry, M.E., J.G. Mears, P. Patel, K. Schaefer-Rego, L.D. Carmichael, G. Martinez, and R.L. Nagel. 1984. Dense cells in sickle cell anemia: The effects of gene interaction. *Blood* 64 (5): 1042–1046.

FDA. 2008. Guidance for industry and FDA staff: Recommendations for clinical laboratory improvement amendments of 1988 (CLIA) waiver applications for manufacturers of in vitro diagnostic devices. 0910-0598. Bethesda, MD: U.S. Department of Health and Human Services.

FDA. 2014. Blood glucose monitoring test systems for prescription point-of-care use: Draft guidance for industry and food and drug administration staff. 1755. Bethesda, MD: U.S. Department of Health and Human Services.

FDA. 2016. Applying human factors and usability engineering to medical devices: Guidance for industry and food and drug administration staff. 2011-D-0469. Bethesda, MD: U.S. Department of Health and Human Services.

Gardner, L. 2015. Does this picture make you feel sad? Practical questions for ethical photography. Reboot.org. Accessed October 15. http://reboot.org/2015/10/15/picture-make-feel-sad-practical-questions-ethical-photography/.

Griffin, A. and J.R. Hauser. 1993. The voice of the customer. *Marketing Science* 12 (1): 1–27.

Hankins, J. and R.E. Ware. 2009. Sickle-cell disease: An ounce of prevention, a pound of cure. *The Lancet* 374 (October): 1308–1310.

IDEO.org. 2015. *Field Guide to Human–Centered Design*. San Francisco, CA: IDEO.org.

Johansen, E. 2016. Bridging research and action. http://www.slideshare.net/elizjohansen/bridging-research-and-action?qid=928c8eea-c6ef-49c4-b467-a14faeb12139&v=&b=&from_search=2. Accessed on September 1, 2016.

Kingsley, P.A. and C.L. Backinger. 1993. Write it right: Recommendations for developing user instruction manuals for mechanical devices used in home health care. 93-4258. Rockville, MD: FDA.

Kumar, A.A., C. Chunda-Liyoka, J.W. Hennek, H. Mantina, S.Y.R. Lee, M.R. Patton, P. Sambo et al. 2014a. Evaluation of a density-based rapid diagnostic test for sickle cell disease in a clinical setting in Zambia. *PLoS One* 9 (12): e114540.

Kumar, A.A., J.W. Hennek, B.S. Smith, S. Kumar, P. Beattie, S. Jain, J.P. Rolland, T.P. Stossel, C. Chunda-Liyoka, and G.M. Whitesides. 2015. From the bench to the field in low-cost diagnostics: Two case studies. *Angewandte Chemie* 54 (20): 5836–5853.

Kumar, A.A., M.R. Patton, J.W. Hennek, S.Y.R. Lee, G. D'Alesio-Spina, X. Yang, J. Kanter et al. 2014b. Density-based separation in multiphase systems provides a simple method to identify sickle cell disease. *Proceedings of the National Academy of Sciences of the United States of America* 111 (41): 14864–14869.

Laksanasopin, T., T.W. Guo, S. Nayak, A.A. Sridhara, S. Xie, O.O. Olowookere, P. Cadinu et al. 2015. A smartphone dongle for diagnosis of infectious diseases at the point of care. *Science Translational Medicine* 7 (273): 273re1.

Langhan, M.L., A. Riera, J.C. Kurtz, P. Schaeffer, and A.G. Asnes. January 2015. Implementation of newly adopted technology in acute care settings: A qualitative analysis of clinical staff. *Journal of Medical Engineering & Technology* 39 (1): 44–53.

Maidique, M.A. and B.J. Zirger. 2013. A study of success and failure in product innovation: The case of the U.S. electronics industry. *IEEE Transactions on Engineering Management* EM-31 (4): 192–203.

Mallette, T. 2016. Medical device development—How to define requirements. Accessed September 19. http://www.kmcsystems.com/blog/bid/103309/How-to-Define-Your-Medical-Device-Requirements.

Oden, M., Y. Mirabal, M. Epstein, and R. Richards-Kortum. 2010. Engaging undergraduates to solve global health challenges: A new approach based on bioengineering design. *Annals of Biomedical Engineering* 38 (9): 3031–3041.

Odima, P.A., J.J. McDermott, and E.R. Mutiga. 1994. Reproductive performance of dairy cows on smallholder dairy farms in Kiambu district, Kenya: Design, methodology and development considerations. *The Kenya Veterinarian-A* 18 (2): 366–368. http://agris.fao.org. http://agris.fao.org/agris-search/search. do?recordID=KE9642614.

Peace Corps. 2007. Participatory Analysis for Community Action (PACA) training manual. Washington, DC. http://metacamp.info/Contents_files/Peace%20 Corp_Participatory%20Analysis.pdf. Accessed on September 1, 2016.

Peng, Y.-N. and S.W. Sanderson. 2014. Crossing the chasm with beacon products in the portable music player industry. *Technovation* 34 (2): 77–92.

Phillips, K.A., S. Van Bebber, and A.M. Issa. 2006. Diagnostics and biomarker development: Priming the pipeline. *Nature Reviews. Drug Discovery* 5 (6): 463–469.

Piel, F.B., A.P. Patil, R.E. Howes, O.A. Nyangiri, P.W. Gething, M. Dewi, W.H. Temperley, T.N. Williams, D.J. Weatherall, and S.I. Hay. 2013. Global epidemiology of sickle haemoglobin in neonates: A contemporary geostatistical model-based map and population estimates. *The Lancet* 381 (9861): 142–151.

Plattner, H. 2011. Bootcamp bootleg. Stanford, CA: Institute of Design at Stanford. https://dschool.stanford.edu/wp-content/uploads/2011/03/Bootcamp Bootleg2010v2SLIM.pdf.

Prestero, T. 2010. Better by design: How empathy can lead to more successful technologies and services for the poor (Discussion of design case narratives: Rickshaw Bank, Solar-Powered Tuki, FGN Pump). *Innovations: Technology, Governance, Globalization* 5 (1): 79–93.

Saad Bhamla, M., B. Benson, C. Chai, G. Katsikis, A. Johri, and M. Prakash. 2016. Paperfuge: An ultra-low cost, hand-powered centrifuge inspired by the mechanics of a whirligig toy. *bioRxiv*, August 30, 2016. doi:10.1101/072207.

Sanders, E.B.N. 2002. From user-centered to participatory design approaches. In Frascara, J., ed., *Design and the Social Sciences: Making*. London, U.K.: Taylor & Francis. http://books.google.com.

Serjeant, G.R. 2010. One hundred years of sickle cell disease. *British Journal of Haematology* 151 (5): 425–429.

Seshadri, P., T.N. Reid, and J.W. Booth. 2015. Framework for fostering compassionate design thinking during the design process. *Proceedings of the 121st ASEE Annual Conference and Exposition*, American Society of Engineering Education, Indianapolis, IN, June 15–18, 2014. Paper ID 10180. http://www.asee.org/file_server/papers/attachment/file/0004/4288/ Final_ASEE_Paper_DfC.pdf.

Stout, W. 2003. *IDEO Method Cards: 51 Ways to Inspire Design*. Palo Alto, CA: IDEO.

Taylor, S.J., R. Bogdan, and M. DeVault. *Introduction to Qualitative Research Methods: A Guidebook and Resource*. New York: Wiley, 2015.

Thorpe, W., H.G. Muriuki, A.O. Omore, and M.O. Owango. 2000. Dairy development in Kenya: The past, the present and the future. https://cgspace.cgiar.org. https://cgspace.cgiar.org/handle/10568/1723. Accessed on September 1, 2016.

UX Mastery Community. 2016. Empathic design, definition and framework. Accessed September 19. http://community.uxmastery.com/t/empathic-design-definition-and-framework/868.

Varricchione, T. 2016. Shades of gray in human research: 3 steps to determine if human factors & usability studies need IRB review. Ximedica Living Innovation Blog. Accessed September 20. http://www.ximedica.com/index.php/about/entry/shades-of-gray-in-human-research-3-steps-to-determine-if-human-factors-usab.

Waithaka, M.M., J.N. Nyangaga, S.J. Staal, and A.W. Wokabi. 2002. Characterization of dairy systems in the western Kenya region. https://cgspace.cgiar.org. https://cgspace.cgiar.org/handle/10568/1859. Accessed on September 1, 2016.

Wong, A.P., M. Gupta, S.S. Shevkoplyas, G.M. Whitesides, and M. George. 2008. Egg beater as centrifuge: Isolating human blood plasma from whole blood in resource-poor settings. *Lab on a Chip* 8 (12): 2032–2037.

Index

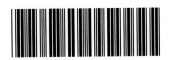